D1060942

DISCARD

Typhoid Mary

Typhoid

Mary

Captive to the Public's Health

Judith Walzer Leavitt

Beacon Press

Boston

Beacon Press
25 Beacon Street
Boston, Massachusetts 02108-2892

Beacon Press books are published under the auspices of
the Unitarian Universalist Association of Congregations.

00 99 98 97 96   8 7 6 5 4 3 2 1

Text design by Christopher Kuntze
Composition by Wilsted & Taylor
∞ Printed on acid-free paper

Library of Congress Cataloging-in-Publication Data can be found on page 332.

For Lewis

זֶ֣ה דוֹדִי֮ וְזֶ֣ה רֵעִ֔י

SONG OF SONGS 5:16

Contents

Illustrations

Acknowledgments

IT IS ALWAYS A GREAT PLEASURE, UPON completing a project such as this one, to remember all the people whose efforts helped make it possible and to have an opportunity to thank them publicly. In this case there were many, and their efforts mighty.

I begin with the students in my course, The Development of Public Health in America, at the University of Wisconsin, Madison. Since 1976, undergraduate and graduate students alike have demonstrated their fascination with Mary Mallon and the ways they could use her story to illuminate continuing issues in the field. I cannot name all of the students whose excitement with this subject finally ignited my own to the point that I began this project, but I understand my debt to them. Like all professors, I learn much from my students.

I would like to thank many graduate students in the history of medicine at the University of Wisconsin for the role they played, first in the classroom, and continuing beyond, in helping to shape my ideas and to sharpen my thinking. To Jon Harkness I owe a special thanks. Over the years, Rima Apple, Bob Bartz, Beth Black, Charlotte Borst, Marc Dawson, Diane Edwards, Eve Fine, Liz Hachten, Patty Harris, Judith A. Houck, Mary V. H. Jones, Susan Eyrich Lederer, Lian Partlow, Leslie Reagan, David Sandmire, Lisa Saywell, Rennie Schoepflin, Susan L. Smith, Diana R. Springall, Karen Walloch, John Harley Warner, and Tom Wolfe have pushed me even as I tried to push them. I am grateful to them all.

My colleagues at the University of Wisconsin have been equally important in helping me develop and continuing to challenge my ideas about what meanings we can derive from Mary Mallon's experiences. I would like to thank, in the history of medicine, Thomas Broman, Harold J. Cook, Vanessa Northington Gamble, and Ronald L. Numbers for putting up with this project and, more significant, for putting up with me as I obsessed about it. I would also like to thank all the graduate students and fellow faculty in the history of science and in women's studies for their considerable interest in this project.

My family, of course, has had to put up with more than anyone else. I am ever grateful to my children, Sarah A. Leavitt and David I. Leavitt, who, now adults, offer a special blend of intellectual and familial encouragement. Both of them provided practical help to this specific project as well as general goodwill about difficult schedules and delayed activities. My mother, Sally H. Walzer, who moved to Madison in the middle of this undertaking, has been ever-eager and supportive of my work on Mary Mallon as she has been of each of my career steps since I was too young to notice. Without her encouragement, and that of my father, Joseph P. Walzer, which I continue to feel through her, I would not be in a position to write this book. To Lewis A. Leavitt I owe more than can ever be written on the page. For his loving support over thirty years, and in anticipation of many more ahead, I dedicate this book.

This project benefited greatly from the research assistance of a number of people. I would like to thank Dawn Corley, Irving Ishado, Sarah A. Leavitt, Jennifer Munger, Lian Partlow, and Sarah Pfatteicher, all of whom were creative and resourceful—and persistent—in tracking down sources. For special contributions and consultations, I am happy to acknowledge the help of Nina Ackerberg, Peter Ackerberg, John Q. Barrett, Joan Jacobs Brumberg, Ann Carmichael, Bob Conlin, Gerard Fergerson, Vanessa Northington Gamble, Bert Hansen, Dirk Hartog, Greg Higby, Saul Jarcho, Robert J. T. Joy, David I. Leavitt, Barron H. Lerner,

Gerda Lerner, Stephanie Mathy, John Parascondola, Sarah Potts, Carolyn Shapiro, Robert Skloot, and Rebecca Walzer. These people were willing to put aside their own work to offer help at very important moments in the project, and I am extremely grateful to them all.

I am grateful for the responses of many people to my Author's Query in the *New York Times* Sunday Book Review section and the *Irish Echo*. These letters not only answered many of my questions, they also provided the comfort of knowing there were people out there who might be interested in reading this book.

I am in great debt to my colleagues who took the time to read a draft of the complete manuscript and offer detailed and informed opinions about what they read. I want to thank Thomas D. Brock, Susan Stanford Friedman, Linda Gordon, R. David Myers, and Ronald L. Numbers. While I know I did not answer all their concerns, I benefited from their insights, and I tried to do justice to their comments. I know some of their collective wisdom is reflected in the pages that follow, but these wonderful scholars are in no way responsible for the mistakes and shortcomings that remain.

I am happy to acknowledge the financial support that allowed this project to come to fruition. Foremost, I am grateful to the National Endowment for the Humanities, and to project officer Daniel Jones, for generous grant support, and to the University of Wisconsin Foundation for its matching grant. The University of Wisconsin, Madison, sabbatical program provided one semester free of teaching duties. The Institute for Research in the Humanities at the University made a home for me for one semester, and I benefited from the experience there of trying out my ideas in an interdisciplinary group. My tenure as Evjue-Bascom Professor of Women's Studies (1990–1995) provided added support for this project. Without all of this help, this book would not have become a reality.

I especially want to thank three people whom I have come to know quite recently. They have made it possible for me to have access to materials otherwise hidden, and their cooperation and enthusiasm for my project have been of ultimate importance. I am ever grateful to John S. Marr, M.D., M.P.H., now of the State Department of Health in New York; Ida Peters Hoffman, now retired from the City Health Department; and Emma Rose Sherman, also retired from her work first in bacteriology and then in education for the City of New York. These people were generous with their time and their knowledge; they opened their homes and their archives to me and shared their research, experiences, and memories. Only scholars and writers who have received similar help in their research from such personal and open communications can understand my debt and my gratitude to these three people. I only hope they get some pleasure out of the completed project.

Parts of chapter 1 and chapter 4 are reprinted and used here with permission: " 'Typhoid Mary' Strikes Back: Bacteriological Theory and Practice in Early Twentieth-Century Public Health," *Isis* 83 (1992): 608–29; "Gendered Expectations: Women and Early Twentieth-Century Public Health," in *U.S. History as Women's History: New Feminist Essays*, ed. Linda K. Kerber, Alice Kessler-Harris, and Kathryn Kish Sklar (Chapel Hill: University of North Carolina Press, 1995), pp. 147–69.

I also am pleased to acknowledge the help of a team of editors at Beacon Press. First and foremost is Lauren Bryant, no longer at the Press, who convinced me to sign and who gave the full manuscript her close attention in her capacity as free-lance editor even while her brand-new twins demanded her time and energy. I am grateful for her contributions. Marya Van't Hul took over the project graciously and with enormous enthusiasm. I am particularly grateful for her insistence on certain changes that I only over time came to appreciate. Beacon has been small enough to be welcoming and generous with attention and big enough to do a super job, and I thank all the people there who helped this book emerge.

October 1995
Madison, Wisconsin

Prologue

SHE WAS AN IMMIGRANT WOMAN WHO made her way as a cook. Born in Ireland, she boarded a boat for America when she was a teenager. She lived with an aunt for a time, but as an adult she settled down in domestic service in New York City. She cooked in the homes of the city's elite, in their Park Avenue brownstones and in their summer estates on Long Island or the Jersey shore.

She was by repute an excellent cook and did not go unemployed for long periods. Sometimes she boarded with her employers, sometimes she lived with friends in the city—often with one particular male friend. We do not know how happy she was in her personal life, but in her work she was said to demonstrate a certain pride and satisfaction. Some families who employed her praised her accomplishments in the kitchen and her care of the children.

We do not know when she contracted typhoid fever, except that it must have been during or before 1900. She denied ever having been sick with the disease, and it is likely she never knew she had it, suffering only a mild flu-like episode. But between 1900 and 1907, she infected some twenty-two people with typhoid fever through her puddings and cakes. They suffered more serious disease symptoms; one of them died from the illness.

The authorities decided she was too dangerous to be allowed to continue to earn her living by cooking. In fact, they decided she should not even be allowed to walk the streets of the city. They put her in a small bungalow on the grounds of a large isolation hospital on North Brother Island in the East River. She was thirty-seven years old. She lived alone in the cottage for more than two years and then came before a judge to plead for release from her banishment. The judge was sympathetic, but did not want to be responsible for letting the Irish woman return to New York City and continue infecting people through her cooking, so he declared her a menace to the public's health and sent her back to the small island.

Another lonely year passed. Finally a health department official decided it was not right to keep her isolated any longer, and he allowed her to go free. She worked in a laundry for a while, but she could not make a living away from her profession.

Eventually, she returned to cooking. When the health authorities found her the next time, it was estimated she had spread typhoid fever through her cooking to at least twenty-five more people, another two of whom died from the exposure. This time officials isolated her back on North Brother Island for the rest of her life. She lived twenty-three more years, in the one-room cottage on the small island, alone. She worked in the island's bacteriology laboratory for a while. She died on November 11, 1938.

Mary Mallon was her name. This book tells her story— rather, her stories, for there are many, depending on the teller's perspective and stance—to illuminate the many dimensions of sickness and sickness control that confronted Americans early in this century and continue to challenge us at the century's end. There will be no easy answers here to our country's present dilemmas with AIDS and tuberculosis. There will be, I hope, some insights that give meaning to our present concerns about controlling epidemics and force us to focus on the social dimensions of our efforts to combat the devastation sent our way by microbes. The many stories of Mary Mallon are the stories of the sufferers, of those who try to help the sufferers, of those who demonize the sufferers, and of those who try to prevent the suffering. They are the stories of the human side of disease and its control.

Typhoid Mary

"A Special
Guest
of the
City of
New York"

*M*any, perhaps most, American adults have heard of "Typhoid Mary." The phrase connotes a polluted woman, someone who carries and gives disease to others. But although many people have heard of "Typhoid Mary," most are vague about who she actually was, and almost no one knows her name. Some may conjure up the image of an Irish immigrant woman, heavy and ugly, who spread typhoid fever through her cooking. Many people cannot pinpoint the period in history in which she lived, and some believe her to be fictitious.

This book centers on Mary Mallon, the woman known as "Typhoid Mary,"[1] not only because of her familiarity and meaning in American culture, but also because of the important issues raised by the stories of her capture and captivity, which have not been examined previously in any depth.[2] The dilemma Mary Mallon posed for health officials in the early twentieth century —namely, how to protect the health of the public when it is threatened by an individual carrier of disease and at the same time preserve that individual's civil liberties—is one that is very much still with us. Moreover, Mallon's case illustrates the intertwining of science and culture. Through the lens of Mary Mallon's experiences, we can view how the values of American public

1

health during the first third of the twentieth century interacted with scientific activity. Knowledge of those values and events can enhance our understanding of and responses to the HIV epidemic and the resurgence of tuberculosis at the end of the century. One individual introduces us to a world of the past and offers a vital perspective on our own world of the present.

How far have Americans been willing to go to protect the public's health? Mary Mallon's experiences indicate the lengths to which officials in the past carried their obligation. Because they believed she threatened the health of those around her, New York City officials tracked Mary Mallon down and arrested her on two separate occasions, and forcibly isolated her for a total of twenty-six years of her adult life, beginning when she herself had no disease symptoms and was only thirty-seven years old. Her example reveals that the United States indeed holds the value of health dear. Americans want to be healthy and want to be protected from any neighbors who might threaten their health. Over the course of the nation's history, people have searched for health, have instructed the government to protect health, and have asked scientists to solve health problems when they arise. The government has used immigration policy to set United States residents apart from those of other nations in attempts to keep Americans free from disease. Elected officials have spent enormous amounts of money in the cause of a healthy citizenry. As I write, our nation's "health care crisis" remains unresolved and recurs at the center of political debate.

In addition to a strong commitment to preserving health and preventing disease, Americans also hold dear the value of individual liberty, and our constitution and laws reflect this commitment. Americans see themselves as defenders of liberty, at home and sometimes abroad. The laws of the United States and the nation's articulated values demand that government protect citizen liberty even while representatives carry out their duties to watch over citizen health and welfare. Thus, our laws guarantee the rights and immunities of all citizens against interference with the rights and privileges of citizenship. There are, of course, situations under which the nation agrees to abridge citizens' liberty: for murder, crimes against persons and property, and some civil infringements. Is sickness or carrying disease one of the situations in which most Americans can accept depriving people of their liberty?

In exploring the meanings of Mary Mallon's experiences early in the twentieth century with this question in mind, I examine in this book how American society, as a nation and as individuals, has approached taking away the liberty of someone who is sick or a carrier of sickness in the name of protecting the public's health. In so doing, I pose the question of how we have weighted the two values of health and liberty when they come into conflict and address what might be at risk in the balancing.

If science could always be depended upon to find cures and preventive vaccines for all our ills, we still would not be able to avoid this dilemma. There is a cure for syphilis, to cite but one example, yet syphilis continues to plague Americans. A medical magic bullet cannot, as much as we might wish it, solve our medical problems. No single factor can address our difficult health concerns. Because health and disease are deeply embedded within the social and changing world, it is imperative that we learn to consider the full range of contexts in which disease ravages. The challenge before us today, as in the past, is to determine how to protect the individual liberties of the sick or those identified as carriers of sickness and at the same time actively protect the public's health.

It is very difficult for most healthy Americans to envision themselves as the ones whose liberty might be threatened in the effort to protect the health of the community. As a society, we have become masters of stigmatizing the sick and the contagious; we label them as separate from the mainstream. As we did so easily in the past, Americans are again considering isolating—

locking up—those who threaten public health. But any complacency about this subject is grounded in illusion. The liberty not just of people who are now sick or infected but of each individual citizen is at stake; indeed, our cultural ethos itself may be threatened in this dilemma. Because these are such important issues for our own times, we must, as individuals and as a society, try to come up with some answers to these difficult questions.

The quandary posed is, of course, not hypothetical or merely theoretical, but as real in our end-of-the-century world as it was earlier in the century. Public health officers and the courts today must often decide whether to remand specific individuals to the hospital or to isolation because they threaten the health of those around them. As I write, headlines in a local newspaper read, "Woman with HIV Sought as a Threat to Public Health." A Milwaukee woman, infected with the virus, "reportedly engaged in highly risky, unprotected sex," and has become the "focus of unprecedented attention by state and city public health officials who are trying to figure out how to stop her potentially lethal activity."[3] Officials and the society they represent need help thinking about the issues involved in locking up, for example, a person with AIDS who persists in behaviors that place others at risk. They need help determining when and if isolation may be advisable for this woman or, for example, for another Wisconsin woman who suffers from a drug-resistant case of tuberculosis.[4] Medicine cannot answer all of their questions, nor should we seek the answers in medical control alone. It is my hope that the historical example explored in this book, the case of Mary Mallon, can illuminate the issues that most concern us today and help us find present-day solutions to our present-day problems.

The book is organized in two ways. Readers will find a chronological narrative of Mary Mallon's life and experiences woven throughout the text, with a full outline previewed in chapter 1. Each chapter unfolds more details about Mary Mallon's experiences and moves the narrative forward. A second, and stronger, organizing principle is my attempt to immerse the reader at separate times in a number of different perspectives on Mary Mallon; that is, I have purposefully disentangled the strands of her history to force us to see, and to understand, that there are various ways to tell Mary Mallon's story and that while they differ, they are all relevant. The physicians who cared for Mary Mallon made one set of observations about her, newspaper journalists brought quite another point of view to her story. Officials trying to determine public policy using her example approached her from yet another perspective. The interpretations are different; some exist comfortably alongside one another and some are in significant conflict. I will not make it easy for the reader to choose only one perspective as the best view on the past or to choose only one way in which to use these stories in the present. Instead, I encourage readers to engage, as I have, in the process of interpretation, and to find their own integrated meanings in these stories, meanings that I hope will help us as a society to come to terms with our health dilemmas and force us as individuals to remember and use all the pasts we can recover.

Memory about the past helps construct our present. But whose past, or which past, shall we remember? And who shall decide how we use the past in understanding our present? Our reading of the past is by necessity mediated through our present world. Because the road from and to the past is a two-way street, we must be alert to how the realities of the present have an impact on how we construct and reconstruct the past. Present-day experiences with new viruses and old diseases reappearing in drug-resistant forms influence us as we try to figure out what Mary Mallon's experiences mean. If we are aware of our present sensitivities, they can help rather than hinder our understanding of history, just as history can help us comprehend our options in the present.

Remembering Mary Mallon helps us keep in mind the complexity of the past as it helps to shape our present-day ideas about people who are sick or who may carry sickness to others. In this book I retell Mary Mallon's many stories and explore the perspectives and motives of Mary Mallon and the people who encountered her—the people who became ill because she exposed them to pathogenic microbes, the people who kept her isolated as a "special guest of the city of New York" for twenty-six years,[5] the people who tried to set her free from her quarantine, the people who studied typhoid through the evidence she provided, the people with whom she personally interacted, the people who condemned her during her lifetime, and those who continue to use her memory into the present.

The first perspective on Mary Mallon's story comes from medicine and the authority of the new science of bacteriology. The turn of the twentieth century represents one of the most exciting and dramatic periods in all of medical history. At the end of the nineteenth century, medical scientists had come to accept germ theory, a new theory of disease causation, brought to medicine through basic science research. Laboratory experiments established that microorganisms could cause disease, a realization that radically altered previous views that undifferentiated filth and air contaminated by rotting organic material (miasmas) caused disease. The optimism spurred by the study of microorganisms led public health physicians, who were in direct confrontation with infectious disease in the cities where death rates soared along with the population, to search out answers from the new science and from the laboratory whenever possible.

Typhoid fever was one of the nineteenth century's worst killers. Though it abated somewhat with urban sanitation measures, it remained a significant public health problem. Turn-of-the-twentieth-century bacteriologists tried to understand how this bacterial infection continued to thrive in relatively clean city environments. The answer came through bacteriological studies in

Europe and the United States that led to the realization that typhoid, along with a few other diseases, could be transmitted by healthy people.

Mary Mallon was the first healthy carrier of typhoid to be carefully traced in North America. She was the first of hundreds of New Yorkers whom the health department accused of sheltering typhoid bacilli in their gallbladders and of transmitting the germs to susceptible people through their urine and feces via unwashed hands. She was not sick herself, but the presence of the pathogenic bacilli in her body defined her as hazardous to others. "A bacteriological examination revealed the fact that fully thirty percent of the bacteria voided with the feces were of typhoid bacilli," claimed the scientists during her habeas corpus hearing.[6] They were identifying health dangers using a brand-new method, a bacteriological marker possible to establish only through the use of laboratory tests. The medical view of her life, which focused on this laboratory finding and its exciting implications, is thus characterized by optimism and faith in science: her capture demonstrated that it was possible for humankind to conquer disease.

The second narrative of Mary Mallon's story comes from the point of view of public policy makers. This perspective built directly on the scientific one. The people responsible for devising health procedures that would truly protect the public in the early twentieth century saw the case of Mary Mallon as a very important turning point. Because of the new science, it was possible to find individuals who although healthy themselves put the general public at risk for disease. Having located such carriers, the health policy makers defined them as menaces to the public health. According to this viewpoint, it was necessary to keep Mary Mallon under lock and key for twenty-six years because she was responsible for three deaths and at least forty-seven cases of typhoid fever. To people like Hermann Biggs, the medical officer of the New York City Department of Health, Mary Mallon represented a clear-cut case of the necessity of infringing on individual rights in order to protect the public.

This public policy telling of the story portrays Mallon as a cog in a machine much larger than herself. Health officials used what they learned from Mallon, in the laboratory and in her isolation, to create rules and regulations that they could use to control other healthy carriers. She was the worst case who prepared health officers to cope with other healthy carriers and provided them with an argument to use to increase their authority. The story of Mary Mallon as a prelude to new public health policy is one in which she herself plays a relatively unimportant part, one that emphasizes her expendability to a greater good.

The third perspective on Mary Mallon's case emanates from the law and the lawyers who defined and defended it. While following closely on the tails of public policy, the legal story provides a different arena in which the supremacy of the new medicine was tested. The police powers left with the states under the U.S. Constitution mandate that states must operate to protect the health and welfare of their citizens. This is not just a right of the states, but an obligation. Over the course of United States history, various governmental activities evolved to meet this obligation. One of them was for authorities to remove, whenever possible, the causes of fatal disease that were present in the environment. By the beginning of the twentieth century most Americans agreed that government should act to prevent disease even when that meant the occasional infringement on the liberty of those who might have stood in the way of such disease prevention. Most such infringements—for example, forcible quarantining of individuals sick with diseases such as smallpox, so that they could not easily infect their neighbors—were viewed as the cost of health for the majority. The questions Mary Mallon's experiences raised involved whether forcible quarantines could be extended to healthy people and whether such people could be kept isolated indefinitely.

Mary Mallon's lawyer, George Francis O'Neill, argued that Mary Mallon had never been sick with typhoid and was thus not a menace to the health of society. He also noted that she had been arrested without proper warrants or due process. O'Neill organized Mallon's court hearing around the question of whether or not the health department had a legal right to banish a healthy person to lifetime isolation. The legal perspective focuses on individual rights and issues of justice. Ideas about these issues have changed over time—today they differ from earlier in the century especially with regard to interpretation of due process requirements—and the law can be two-sided: on the one hand is the commitment to protect the public's health; on the other is the fear of arbitrary power and the loss of individual freedoms. When the lawyers tell Mary Mallon's story, her long-term forced incarceration becomes a complex legal dilemma.

The fourth perspective on Mary Mallon's experiences derives from the social expectations and prejudices of the period. We see them at work in the language a diverse group of people used to talk about her—language that went beyond factual scientific description to focus on Mallon's appearance and behavior, for example. Clearly, who she was and what she represented significantly affected the story people told about Mary Mallon.

There were those who argued during the years of her incarceration that Mallon got what she deserved. Their point of view was based in part on judgments about her culpability for her actions, assuming that she knowingly transmitted typhoid fever and that she acted from free will. These assumptions about Mallon's personal responsibility need to be analyzed in terms of the expectations people brought to their understanding about who Mary Mallon was and how she should act. Her lower class and immigrant status, at a time when so many Americans championed native-born, middle-class behavior patterns, seems to have influenced public as well as scientific opinion about her, especially since she did not seem to aspire to middle-class behavior patterns herself. Many people, including some of the bacteriologists and physicians in whose care she found herself, came to think of her as expendable in the fight to protect the public health of all New Yorkers. Influenced by social prejudices, they blamed Mallon for her own fate. The microbe was not at fault, its carrier was.

The fifth perspective on Mary Mallon is the one constructed by the media in newspaper and journal representations. These public descriptions first emphasized, for dramatic purpose, the personal misfortune of a woman who was forced to give up a productive life to languish on an island. But by 1915, when Mallon returned to cooking after having promised she would not, the press more often demonized and blamed her. Reporters presented Mary Mallon to the world as someone to be dreaded, a carrier of sickness and death, someone to be shunned, ridiculed, "as a fiend dropping human skulls into a skillet."[7] Their words and editorial cartoons stripped Mallon of her human qualities. "This human culture tube," wrote one reporter, "has worked for prominent families in this city and communicated the disease to some of its members."[8] The news media accounts of the story dehumanized the carrier, using her life as a lesson to be learned and turning her into a uni-dimensional character.

Understanding how the media creation of Typhoid Mary gradually took the place of Mary Mallon is a crucial step in understanding the full dimensions of her story. Both the medical world and the American public have lived with Typhoid Mary for a long time, and although her meanings vary, she has not yet disappeared as a useful concept. Why did her medical story resonate in the public mind and in what ways was it purposely stylized? The public representation of a dangerous woman must be analyzed, especially in light of our recent exposure to yet another epidemic and new groups of stigmatized people who are labeled and sometimes treated as our generation's Typhoid Marys. Going back to the roots of this particular creation of Typhoid Mary can illuminate its present-day meanings and help sensitize us to our experiences with HIV infection, AIDS, drug-resistant tuberculosis, and the people who suffer from these diseases.

The sixth perspective on Mary Mallon is her own. An Irish immigrant cook, with limited career opportunities, but with quite a good reputation among New York's finest families, Mary Mallon deeply resented her incarceration from the beginning. From the day in 1907 when her employment came to an abrupt end, when the health officials knocked at her door and literally dragged her, kicking and screaming, into a city ambulance, and ultimately deposited her in a small cottage on an island on the grounds of an isolation hospital, Mallon claimed never to have understood the basis on which she, a healthy woman in mid-career, could be isolated and locked up for life. As she put it to a reporter, "I never had typhoid in my life, and have always been healthy. Why should I be banished like a leper and compelled to live in solitary confinement with only a dog for a companion?"[9]

Focusing on the woman and her life experiences, we come to understand the human dimension of public health policy, especially when it is based on still-new scientific propositions. Here was a woman who had never experienced any symptoms of typhoid and whose life was transformed for the worse because scientists insisted that microbes she could not see and in which she had no reason to believe had lodged in her gallbladder. Is it any wonder that she was incredulous and belligerent when first approached by health officials? Although possibly never convinced that she was in fact a public health danger, Mallon, after her second isolation, became resigned to her fate and died in captivity in 1938. From her own perspective, Mary Mallon's story is one of oppression, isolation, and injustice, of state authority run amuck.

The seventh, and final, perspective on Mary Mallon's story comes from its frequent retelling since her death. In what forms did her life continue to have cultural meaning after 1938? Why do we, to this day, see references to Typhoid Mary, a mark of her enduring meaning to our society? The post-1938 stories—in newspapers, journals, radio plays, novels, short stories, and theater—show compassion for Mallon's personal misfortune at the same time that they separate the historical figure from what she has come to mean.

Reflecting the advantages of hindsight and the perspectives of a more modern era, many recent accounts give more agency to Mary Mallon than the media at the time mustered. In emphasizing a positive view of her strength and feistiness, some modern-day writers depict a complex interaction between individual and society and a more analytical sense of what Mallon represents in our culture today. Paradoxically, even though these recent retellings seek to humanize Mary Mallon, they also make an explicit connection between Mallon and some of our current fears about AIDS and other "microbes into infinity."[10] In so doing they perpetuate the notion of Typhoid Mary as a metaphor for contagion and fear of contamination in some of the same ways the media used Mary Mallon's story in the past.

The phrase *Typhoid Mary* has modern-day resonance beyond attempts to recapture Mary Mallon's history. It has an independent life of its own, as a metaphor for contamination and the transmission of harm or death. Used now by people who have no memory or knowledge of Mary Mallon, the epithetical or metaphorical *Typhoid Mary* carries different implications at the end of the century than it did at the beginning. The process of the construction of meaning of *Typhoid Mary*, which began during Mary Mallon's lifetime, continues after her death, transformed yet again in a specific historical context, by end-of-the-century experiences with new epidemics.

These multiple perspectives on Mary Mallon's story lead to different conclusions about her significance and meaning. There are many ways in which to read the lives of people in the past and no one right way to tell the past's stories, just as there is no one way to experience events in the present. The diversity with which humans interpret life's meanings helps illuminate where we have been, where we are, and where we are going. I hope the stories presented here weave a tapestry that is both rich with past memory and useful in searching for today's answers to our pressing public health problems.

"The Rigorous Spirit of Science"

The Triumph of Bacteriology

ary Mallon, born in 1869, had the distinction, at the age of thirty-seven, of being the first person in North America to be identified, charted, and reported in the literature as a healthy typhoid fever carrier.[1] An Irish-born cook who immigrated to the United States as a teenager, she found work as a cook for wealthy New Yorkers and during the summer of 1906 was working in the rented summer home of a New York banker, Charles Henry Warren, in Oyster Bay, Long Island. When typhoid fever struck six people in the household of eleven, the owners of the home, Mr. and Mrs. George Thompson of New York City, hired investigators to determine the source of the epidemic.

It was not unusual for cities, states, or private citizens to seek such an inquiry into household typhoid fever outbreaks. The common sources of the infection included water or food supplies, and homeowners could correct the defects and assure themselves and their families safety against further infection. In this case, however, the studies proved inconclusive. Thinking they would be unable to rent the property again unless the mystery of these cases could be solved, the Thompsons hired George Soper, a civil engineer they heard about through social connections, to investigate the outbreak further. Soper was known for his epidemiological analyses of typhoid fever epidemics.[2]

14

George Soper had been born and raised in New York City. He attended the Rensselaer Polytechnic Institute in Troy, New York (B.S. 1895), and returned to the city to attend Columbia University (A.M., 1898; Ph.D., 1899) in sanitary engineering. He was well launched on a successful engineering career by the time the Thompsons hired him to investigate the Oyster Bay outbreak. He had already worked for the Boston Water Works and had successfully investigated typhoid fever outbreaks in Ithaca, New York, and other U.S. cities.[3]

Soper began his investigation by reviewing the facts already known. The outbreak's first case had been discovered on August 27 when one of the Warrens' daughters became ill. Next, two maids and Mrs. Warren were affected, followed by another daughter and the gardener. Soper studied the records and ruled out the common causes of such typhoid fever outbreaks, contaminated water and milk. He systematically discarded other possible sources of infection, including clams from the bay and other foodstuffs consumed in the house and any contacts between family members and people outside who might have had the disease. When none of these alternative explanations proved viable, Soper pressed family members to remember any other distinctive events that might have taken place during the summer weeks when some members contracted typhoid. Through close scrutiny, Soper found his clue: he learned that the family had changed cooks shortly preceding the weeks in question.

Believing the cook, named Mary Mallon, who had left the family three weeks after the outbreak, to be a prime suspect, Soper turned his attention to tracking her down. Although the family claimed the woman had been in perfect health, Soper, who undoubtedly knew about healthy carriers of other diseases and might have been reading (as he later claimed) literature from Germany and elsewhere in Europe about healthy typhoid fever carriers, expressed confidence that such a person was most likely to have caused this particular household outbreak. Soper was encouraged in his theory about the cook when he learned that she often prepared for the family an ice-cream dessert served with fresh sliced peaches, which would have been an excellent medium for typhoid infection.[4]

Soper gathered his strongest evidence of the cook's involvement by tracing her job history before her arrival in Oyster Bay in August, 1906. This kind of "shoe leather" epidemiological study, tracking down cases and patterns, was not new in the twentieth century. When he made the rounds and followed leads to find his target, Soper was following traditional methods dating to prebacteriological days.[5] Relying heavily on information provided by Mary Mallon's employment agencies, he found eight families who had previously employed her, the earliest beginning in 1897. In seven of these families typhoid fever had developed.[6] The following is an expansion of the chronology Soper uncovered.

1. Summer, 1900, Mamaroneck, New York. Mary Mallon had worked for a New York family with a summer home on Long Island for three years when one case of typhoid fever developed in a young male visitor about ten days after his arrival. There were no other reported cases during her tenure with this family, and, Soper reported, "It was believed at the time that the young man had contracted his typhoid before he came to visit the family."[7]

2. Winter, 1901–1902, New York City. Mary Mallon cooked for a New York City family for eleven months. One month after her arrival, the family's laundress came down with typhoid fever. At the time there was no investigation of this case.

3. Summer, 1902, Dark Harbor, Maine. In the early summer of 1902 the family of New York lawyer J. Coleman Drayton suffered a severe outbreak of typhoid fever. The Draytons had hired Mary Mallon to accompany them to their summer residence in Dark Harbor, Maine, just before leaving New York City in June. Beginning with the footman, seven of the nine (family of four and five servants) became infected.[8] Only Coleman Drayton and Mary Mallon escaped the disease. The cook stayed on to help nurse the

sick, for which Mr. Drayton was so grateful that he gave her a bonus for her trouble. The outbreak had been investigated by Dr. E. A. Daniels of Boston and Dr. Louis Starr of Philadelphia, who had concluded that the footman had brought the illness into the house.[9]

4. Summer, 1904, Sands Point, New York. Nine months following Mary Mallon's employment, an outbreak of typhoid fever affected four newly employed servants in the Long Island summer household of Henry Gilsey. The servants lived in a house apart from the family, and the family members were not infected. The episode was investigated by Dr. R. J. Wilson, superintendent of hospitals for communicable diseases in New York City, who believed that the laundress (the first infected) brought the fever to the servants' quarters.[10]

5. Summer, 1906, Oyster Bay, New York. Six persons in the Charles Henry Warren household of eleven were infected with typhoid fever. They included three family members—Warren's wife and two daughters—and three servants—two maid servants and the gardener. Before Soper began his investigation of this outbreak, two other experts, E. E. Smith and D. D. Jackson, had concluded that the water supply "must have been contaminated," possibly by the cleaners of the tank who "perhaps carried typhoid excreta on their boots."[11]

6. Autumn, 1906, Tuxedo Park, New York. Two weeks following Mary Mallon's arrival as cook to the George Kessler family, a laundress was taken ill. The cause of her illness remained unclear.

7. Winter, 1907, New York City. The Walter Bowen family of 688 Park Avenue hired Mary Mallon during the winter of 1906–1907. Two months after her initial employment, a chambermaid in the household became sick with typhoid fever, and soon after the daughter of the family became ill and died. It was within this house that George Soper conducted his first meeting with Mary Mallon.[12]

About his findings, Soper noted, "There is a remarkable resemblance between these seven fragments. In each instance one or more cases of typhoid have occurred in households from ten days to a few weeks after the cook has arrived or among people who have, within that period, come to live near her and eaten the food which she has prepared."[13] Soper identified twenty-two cases of typhoid in his search of Mary Mallon's employment between 1900 and 1907, although his enumeration, which is the one quoted by all those who used his evidence, was twenty-six. This number is actually quite small and indicates that many of the people for whom Mallon cooked during these years may have been already immune to typhoid by virtue of having recovered from the disease. During these same years, between 3,000 and 4,500 new cases of typhoid fever were reported each year in New York City, and most of these people would have been exposed to the disease through contaminated water supplies or other sources more common than an individual healthy carrier. (Immunization became available after 1911.)[14]

Fourteen of the initial twenty-two infected people traced to Mary Mallon were domestic servants and eight were members of the families who employed them. Soper called attention to the class of those infected in his first paper and later repeated his observation: "The social position of the persons attacked differed decidedly." Soper's audience at the Biological Society of Washington, D.C., when he first publicly presented his evidence on April 6, 1907, emphasized the servants' susceptibility. Some believed with Dr. C. W. Stiles that more servants got sick because "personal cleanliness has an important bearing," implying that servants were dirtier than their employers. In the discussion, Soper muddied the water somewhat by explaining that more servants became ill because cooks handled their salads, fruits, and other raw food items more often than they did for family members and thus had greater opportunity to infect other servants, an observation that was not necessarily true.[15] The resultant perception that servants were uniquely sensitive to typhoid infection from healthy carriers has lasted in the literature to the present.[16]

Although almost all of the outbreaks with which Soper linked Mary Mallon's name had been investigated and other sources identified as their cause, Soper remained unpersuaded by the previous reports.[17] The twenty-two cases in families with which he could connect Mary Mallon convinced Soper that it was the cook who constituted the danger. We have no independent source through which to verify Soper's accounting of Mallon's employment history, and internally, his tellings of the story disagree on small details. The account, nonetheless, was consistent in connecting Mary Mallon and typhoid fever. Being himself so skeptical of others' investigations, Soper knew that in order to convince others of his own arguments about Mallon's involvement, his epidemiological conclusions had to be thorough and backed with laboratory proof. This need for laboratory certainty explains why Soper was so persistent in his investigation and, once he found her, insistent on obtaining specimens of urine and feces from Mary Mallon.

Mary Mallon's apprehension in March, 1907, in the Park Avenue home in which she was then employed, was dramatic. George Soper appeared without warning and explained to her that she was spreading disease and death through her cooking. He wanted samples of her feces, urine, and blood to test them in the laboratory. The story seemed preposterous to the healthy Mallon, who promptly threw him out of the house. Mallon's response was not unreasonable in an era before the idea of a "healthy carrier" was known to the general public and even before many in the medical profession understood it. Soper persevered. He took a medical colleague and visited Mary Mallon in her home, where, again, she evicted him.[18]

When he could not obtain the necessary samples for laboratory testing himself, on March 11, 1907, Soper presented his evidence to Hermann Biggs, medical officer of the New York City Health Department, so that he could pursue the case. As an independent investigator, Soper did not have the authority to demand compliance. Biggs and his health department colleagues found Soper's epidemiological evidence sufficiently compelling to follow through on his suggestions. Soper's evidence convinced them that if Mary Mallon could be found, and her feces and urine tested, the laboratory would prove what Soper's epidemiological study had already shown—that Mary Mallon, although healthy, had transmitted typhoid fever to those who had eaten the food she prepared.

When approached by the official city health inspector, Dr. S. Josephine Baker, Mallon still did not understand the demands for laboratory specimens and refused to provide the evidence. Dr. Baker called in the police to help and the officers took Mallon by force and against her will to the Willard Parker Hospital, New York's receiving unit for those suffering from contagious diseases. There they subjected her excreta to careful laboratory analysis.[19] Finding high concentrations of typhoid bacilli in her feces, authorities kept Mallon in health department custody, moving her to an isolation cottage on the grounds of the Riverside Hospital on North Brother Island in New York.

The city kept Mallon in her isolation retreat for two years before she sued the health department for release in 1909. Her lawyers argued before the New York Supreme Court that she had never been sick and could not be the "menace" to society that the health department claimed. The judge, while voicing sympathy, sided with the health department and sent Mary Mallon back to her island cottage.[20] After another year of isolation, a new health commissioner released her on the promise that she would not cook again. Ultimately she reneged on this agreement, and in 1915 the health authorities found her cooking at the Sloane Maternity Hospital, the site of an outbreak of twenty-five new cases of typhoid fever. This time they sent her back to her island isolation for the rest of her life. On November 11, 1938, Mary Mallon died, having been "a special guest of the City of New York" for more than twenty-six years.

The details of Mallon's experiences beginning with her 1907 detention are further explored in the other chapters of this book. For the remainder of this chapter, I want to examine how and why it came to be that health officials in 1907 were eager and able to locate healthy carriers of typhoid fever and what Mary Mallon, as the first such carrier to be carefully traced, represented to the followers of the new science of bacteriology. The perspective of the bacteriologists, which emphasizes the triumph of scientific and laboratory methodology and has become the commonplace narrative in the medical literature, is but the first of multiple viewpoints on Mary Mallon that this book analyzes.

Throughout the nineteenth century, epidemics of infectious diseases, many of which already had threatened and scourged America in the colonial period, increased in their destructive powers. As the population in major cities exploded through immigration, epidemics of cholera, smallpox, and yellow fever took increasing numbers of lives. Today at the end of the twentieth century, even while epidemics of HIV infection and drug-resistant tuberculosis threaten hundreds of thousands, even millions, of Americans, we cannot easily comprehend the high threat of disease with which nineteenth-century urbanites lived.

On top of the ever-present childhood diseases that may have accounted for 60 percent of total urban deaths and carried away more than one in ten infants before their first birthdays, as well as various other endemic problems affecting adults, fatal epidemics periodically swept through America's cities. These outbreaks —for example, cholera, which left an emaciated shell of a person if it did not kill, or the permanently scarring smallpox, which sometimes carried a high death rate—left behind extraordinary debility, and, often, complete civic disarray. Urbanites who could afford it fled their homes for the hoped-for safety of the less crowded rural areas. The exodus sometimes included government officials who abandoned the city to fend for itself at the height of the crisis.[21] Too familiar was the sight of the horse-drawn ambulance or the disinfecting van, and the hearse.

In response to the devastation from disease, especially epidemic disease, cities and states organized health departments whose functions included planning programs to obviate the worst of the disasters.[22] Before the nineteenth century, health work remained haphazard and usually limited to epidemic emergencies: when an epidemic ended, health boards would be disbanded until the next one threatened. In the nineteenth century, however, urbanites, faced with increasing sanitation crises and devastating epidemics, began demanding a more systematic approach to disease control. Much of the work early in the century rested on the prevailing medical theory that dirt caused disease and emphasized keeping the city environment clean. The so-called "filth" theory of disease posited in a very general sense that undifferentiated urban pollution—deriving from waste material from the horses, cows, and pigs that roamed freely around America's burgeoning cities and other rotting organic refuse and garbage left uncollected on city streets—caused bad air, or "miasmas," which could lead to disease. In response to this perceived health reason to clean up the environment, health officers developed large-scale sanitation projects to bring clean water into the cities and allow efficient sewage disposal and garbage collection and disposal. In addition, nineteenth-century health departments operated vaccination programs, isolation hospitals, and dispensaries to help bring health to urban residents.

The results of some of these nineteenth-century responses to the threat of disease are with us still today. The city of Chicago, for example, built upon low-lying flatlands, literally raised its buildings above the water table in order to provide for sanitary sewerage and clean water.[23] New York and Boston sought clean water miles from the city and spent considerable sums constructing pipes and aqueducts to transport it. All major cities engineered massive waterworks and intricate networks of pipes to carry clean water to city-dwellers. Creative solutions to the garbage disposal problems evolved as public works and public health departments cooperated to diminish the dangers from disease. Local governments spent large proportions of their budgets on these infrastructure necessities in response to the public demand for aid against the risks to health abounding in the city environment.

By the last decades of the century, the experimental work from the laboratories of Louis Pasteur in France and Robert Koch in Germany had revolutionized medical theory about the causes of epidemic disease, substituting microorganisms for undifferentiated filth as the culprit. Narrowing the etiology of disease from the whole urban environment to microscopic germs seemed to pinpoint the public health activity needed to eliminate the problems. Medical scientists, some of whom completely abandoned the old theories, were convinced that the identification of microorganisms as a single cause of infectious diseases would allow them to target specific public health activity to find and eliminate those germs.[24] The new science promised to eliminate some of the worst scourges of urban life and bring health to all who followed its precepts.

The effects of bacteriology on public health theory and practices can be understood vividly through the activities of Charles V. Chapin, whose forty-seven-year career as superintendent of health for Providence, Rhode Island, spanned the turn of the twentieth century. Chapin's enthusiasm for bacteriology turned him against many of the old practices that had derived from the notion that filth caused disease. Through his one-sided approach, we can best understand the lure of the new science. James H. Cassedy, Chapin's biographer, has portrayed the excitement of those years for people engaged in efforts to protect and promote the public's health.[25] Laboratory experiments led to frequent announcements of new microbes, which in turn provided links to understanding diseases that had baffled scientists and decimated populations. The hope and promise of these revelations carried Chapin and many public health workers on a wave of optimism, as they scrambled to incorporate the findings into their daily tasks. Chapin became the nation's leading proponent of using the new science to change the focus of public health work away from broad environmental sanitation to a narrower search for microbes to destroy. In 1902, he wrote an impassioned article claiming that bacteriology "drove the last nail in the coffin" of the old filth theory of disease. Sanitary reforms, such as cleaning streets and collecting garbage, were no longer necessary, Chapin claimed, because it would "make no demonstrable difference in a city's mortality whether its streets are clean or not, whether the garbage is removed promptly or allowed to accumulate, or whether it has a plumbing law."[26]

While today we recognize a link between poor sanitation and germ propagation, Chapin, in his eagerness to get people to accept invisible microorganisms as the single cause of disease (an idea some medical and many lay people initially distrusted), appeared to discard notions about filth—which he agreed might be aesthetically distasteful but not itself dangerous to health—and attacked the old practices one after another. For example, in one of his most influential papers he decried as a "fetich" the common practice of fumigating with steam or formaldehyde the rooms in which the sick had suffered or died.[27] Chapin worked to replace city-wide clean-up programs with ones focusing on living human germ carriers (those persons sick or carrying infectious diseases) and encouraging personal habits that would protect individuals from the people around them. While Chapin remained optimistic about what the new science of bacteriology could offer, he never promised that bacteriology alone could "stamp out" disease.[28] He understood how hard it would be to implement what were to a large extent changes in personal behavior.

Chapin emphasized a new worry that had been uncovered by recent bacteriological studies: the risk posed by healthy carriers, people who themselves were not sick but who could nonetheless infect others. The Providence health officer became the nation's preeminent leader in educating the public (and his peers) about these hidden dangers:

Neither you, nor I, nor the Board of Health, know where these [carriers and missed cases] are. The occupant of the next seat may, for all one knows, be a diphtheria carrier, so may the saleslady who ties up the package, the conductor who gives the transfer, or the expressman who leaves a parcel at the door. The dirty man hanging on the car strap may be a typhoid carrier, or it may be that the fashionably dressed woman who used it just before was infected with some loathsome disease. If these people were sick in bed we would avoid them. As it is we cannot. Science has shown this new danger.[29]

Chapin believed that as experimental and laboratory studies revealed new sources of exposure to infectious diseases, citizens had to assume an increasing responsibility to try to avoid them:

Contact with the fresh secretions, or excretions, of human beings, is the most important source of infection for most of our common contagious diseases. By turning the face from the coughing and loud talking of our neighbors; by putting nothing in the mouth except clean food and drink; by never putting the fingers in the mouth, or nose; most contagious diseases can be avoided. Wash the hands well before eating and always after the use of the toilet. Teach this to the children by precept and especially by example.[30]

Chapin not only preached the new gospel of individualized public health, he also put the new science into practice by newly prioritizing public health procedures.[31] He pleaded with his fellow health officers to adopt a "more rational perspective" by directing their efforts toward the isolation of infectious diseases, medical inspection, vaccination, and laboratory investigation of milk supplies, instead of to abatement of nuisances and municipal housekeeping.[32]

Over time, other health officers and health departments around the country adopted many of these precepts. The health department in Milwaukee, Wisconsin, for example, had given up control over water and garbage to the department of public works by 1911.[33] The emphasis of local health work changed from city-wide sanitation and disease control to closer observation of individuals, their habits, and their potential to carry disease. Most health officers believed that it was possible and even financially necessary to keep many older sanitation activities and adapt them to coexist with the new bacteriological programs rather than to begin anew, as Chapin's rhetoric suggested. Indeed, since microbes bred in unsanitary environments, the two theories seemed compatible.

Concomitant with the shift in emphasis in public health work, bacteriological laboratories with their microbe-identifying capabilities became the single most crucial tool in identifying the people and the problems to which health departments should attend. During the "golden age of bacteriology," in the words of one of the country's leading public health theoreticians, Charles-Edward Amory Winslow, "the laboratory . . . [was] the scientific foundation of the public health campaign in America."[34]

Typhoid fever was one of nineteenth-century America's most serious health problems, and its history illustrates how the new science of bacteriology worked alongside the old filth theories to contribute to curtailing the incidence and deaths caused by the disease. (Today, clean water supplies and antibiotics have made typhoid fever a minor statistic in the full picture of disease dangers.)[35] Science's understanding of microorganisms and their role in disease transmission added to efforts already begun in the prebacteriological era to alleviate the worst of typhoid fever's devastation. In the minds of bacteriologists and medical scientists of the period, the disease provided an excellent example of how science could save lives.

In the mid-nineteenth century, when scientists first distinguished typhoid fever from typhus as two distinct diseases (caused by different microorganisms), the former was already causing significant public health problems in American cities.[36] A water- and food-borne systemic bacterial infection, typhoid brought sustained fever, headache, malaise, and gastrointestinal problems (constipation or diarrhea) to its victims. A few days following exposure, the patient experienced headache, loss of appetite, and chills. The body temperature slowly rose—to 104 or 105 degrees—and could remain high for two weeks; with only cold baths to relieve the fever, it often did not disappear for four weeks or more. Victims developed a characteristic rash on the abdomen and chest, which lasted for a few days. Severe cramping, tenderness, and diarrhea added to the patient's woes. Sick for over a month, the patient weakened and became susceptible to complications. Although many mild cases occurred, typhoid fever carried a case fatality rate of about 10 percent.[37]

Typhoid struck most harshly in those cities that sent untreated lake or river water through the pipes; thus it responded well to water filtration systems and sanitation efforts instituted in many cities during the last third of the nineteenth century or in the early years of the twentieth century.[38] Often it took repeated epidemics to convince legislators or taxpayers to spend the large sums necessary to clean up the water supply. Milwaukee, for example, did not eliminate the "typhoid highball" drawn from the city water pipes until citizens, after suffering from a major bout of diarrhea in 1916, finally approved a bond for a new sewage-treatment plant.[39]

New York City brought clean water from the Croton watershed in the 1840s, but by the 1880s population density had severely taxed the system and led to serious pollution problems. Minor patching to the system sufficed until the turn of the cen-

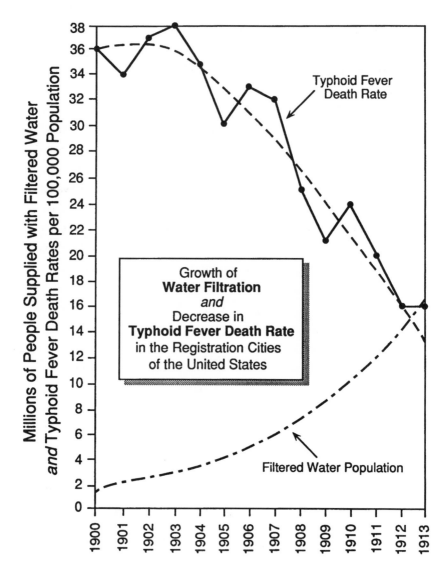

Fig. 1.1. *Water Filtration and Typhoid Fever Death Rates, U.S., 1900–1913.*

tury. In 1907, the year of Mary Mallon's first move to North Brother Island, continuing high typhoid fever rates convinced many New Yorkers that they could wait no longer to filter the water flowing in the city pipes. While advising citizens to boil their water, city leaders put in process plans for a new sewer system and in 1911 finally appropriated almost $9 million to construct a filtration plant.[40]

Typhoid fever exemplified the effectiveness of sanitation practices based both on the old filth theory of disease and at the same time incorporating the new tenets of bacteriology. When the *salmonella typhi* bacillus was identified (1880) and traced to contaminated water supplies, it underscored the necessity of providing clean water in urban environments. William T. Sedgwick, the Massachusetts state bacteriologist, and the Lawrence Engineering Laboratory pioneered an effective sand filter in the 1890s and paved the way for safe drinking systems. As more and more cities responded by adding filtration to their water systems in the early twentieth century, typhoid fever diminished nationwide as a major cause of morbidity and mortality (see fig. 1.1).[41]

Yet typhoid fever did not disappear. In 1900, over 35,000 deaths in the United States were attributed to typhoid.[42] In the first decade of the twentieth century, thanks to bacteriological investigations, medical scientists began to understand why there were still cases of typhoid after sanitation efforts had significantly lowered the incidence of the disease. "Residual" typhoid seemed to be caused by apparently healthy persons, either those recovered from a case of the disease or those who could not remember being sick at all but who nevertheless harbored the bacillus and transmitted it to others. Labeled "germ distributors," "chronic carriers," or "healthy carriers," these individuals became important foci for bacteriologically oriented public health officials, potent illustrations of how the new science, by creating a new taxonomy, both aided and complicated the fight against disease. By 1907 when bacteriologists identified Mary Mallon as a healthy typhoid carrier, scientists had already firmly established that healthy people could carry *salmonella typhi* in their excreta and transmit the disease to others.[43]

Researchers slowly elaborated the details of how healthy people harbored and transmitted the disease to others. American scientists, familiar with European research on typhoid carriers, shared data from various centers around the country, including San Francisco, St. Louis, Syracuse, Boston, Chicago, Wisconsin, and Minnesota. In the early decades of the twentieth century, American bacteriologists came to understand that the carrier state could follow either mild, even subclinical, cases or acute illnesses; that it seemed to last more than six weeks in approximately 3 percent of recovered cases; and that more women than men seemed to be chronically affected, especially when those women had been infected during their middle years. *Salmonella typhi* could be isolated from blood, urine, or feces; the bacilli often lodged in the gallbladder. Carriers transmitted the disease in the same ways as typhoid victims might infect others, through water or food contaminated by their feces or urine.[44]

Many scientists believed that Mary Mallon's apprehension in 1907 was a momentous event, one in which the new science of bacteriology played a heroic role. They championed bacteriology's new key function in streamlining the efforts of the health department by reducing the attack on typhoid to those individuals who could be identified by laboratory methods as dangerous. Mallon's example demonstrated the vital importance of the laboratory as a supplement to or even a substitute for physical examinations. The laboratory would help the health department get people like Mary Mallon off the streets and out of the homes of healthy citizens. Scientists and health officials believed the new science would help protect the public's health in the best possible way.

The laboratory to which Mallon's specimens were brought,

part of the division of pathology, bacteriology, and disinfection within the health department, had been the dream of Hermann Biggs, probably the premier public health officer in the country.[45] It early achieved a national reputation. Charles Chapin described the New York laboratory as "perhaps the most important step in modernizing public health practice in the United States."[46] In 1893 Biggs had hired William Hallock Park, a physician trained at Columbia University College of Physicians and Surgeons and in the scientific laboratories of Vienna, to organize the bacteriological laboratory, and Park remained as its director until 1936. He and his colleagues carried out studies that put New York in the forefront of bacteriological investigations in the United States. Among their more important works were their studies of healthy carriers.[47] Mary Mallon, because of her long stay under department auspices, provided much of their longitudinal data on typhoid fever carriers. As Charles F. Bolduan, Park's associate at the laboratory, put it, Mallon "gave Park a splendid opportunity to develop laboratory methods for the detection and isolation of typhoid bacilli in stools."[48]

Mary Mallon's feces received close laboratory scrutiny from March 20, 1907, the day after she was first brought to the hospital, until she sued for release, the last examination recorded in the court records occurring on June 16, 1909. More examinations were made after her second incarceration in 1915; unfortunately the data from these are less detailed and probably incomplete. The laboratory investigations proved of major importance in the legal investigation and the health department's public justification of subsequent events. They were basic to the bacteriologists' claim that Mallon was a "menace" to the public's health.

During the twenty-eight months between March 1907 and June 1909, health officers collected 163 fecal specimens from Mallon, an average of more than one a week.[49] In Mallon's words: "When I first came here they took two Blood Cultures and feces went down three times per week say Monday Wednesday & Friday respectfully [sic] until the latter part of June after that they only got the feces once a week which was on Wednesday."[50]

The laboratory analyses revealed that Mallon was an intermittent carrier of typhoid fever. Repeatedly over these months, her feces contained no typhoid bacilli at all, the laboratory reports showing negative for twelve consecutive examinations, from September 16 through October 14, 1907. In a sporadic pattern over the twenty-eight months, 120 of the 163 cultures tested positive, 43 negative in this period. Her urine consistently tested negative.

Soper, no doubt trying to make his case stronger, somewhat misrepresented the laboratory results in his accounts. He claimed that the 1907 examinations revealed "only a few instances [when] the typhoid organisms [were] not found."[51] In fact the year's totals indicated fifty-five positive cultures and thirty-four negative.

While the city was conducting its laboratory tests, Mallon arranged for her urine and feces to be analyzed by a private company, the Ferguson Laboratories. The specimens were brought to them by Mr. A. Briehof, a friend of Mallon's, with whom she lived before her detention.[52] George Ferguson conducted ten tests on Mallon's urine and feces between August 1, 1908, and April 30, 1909, concluding, "I would state that none of the specimens submitted by you, of urine and feces, have shown typhoid colonies."[53]

Comparing the dates of Ferguson's analysis with the health department's analysis reveals that of the ten negatives the private laboratory found, eight were reported during weeks when Mallon's feces tested positive in the city laboratory. There are a number of possible explanations for the discrepancy between the city and private laboratory reports. We do not know the manner in which Mallon's feces were transported to the private laboratory, and it is possible that the specimens were not fresh when they reached the laboratory. There is also the possibility that the laboratory did not itself carry out the work expeditiously or carefully, or that it had incentives to carelessness. Since Mallon was an intermittent carrier, there were bound to be both times during which her feces carried the bacteria and times when they did not.[54]

Mallon denied the validity of the health department's laboratory tests when they confirmed the presence of bacteria associated with a disease that she insisted she had never suffered. She repeatedly voiced her skepticism about the reliability of these positive bacteriological findings. Nonetheless, she accepted and used the negative laboratory results from the Ferguson Laboratory to bolster her case in court. Although she may have felt herself to be a victim of bacteriology, she apparently did not mind enlisting the laboratory—the emblem of the new science—to present her side and fight for her liberty.

The health department used its predominantly positive laboratory reports to make its 1909 legal case, to insist to the court that it was necessary to isolate Mary Mallon. Dr. Fred S. Westmoreland, the resident physician at Riverside Hospital on North Brother Island, in whose care Mallon was placed, offered the following conclusion before the judge:

A bacteriological examination revealed the fact that fully thirty per cent of the bacteria voided with the feces were of typhoid bacilli; the urine was negative.... Weekly examinations of the stools have usually revealed large numbers of bacilli.... In view of the foregoing and owing to the large quantities of typhoid bacilli existing in the alimentary tract, or gall bladder of the patient and her occupation as a cook or the fact that she may at any time come in contact with people wherein they would be likely to be infected with the typhoid bacilli, the Department of Health concluded that the patient would be a dangerous person and a constant menace to the public health to be at large; and, consequently, ... decided, after careful consideration and acting upon their examination of the patient, to place her in a contagious hospital and isolate her from the general public.[55]

The laboratory reports formed the central argument in the health officials' 1909 case as they had for Soper's initial identification. Without them, the court probably would not have kept Mary Mallon in isolation; with them, the case seemed clear to the Honorable Mitchell L. Erlanger, who ordered that the writ should be dismissed and "that the said petitioner, Mary Mallen [*sic*], be and she hereby is remanded to the custody of the Board of Health of the City of New York."[56] Even though the laboratories issued contradictory reports, the seemingly incontrovertible evidence of repeated positive typhoid cultures in the city laboratory data made Mary Mallon's danger as a carrier palpable.

In concordance with the laboratory evidence, the health department addressed the question of how to eliminate Mallon's infectiousness. According to Westmoreland's testimony, "Hexamethylenamin in doses gradually increasing from one hundred to one hundred and fifty grains a day has been given frequently with no apparent benefit. Attention to diet and mild laxative has caused the greatest reduction but not their disappearance."[57] Mallon provided more details of her therapy, which she portrayed as punitive: "In spite of the medical staff Dr. Wilson ordered me Urotropin I got that on & off for a year sometimes the[y] had it & sometimes the[y] did not. I took the Urotropin for about 3 months all told during the whole year if I should have continued it would certainly have Killed me for it was very Severe[.]"[58] She indicated the physicians had also tried brewer's yeast, but "at first I did not take it for I'm a little afraid of the people & I have a good right for when I came to the Department the[y] said [the bacteria] were in my track later another said they were in the muscels [*sic*] of my bowels & laterly the[y] thought of the gall Bladder." The lack of medical precision convinced Mallon that the doctors did not know what they were doing.

In addition to trying various drugs, health officers urged Mallon to have her gallbladder surgically removed, a suggestion she repeatedly refused.[59] Abdominal surgery was associated with a risk of infection, but the physicians urging surgery on Mallon did not inform her of this or of the procedure's poor record in alleviating the carrier state. Milton J. Rosenau, during the discussion of Park's earliest paper on the subject at an American Medical Association meeting in 1908, opined that "she is perhaps justified in this conclusion [to refuse to submit to surgical interference.]" Mallon's skepticism found support in the medical world. William Park himself concluded in 1914, "Medicinal treatment or surgery seems so far to have yielded only slight results. . . . Removal of the gall-bladder cannot be relied upon."[60] By 1921, the department of health admitted that it followed the history of five carriers who had agreed to the removal of their gallbladders, "all of them without success."[61]

The emphasis on laboratory findings together with the drug therapy and proposed surgery indicate the extent to which health department thinking concentrated on the bacteria themselves rather than on a more comprehensive approach to eliminating the dangers Mary Mallon posed. The energy and commitment of these particular bacteriologically guided health officials was not directed toward social rehabilitation but focused more narrowly on the pathogenic bacilli, illustrating how for them bacteriology reduced the scope of health-related work.

The necessity for keeping Mary Mallon isolated emanated from her laboratory-defined carrier state and from her refusal to accept the authority of bacteriological findings. She persisted in denying that she had ever been sick with typhoid and insisted that she was "in perfect physical condition" and was "not in any way or any degree a menace to the community or any part thereof."[62] Perhaps she denied the validity of the bacteriological findings because her own laboratory informed her that her stools showed no typhoid bacilli, or perhaps because of her rival worldview, one which credited her experience as a healthy woman above a science that defined her as infected. She did not believe the doctors' claims, she said, at least in part because they kept changing them, sometimes telling her the bacilli lodged in her gallbladder and other times locating them in the muscles of her bowels. Eventually, her denial became part of the indictment against her.

The importance of laboratory analysis to the health department becomes even more evident in the record of Mallon's second isolation, which began in 1915 and ended with her death in 1938. The health officials monitored Mary Mallon's feces throughout her life. From the extant records we learn that especially during the 1920s, but periodically during most of the years she was isolated, Mary Mallon continued to provide stool samples to her captors. Only once, on January 3, 1919, did the health department record she "refused to give stools."[63] As offensive and inconvenient as it might have been for a healthy woman regularly to provide stool samples, once as many as fourteen a month and more usually one a week, the process of collection and evaluation continued. The health officers did not permit Mary Mallon to forget why she was isolated, and, more significant, they continued to try to learn through her bodily excretions how carriers' infection patterns might change over time.

Mallon's stool cultures continued to demonstrate the intermittent character of the woman's pathogenicity. The samples for which we can find information—for some years quite complete and for others very scant—indicate a predominance of positive cultures during the second incarceration, among which were occasional negatives. In 1915 and 1916 all of the tests for which we have evidence (fourteen and seven, respectively) proved positive for *salmonella typhi*. However, of the six recorded during 1917, only two tested positive, and four negative. During 1923, fifty-one of fifty-four tested positive, and during 1924, fifty of fifty-eight samples taken likewise contained the typhoid bacteria. Between 1907 and 1909, Mallon produced 120 positive stool samples and 53 negatives (including the specimens tested by the Ferguson

Laboratory); between 1915 and 1936, we have evidence of 207 positives and 23 negatives.[64]

The laboratory and its ability to identify danger were elevated to new heights of importance in this persistent examination of Mary Mallon's stools. After 1915 the repeated tests were no longer based on the need to prove that she carried typhoid; that had already been accomplished. The repetitive procedures nonetheless remained important to the laboratory and health department officials. Undoubtedly, the bacteriologists felt it was essential to scientific knowledge to document a long-term record of the carrier state. In more practical terms, without the laboratory proof that Mallon remained contaminated, how could they continue to isolate a healthy woman?

Since 1888, when Charles Chapin established the first municipal laboratory in the United States, the proof of laboratory results had steadily gained significance in public health investigations.[65] Laboratory verification had become the hallmark of the new science of bacteriology and vital to what became identified as the "new public health" in the early years of the twentieth century. Writing in 1923, C.-E. A. Winslow claimed, "The laboratory has become the scientific foundation of the public health campaign in America, developed to a point perhaps unequaled in any other country. The activities of the chemist and the bacteriologist . . . impart throughout the whole range of the work of the health department the rigorous spirit of science."[66]

Mary Mallon's capture epitomized what the new laboratory science could provide and the hope for the future. It had now become possible to isolate the germs that caused disease in the laboratory, bacteriology's major tool. Having done that, it would be possible to discover how the microorganisms were spread and, scientists believed, to stop that dissemination. Those who saw the story of Mallon's pursuit and capture as a triumph of the new science were convinced that the bacteriological success alone was what made the story important. She could not have been found without Soper's careful epidemiological work and could not have been isolated without the subsequent laboratory proof of the dangers she posed. It seems probable that she could not have been held twenty-six years in isolation without the continuing laboratory substantiation. Finding and isolating Mary Mallon represented the scientific optimism of the early twentieth century and the faith that science would serve humanity by curbing disease.

Mary Mallon's story, when understood from this scientific perspective, is a compelling and clear testimonial to scientific advancement. Hundreds and thousands of other healthy carriers of typhoid fever identified in New York City and around the country in the years following 1907 were found through similar epidemiological studies, with the laboratory adding proof that they shed typhoid bacilli in their feces or urine. Medical science proved its worth in the case of healthy carriers of typhoid fever.

However important the advancements of understanding the carrier state and locating carriers were, these steps did not themselves answer the challenge of disease control. Bacteriology had addressed the question of why typhoid fever continued to threaten the population, but it could not alone provide the means by which people could be protected. Given the sheer volume of hundreds or thousands of carriers in major cities and states around the country, health departments needed to find ways to adapt the scientific findings to practical public health policy. In determining their actions, health officials relied on a combination of factors, including but not limited to scientific findings. If we are to remember and give deeper meaning to Mary Mallon and this important episode in medical history, and to use it to increase our comprehension of present-day health problems, we need to look beyond the "shoe leather" epidemiology and the laboratory findings to uncover other perspectives on her story.

"Extraordinary and Even Arbitrary Powers"

Public Health Policy

$\mathcal{F}$or the city and state officials responsible for developing and executing health policy, Mary Mallon posed a challenge beyond the single individual. Their perspective accepted the bacteriology laboratory findings identifying Mary Mallon as a menace and emphasized the very practical question of how to stop her from endangering the health of others. The public officials who encountered her also needed to determine health policies that would put this one carrier's story to use against the threat that all healthy carriers seemed to pose to the public. To investigate Mary Mallon's story in terms of health policy from the perspective of the people officially responsible for the protection of the public's health, we need to examine public health authority in this period and to try to understand the dimensions of the healthy carrier problem as they saw it.

In the early twentieth century, as now, every state in the nation supported a board of health, whose job was to protect and promote the public health. These departments had evolved over the second half of the nineteenth century, and their actual structures and capabilities, and especially their budgets, varied considerably from state to state by the beginning of the twentieth century. Available funding, in part, defined their duties, and some were extremely limited in what they could accomplish. Those states that contained large cities usually delegated to those cities their own public health work and responsibility. Such was the case in New York.[1]

The New York City Health Department began operations formally at the turn of the nineteenth century, but it was not until 1866, when the state legislature approved of a new and greatly expanded Metropolitan Board of Health, that real powers passed to the local level. The local board soon became the nation's leader in terms of defining municipal programs to promote health and prevent disease, and its accomplishments were adopted as models across the country.[2] In addition to its vast sanitation projects, like water works and sewer systems, the board successfully launched programs to combat disease, such as vaccinating to prevent smallpox and establishing isolation hospitals. With time and experience, the policy-making board of health and the city department of health, which carried forward board policy, found ways to increase operating budgets and expand services.

The health department's bacteriology laboratory where Mary Mallon's fecal samples were examined was the most influential public laboratory in the country, and, amid much publicity, gained the cooperation of physicians in reporting infectious diseases, even cases of the controversial tuberculosis.[3] Hermann Biggs, who trained at Cornell University and the Bellevue Medical College as well as in the scientific laboratories of Berlin before joining the department in the 1880s, became New York's chief of the division of bacteriology and disinfection in 1892. He hired William Hallock Park to run the laboratory and assumed the position of general medical officer in 1902, a position he held until he moved to the state health department in 1913. His twenty-six years with the city department and his later career as state commissioner of health during the crucial early years of bacteriology made Biggs, along with people like Charles Chapin who served in

Rhode Island for forty-seven years, one of the most important health officers in the country.[4]

Biggs understood what was possible in health department work. He maneuvered the politics of city health work and succeeded as an effective bridge between the private physicians and the politicians. His vision was perhaps best epitomized in the oft-repeated health department motto, "Public health is purchasable. Within natural limitations a community can determine its own death-rate." He summed up his philosophy:

Disease is largely a removable evil. It continues to afflict humanity . . . because it is extensively fostered by harsh economic and industrial conditions and by wretched housing in congested communities. These conditions and consequently the diseases which spring from them can be removed by better social organization. No duty of society, acting through its governmental agencies, is paramount to this obligation to attack the removable causes of disease. The duty of leading this attack and bringing home to public opinion the fact that the community can buy its own health protection is laid upon all health officers. . . . It means the saving and lengthening of the lives of thousands of citizens, the extension of the vigorous working period well into old age, and the prevention of inefficiency, misery and suffering.[5]

Biggs's philosophy combined older hygienic ideas with the newer bacteriological concepts. He defined the goals of public health work in the early twentieth century and at the same time illustrated the optimism of health workers in this period. Human intervention could make the world a healthier place. Typhoid fever appeared to be one disease that approached, in the words of another public health optimist, "absolute preventability."[6]

Biggs held an expansive view of the importance of public health; he also espoused an expansive idea of health officials' authority to accomplish the goal of protecting the public from preventable diseases. When he traveled to Edinburgh to read a paper at an international tuberculosis conference in July, 1910, three years after Mary Mallon's first apprehension and four months after her release, Biggs described for his international colleagues the broad scope of health authority in New York City:

The Board of Health of New York City has legislative, judicial, and executive powers. Its regulations on all matters pertaining to the public health are final, and there does not exist in any individual or in any body any power of review or revision of the action of the Board of Health excepting in the courts. . . . I do not think that any sanitary authorities anywhere have had granted to them such extraordinary and even arbitrary powers as rest in the hands of the Board of Health of New York City.[7]

Even allowing for some hyperbole in Biggs's address before an international audience, his statement provides a context in which to examine the policies developed to cope with Mary Mallon and other healthy carriers in New York City. New York health officials did have substantial authority to determine public health actions, in the definition of the problem, in executing its solutions, and in its presentation to the public.

Noting Biggs's political skills in working well with both Tammany and reform governments, Johns Hopkins physician William Welch wrote that Biggs had "unsurpassed persuasiveness and skill in the presentation of his arguments to the authorities in power. Not less skilful was he in securing the support of the press and of the general public. . . . Biggs had a genius for leadership and has been justly called a sanitary statesman."[8] In the hands of Biggs and his colleagues, New York City Health Department activities aimed at stemming the damage from typhoid fever and its carriers can be seen to represent the most (and perhaps the best) of what was possible in American public health policy.

Before health authorities apprehended Mary Mallon in 1907, public health officials had not implicated healthy people in causing outbreaks of typhoid fever; as we have seen, their activity had centered upon the environment and the sick as possible causal agents. Even the decade-old bacteriological knowledge that recovered typhoid patients could harbor the bacilli in their urine and feces for years after recovery had not yet in the United States been applied to an actual carrier, and the general public was not aware of this knowledge at all. Thus, when George Soper appeared on Mary Mallon's doorstep convinced that she was a carrier, a new interaction was taking place.

Soper described what happened when he located Mary Mallon in the Walter Bowen home at 688 Park Avenue in March, 1907:

I had my first talk with Mary in the kitchen of this house. . . . I was as diplomatic as possible, but I had to say I suspected her of making people sick and that I wanted specimens of her urine, feces and blood. It did not take Mary long to react to this suggestion. She seized a carving fork and advanced in my direction. I passed rapidly down the long narrow hall, through the tall iron gate, . . . and so to the sidewalk. I felt rather lucky to escape.[9]

Unable to obtain Mallon's cooperation at her place of work, Soper tried her at home in an encounter which, he said, he "staged more deliberately." Soper and an assistant, Dr. Bert Raymond Hoobler, "waited at the head of the stairs in the Third Avenue house."[10] When Mary Mallon arrived,

Dr. Hoobler and I described the situation with as much tact and judgment as we possessed. . . . We wanted a small sample of urine, one of feces and one of blood. . . . Indignant and peremptory denials met our appeals. We were unable to make any headway. Mary's position was like that of the lawyer who, on being told by the judge that the facts were all against his client, said that he proposed to deny the facts. Mary denied that she was a carrier. . . . Nothing could alter her position. As Mary's attitude toward us at this point could in no sense be interpreted as cordial, we were glad to close the interview and get down to the street. We concluded that it would be hopeless to try again.[11]

Soper later described this second encounter even more starkly: "Mary was angry at the unexpected sight of me," he wrote. Insisting she knew nothing about typhoid and had not caused it, "she would not allow anybody to accuse her." Soper left her, "followed by a volley of imprecations from the head of the stairs."[12]

Believing that his epidemiological evidence implicated Mallon in the transmission of typhoid fever, Soper reported his findings to Hermann Biggs and the New York City Health Department, who, he felt, had the authority to take the case further. The city's public health officials, convinced by Soper's data, immediately investigated. Dr. Walter Bensel, sanitary superintendent, sent his assistant, Dr. S. Josephine Baker, to the Bowens' Park Avenue house to collect specimens of Mary Mallon's blood and urine.[13]

Baker had been born and raised in Poughkeepsie, New York, in a privileged family. Her father's death (from typhoid fever) when she was sixteen, however, put some brakes on her ambitions. Although unable to attend Vassar as originally planned, she persevered in getting a medical education with her mother's support. She graduated from the New York Infirmary Medical College in 1898, at a time when not quite 5 percent of American physicians were women.[14] She interned at the New England Hospital for Women and Children in Boston for one year and returned to New York to set up her medical practice. Baker joined the health department in 1901, when it became evident that she, like other medical women in this period, would have difficulty attracting enough patients to make a living in a private practice. In 1907 she was a medical inspector and had not yet begun the work that would make her one of the most influential public health physicians in the country, as head of the division of child hygiene within the health department.[15] (See fig. 2.1.)

The health department showed some sensitivity in sending a woman to collect Mary Mallon's specimens. Soper described Baker as "gentle," but Mallon saw in her only the "red flag" of government authority.[16] She quickly showed Baker the door.

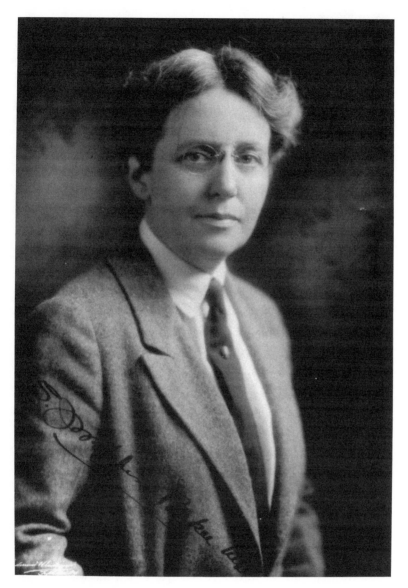

Fig. 2.1. *S. Josephine Baker, 1922.*

Bensel sent Baker back the next day with curt directions, as Baker later recalled being told: "I expect you to get the specimens or to take Mary to the hospital."[17] Worrying how she "would face Dr. Bensel" if she failed in the mission, Baker persisted, accompanied by five police officers and an ambulance. Baker later wrote that when she arrived at the Bowen house the second day,

Mary was on the lookout and peered out, a long kitchen fork in her hand like a rapier. As she lunged at me with the fork, I stepped back, recoiled on the policeman and so confused matters that, by the time we got through the door, Mary had disappeared. "Disappear" is too matter-of-fact a word; she had completely vanished.[18]

The other servants in the house, showing what Baker recognized as "class solidarity," denied any knowledge of Mallon's whereabouts. Baker and the police looked everywhere. They spotted footprints in the snow leading to a chair set up near the fence separating the Bowen property from the neighbor's grounds, and so they searched the neighbor's house as well. For five hours they "went through every closet and nook and cranny in those two houses. It was utter defeat." Finally "a tiny scrap of blue calico caught in the door of the areaway closet under the high outside stairway leading to the front door" betrayed Mallon's hiding place. The police had not previously looked there because of the "dozen filled ash cans . . . heaped up in front of this door; another evidence of class solidarity." Baker described the scene:

She came out fighting and swearing, both of which she could do with appalling efficiency and vigor. I made another effort to talk to her sensibly and asked her again to let me have the specimens, but it was of no use. By that time she was convinced that the law was wantonly persecuting her, when she had done nothing wrong. She knew she had never had typhoid fever; she was maniacal in her integrity. There was nothing I could do but take her with us. The policemen lifted her into the ambulance and I literally sat on her all the way to the hospital; it was like being in a cage with an angry lion.[19]

At the Willard Parker Hospital, bacteriologists examined Mallon's feces and discovered a high concentration of typhoid bacilli, proving in the laboratory that Soper's epidemiological study had been correct. On the basis of this evidence, the health department soon removed Mary Mallon from the hospital to North Brother Island, where she remained for almost three years.

The extant records do not directly reveal the thinking of health officials about this initial isolation of Mary Mallon. Why was quarantine the first response of the New York officials instead of the position of last resort? It seems that Mallon's resistance to being captured defined her as trouble. Certainly cooperation did not mark her behavior. On the other hand, the record is mute on attempts by officials to convince Mallon that what they were doing was reasonable. There is no suggestion that health department officials tried to persuade Mallon that they would release her after either retraining or finding her new employment—an omission Mary Mallon herself noted.[20]

New York City health officials probably regarded their initial isolation of Mary Mallon as a temporary measure that would give them time to determine what long-term procedures could be applied. In 1907, when they first remanded her to North Brother Island, they knew enough to question what they should do, but not yet enough to have developed a policy. As William Park, director of the city's hygiene laboratory, wrote sixteen months into her isolation: "Has the city a right to deprive her of her liberty for perhaps her whole life? The alternative is to turn loose on the public a woman who is known to have infected at least twenty-eight [sic] persons." In framing the question Park considered the large number of people who potentially could be affected, and concluded:

What can we do under these circumstances? It seems to me that any attempt to isolate and treat on bacteriologic examinations . . . is impracticable. When we consider that the presence of the bacilli in the feces of these persons is often only occasional, that numerous contact cases having never had typhoid fever would not come under suspicion, and finally, the impracticability of isolating for life so many persons, we are forced to consider isolation utterly impracticable.[21]

The scope of the problem immediately became clear not only to Park, but to most public health officials who began to grapple with the issue in the early years of the twentieth century. Health departments simply did not have the wherewithal to find and round up all carriers and keep them separate from the general population. Nor would people easily have accepted such mass isolation. Early studies indicated that 2 to 5 percent of all of those people who had suffered from typhoid fever became chronic carriers.[22] If the ill had been reported to health departments, as most jurisdictions required, they could, with adequate budgets and personnel, be followed after recovery. But if their cases were not reported, or if the infected had never identified their illness as typhoid fever (like Mary Mallon), the carriers would be much more difficult to find. Furthermore, many recovered typhoid fever patients would never infect others, so they did not need to be considered as part of a disease prevention program. Perhaps most important, if isolation was to be considered part of the solution, health departments needed to determine if they had the legal authority to incarcerate healthy individuals and, if so, for how long.

Mary Mallon's situation thus illustrated the immediate need for developing a public health policy that would address the problem of stopping transmission of typhoid fever through carriers yet at the same time be feasible in terms of health department budgets and staff abilities and also not overreach the boundaries of health department authority. How could the considerable, but by no means absolute, powers of public health departments be applied to the specific task of regulating the behavior of healthy typhoid fever carriers?

In addressing this basic question, officials needed to determine how many people like Mary Mallon existed in a given population. Health authorities offered wide-ranging estimates of the numbers of typhoid fever healthy carriers, and through these we have an idea of the scope of the problem as it was viewed early in the twentieth century. The number of new carriers was directly related to the number of people ill with typhoid fever, although the total number of carriers in any given population was impossible to estimate accurately because the disease often presents in mild form as a flu-like illness, if it is noticed at all. The numbers of reported sick are always an understatement of the actual numbers of those infected. For estimation purposes, however, the case reports provide a basis for defining the problem.

After studying European and American reports of typhoid fever carriers, Charles Chapin had concluded that the number of new carriers added to a population should be calculated at 3 percent of cases. He suggested in 1910 that there were "probably 200,000 cases of typhoid fever in the United States each year, and 3 per cent of these would be 6,000."[23] Milton J. Rosenau, director of the National Hygienic Laboratory, and later professor of preventive medicine and hygiene at Harvard University, estimated 350,000 cases nationwide in 1900, putting the number of new carriers added each year over 9,000.[24]

On the local level, the numbers of healthy carriers seemed staggering. The state epidemiologist in New Jersey, for example, reasoned that the state of New Jersey alone harbored about 9,000 typhoid carriers at any one time, although in the 1920s, officials knew of only 26.[25] In California, between the years 1913 and 1919, over 9,000 cases of typhoid fever were reported to the state health department; calculating at the rate of 3 percent, 272 new carriers were added to those thousands who already lived in the state. Health authorities tracked only sixteen of them.[26] In Washington, D.C., in 1910, officials believed there might be 1,568 carriers per 100,000 population.[27] The editors of the *American Journal of Public Health* concluded:

The magnitude of the problem [of healthy typhoid fever carriers] is apparent when we consider that even in a healthy city like New York, where nearly 3,000 cases of typhoid fever occur each year, this means the addition of over one hundred typhoid carriers annually. Allowing each carrier only twenty years of life, certainly a conservative estimate, it follows that there must now be over two thousand typhoid carriers at large in New York City.[28]

The problem in New York City, where officials were coping with Mary Mallon, was indeed challenging. In 1907, the year of Mary Mallon's identification, New Yorkers reported 4,426 new cases of typhoid fever (two of which were attributable to Mallon); in 1908, another 3,058. These two years alone, according to the widely accepted formula, combined to generate almost 200 new chronic carriers. The years 1909, 1910, and 1911 followed inexorably with their own high numbers approximating 3,500 new cases each year, each adding close to 100 new carriers.[29]

No one believed it would be possible to find all the healthy carriers of typhoid fever in the population. But health officials, realizing that the dangers from healthy carriers could be greater than from the sick—because susceptible people knew to avoid the sick or to be careful when caring for them, but could not know when they might be at risk of being infected from a seemingly healthy person—determined to find a way to bring most of the carriers within their purview.

As cities' water and milk supplies improved in the early twentieth century, it became increasingly important to formulate a policy for carriers, who as a group emerged as the single most dangerous factor in disease transmission. The Rockefeller Institute for Medical Research concluded that as many as 44 percent of all new cases of typhoid fever reported nationwide were due to carriers.[30] In a five-year study during the 1930s, the state of New York health authorities attributed no typhoid outbreaks to contaminated water, but found carriers responsible for the large proportion of cases.[31] Some investigators concluded that by the 1930s as much as 96 percent of typhoid distribution originated with carriers. A policy to control the danger from healthy carriers became essential: "the difficulty in the eradication of typhoid is not the sick bed patient but rather the healthy carrier who goes blithely on his way distributing his infection."[32]

There were various ways officials could systematically locate carriers. The most promising, although ultimately not the most successful, was to follow recovered sufferers until their stools and urine tested bacilli free. State and local health departments had long required physicians and hospitals to report typhoid fever cases and deaths; thus it was possible to require follow-up laboratory analysis of convalescents' stools and urine and to place restrictions on those persons who carried the bacilli longer than one year. Many health departments followed this path in the early twentieth century, but the success rate for discovering healthy carriers using this method remained small. By following such post-typhoid cases, California officials discovered less than 10 percent of its registered carriers, and New York State almost 20 percent.[33]

A more successful route to locating healthy carriers of typhoid fever was through investigations of actual outbreaks of the disease, either family or community centered. New York found 75 percent of its registered carriers between 1911 and 1932 from such epidemiological investigations.[34] For example, in August, 1909, a "sudden increase in the number of cases of typhoid fever reported from the boroughs of Manhattan and the Bronx attracted attention, and led to an investigation to ascertain the cause of the infections." Investigators implicated a single milk supply in Camden, New York. Officials found the dairy "exceptionally clean and well kept," although it was also home to a recent case of typhoid fever. "With such a history," wrote Charles Bolduan, assistant to Biggs, and W. Carey Noble, city bacteriologist, "one could not help but suspect the presence of a chronic bacillus-carrier." Indeed, stool examinations revealed that the dairyman harbored typhoid bacilli, and the health department connected him to the contaminated milk supply and stopped his work in the dairy. The investigators concluded, "The occurrence of repeated infections in this case shows the danger of having bacillus-carriers in a dairy."[35]

Stephen M. Friedman, in his retrospective study of the 1,004 chronic fecal typhoid fever carriers identified in New York City between 1907 and 1975, reports that such investigation of cases of typhoid fever was the most common method of identifying healthy carriers, accounting for one-third to one-half of all carriers in every decade since 1916.[36] Connecting healthy people to actual cases of typhoid fever identified those already implicated in transmitting disease, the ones the health departments most needed to regulate. Not only was this group already shown to threaten others, but the people found this way often did not know they had ever suffered from typhoid or had had it many years before being connected to an outbreak; thus they would have eluded health regulations based only on following the sick. George Soper followed this method of discovery to find Mary Mallon.

A third method of identifying healthy carriers was one for which health departments had a great optimism: the systematic examination of the stools and urine of food handlers. Once bacteriology established that typhoid could be transmitted by healthy people who prepared the food that others ate, it seemed obvious that if all people who prepared food for others could be examined before they were allowed to handle food outside their own families, epidemics could be stopped. New York City began such a program to identify dangerous food handlers in 1915, the year of Mary Mallon's second incarceration, and made annual medical examinations of food handlers compulsory in 1923.[37] But health departments tracked fewer than 5 percent of carriers in New York and California through this type of program.[38]

Not only was the routine examination program relatively ineffective at identifying potential carriers, it was expensive and cumbersome. Examining the thousands of food handlers annually, officials estimated, cost the city more than $100,000 each year. New York City Deputy Health Commissioner William Best indicated that even if the legislature wanted to increase the department budget to accommodate the certification program, he did not support spending money in this way: "I submit, is such a cost commensurate with the public health benefits obtained?"[39]

The food handler examination policy had even more problems. Private physicians who tested their own patients were reluctant to label them with the stigma of chronic carrier and submitted very few positive identifications to the department. In order for the program to be effective, handlers needed repeated examinations, and even if they could be processed more often than once a year, healthy handlers could still become infected soon after certification. (There is an obvious analogy to HIV testing today.) With all the difficulties associated with the program, New York City discontinued routine testing in 1934.[40]

Health departments were never successful at locating all typhoid fever carriers within their jurisdictions. And the people who were identified presented health authorities with a big question. What should health officials do with them? How could health authorities stop as many carriers as possible from transmitting disease to others? Was isolation necessary or desirable? Embedded within these questions is, of course, the experience of Mary Mallon herself.

Policy developers needed to keep in mind that typhoid carriers menaced other people's health only when susceptible people ingested the pathogenic bacteria that the carriers harbored within their bodies. Passing carriers in the street, sharing public transportation, or sitting beside them in school or at the theater were not dangerous activities. As the state health authorities in New York wrote, "A person of intelligence who is a carrier of typhoid bacilli, but who is willing to observe strictly certain essential precautions, may live and mingle with others and still need not be a source of danger to those about him." The formulation of rules, the officials concluded, thus should "restrict the activities of such persons to the smallest degree consistent with the protection of public health."[41]

Rules already in place by the beginning of the twentieth century forbade any person sick with typhoid fever, or any infectious disease, to handle food. Although rarely enforced, no doubt because of the enormous size of the problem of tracing the activities of the sick who were not hospitalized, this policy provided the precedent upon which regulation of healthy carriers rested. The department determined in 1913 that typhoid fever convalescents who worked in food establishments would not be allowed to return to work until they had been examined for typhoid bacilli and proven to be free of them.[42] A small number of carriers were identified through the execution of this rule. In 1915, for example, the year when Mary Mallon was found cooking at Sloane Maternity Hospital and returned to North Brother Island, 159 food handlers recovered from typhoid fever and were closely examined. The laboratory identified four persistent chronic carriers and refused them permission to return to work.[43]

In 1915 and 1916, the health department instituted new rules clearly related to the reappearance and demonstrated continuing danger of Mary Mallon. These regulations, aimed specifically at more effective control of typhoid fever carriers, were again modified in 1919, 1921, and 1922. First was a more precise definition of when convalescents could be terminated and declared free of carrying bacilli: when both feces and urine could be shown in the laboratory to be free of bacilli if taken at least ten days after the patient's temperature returned to normal. Most significant was the provision that typhoid fever cases (specific coverage of carriers came with the 1921 revisions) should be forcibly removed to the hospital unless the department found "home conditions . . . satisfactory." Health officers would be satisfied that strict quarantine rules could be applied at home if the household provided for the disinfection of all stools and urine of the affected sufferers, agreed to immunize all susceptibles, and insured that those attendant on the sick would have nothing to do with the cooking or care of children for the rest of the family. The sick had to have separate toilet facilities, a stipulation that limited the stay-at-home to the more privileged classes. Health authorities further limited who could remain at home with the stipulation: "The family must be intelligent and willing to carry out rules of the Department of Health."[44]

The names of the unfortunate few who after a bout of typhoid fever continued to test positive for bacilli were entered on a health department list of typhoid carriers. The department kept an individual card for each carrier, on which was entered the specific data available for that carrier. Health officers tried to keep in close contact with these carriers, required them to submit to laboratory analysis on a regular basis, and insisted that they not handle any food. In 1916, New York officials sent their carrier list of twenty-four individuals to the United States Public Health Service.[45] The list grew rapidly, and, by 1918, the health officers wrote: "The problem of supervising typhoid carriers requires constant watchfulness and study. At present we have a record of 70 chronic carriers, three of whom are detained forcibly in Department hospitals [one of these was Mary Mallon], the others being permitted to stay at home under constant supervision."[46]

Despite the obvious difficulty of finding and monitoring healthy carriers, New York City Health Department annual reports optimistically continued to carry the motto "Public health is purchasable."[47] Health officials maintained optimism in part because of frequent carrier cooperation. In New York State, health officer F. M. Meader answered the question "What can be done with these carriers?" with the statement "Inform them that they are carriers. Most persons so informed will care for themselves in such a way that they will not be a menace to the public."[48] In his study of 1,004 New York City carriers, Stephen Friedman similarly concluded:

Most carriers lived with the restriction imposed on them. . . . These restrictions required the carrier to practice good hygiene in his toilet habits, and to keep the Health Department informed as to his address and place of employment. Carriers were forbidden to work as food handlers, nurses or teachers. Thus being declared a carrier sometimes meant economic hardship for that individual.[49]

High-level cooperation might have been predicted by the demographics of the carriers themselves. Most carriers identified were women, and the search for carriers yielded housewives more than any other occupation category. But housewives did not cause most of the typhoid outbreaks. Despite the small number of public food handling carriers identified (only 8.5 percent of the entire city sample), including butchers, bakers, cooks, and waiters, the food handlers accounted for more associated cases of typhoid fever than any other group. Friedman concluded, "The mean number of cases caused by food handlers was therefore about five times the number caused by housewives."[50]

Even with high levels of carrier cooperation, the difficulties of maintaining the program remained enormous. In 1919, one health official estimated that New York City harbored 25,000 typhoid carriers.[51] In that year, the health department restrained two typhoid fever carriers in city hospitals (one of them Mary Mallon), three others had absconded from department purview, and the other sixty-two identified chronic carriers lived under conditions that "in all cases were excellent. They had been carefully instructed how to protect others, and they carefully observe[d] these instructions."[52] Although the majority of healthy carriers under department supervision followed the rules, still a substantial number did not. As the official list of chronic carriers continued to grow—in New York City, in the state, and in the country—so too did the list of those lost to the regulations.

The health department did not have a lot of success in following those people who, although registered, did not show up for the required specimen examination or who did not provide their addresses to the authorities. In 1922, for example, New Jersey officials found Tony Labella, an absconded New York City carrier, a man who had reportedly caused an outbreak of eighty-seven cases (considerably more than Mallon) and two deaths, and blamed him for yet another outbreak that had resulted in thirty-five cases and three deaths.[53] During the year 1922, indeed, six chronic carriers "absconded" from the city list—literally disappeared from the view and control of officials. Four more "refused absolutely to give stool specimens when requested, making it necessary for us to resort to the exercise of police power to procure compliance with the requirements."[54]

During the 1920s, it is clear, many registered carriers refused to cooperate with health department regulations, and some continued to cook after being forbidden by the health department. A few of these found themselves isolated, usually briefly, at Riverside or Kingston Avenue hospitals.[55] None, as far as I can determine, was isolated for life, as Mary Mallon was. We may never understand all the reasons that made health officials put her on North Brother Island, especially in 1907, or even in 1915, but it is instructive to know how they handled similar cases.

In 1924, Alphonse Cotils, a bakery and restaurant owner whose name was on the city list of healthy carriers and who had been forbidden to prepare food in his own business, appeared in court after he had violated the terms of his agreement with the health department. He defied health department rules, his physician said, because officials were " 'annoying' him about working in his own bakery." Cotils knew he was a typhoid carrier, and he knew he was not allowed to prepare food for other people. Like Mary Mallon before him, he refused to cooperate with the regulation and continued his work. But unlike the Mallon case, the judge, while finding him guilty, suspended his sentence "after

Cotils had promised to remain away from his restaurant and keep out of kitchens. He intends to conduct his business by telephone, he said." The judge was quoted in the newspaper: "I am thoroughly impressed with the extreme danger from these typhoid carriers, particularly when they are handling food. I could not legally sentence this man to jail on account of his health . . ."[56]

At the very moment the judge said he could not legally imprison Alphonse Cotils because he was not sick, a healthy Mary Mallon was held on North Brother Island. Both had violated a previously imposed quarantine; only one was detained for it. Was this because she was the first carrier to be traced in New York City? Were her fighting and swearing during her initial arrest enough to explain her unique treatment?

The policies governing healthy carriers answer some of the questions about the particular detention of Mary Mallon. The somewhat ambiguous 1916 guidelines—written after her second incarceration—stated that carriers "need not be retained in hospitals or institutions if not desired. They will be sent home if home conditions are satisfactory." The vagueness of how "satisfactory" was to be determined left room for significant maneuvering and permitted health officials to make decisions about healthy carriers that incorporated a range of considerations. They could, for example, differentiate between Mary Mallon, whom health officials did not trust to behave in the public's interest, possibly because of her blatantly resistant behavior, and other healthy carriers, like Alphonse Cotils, whose resistance was quieter and whose home conditions and personal attributes seemed to predict closer compliance with the health codes.

Although two healthy carriers might have borne equally dangerous pathogenic bacteria as identified in the laboratory, they were not necessarily treated equally in practice. According to the equivocal health department protocols, the carriers' social condition and even their psychological responses could be applied alongside the laboratory reports to evaluate the dangers they presented and to determine ways to protect the public from the dangers they posed. Health officers judged the home conditions, sanitary facilities, and the individual's tractability as they determined the proper regulation of healthy typhoid bacilli carriers.

Once people had been entered on the official list of carriers, officials usually released them to their homes with the hope that they would follow the agreement and not prepare food in the public sphere. But it was not possible for officials to watch all the carriers daily to determine if they actually followed the guidelines. The most officials could accomplish was to require continuing laboratory analysis, usually once every three to six months, and the reporting of address changes, monitored monthly beginning in 1929. If people did not appear for the laboratory tests or if they moved and did not report a forwarding address, there was little the health department could do except wait for the ensuing typhoid outbreaks.

In a California study tracing healthy carriers over a long period of time, investigators reported that about 12 percent of carriers disappeared and a full 25 percent did not cooperate with officials. They noted that males were "lost to the registry more often than females," even though there was a significantly larger number of female carriers.[57] The proportion of the group of carriers labeled uncooperative changed over time. In the years 1910 to 1919 when California's healthy carrier regulation program had just started, 50 percent of the registered carriers did not cooperate with the program. The following decade proved even worse, reaching over 58 percent of carriers who refused to cooperate with the restrictions. But from 1930 to 1939, despite the deepening economic crisis, only 40 percent refused to cooperate. The figure decreased to 20 percent during the 1940s and 12 percent during the 1950s.[58]

There were various reasons why healthy men and women did not cooperate with the healthy carrier restrictions, and it is instructive to compare some of them with Mary Mallon's situation. The most significant reason given in the California study for uncooperative carriers was the need for employment. For those people who prepared food for others as their paid jobs (in contrast to those who prepared food within the home or for occasions like church suppers), being labeled a typhoid carrier meant giving up their means of support and the necessity of learning new skills and seeking alternative employment. Some could make such a transition smoothly; many could not. Some could not find comparable employment outside the food industry. A small percentage of carriers, like Mary Mallon, would not or could not be convinced that they were dangerous to others. Feeling healthy themselves, they did not accept a laboratory finding that they made others ill. Attitudes and employment possibilities could change over time, and occasionally those who had cooperated during the periods they could find work reversed themselves when they could not. As bacteriological understanding spread by the middle of the twentieth century, however, more and more carriers came to accept the fact that they could be transmitting the disease to others even though they felt healthy themselves.[59]

Some jurisdictions, realizing that carriers might lose their jobs and need financial help, instituted a system of temporary stipends for carrier breadwinners who had trouble finding employment. The state of New York, through its local county poor officers, provided some monthly allowances to "supplement the earnings of the patient who can not engage in work which will endanger the food supply."[60] Begun in 1918, the subsidy program never fully maintained those carriers and their families who were inconvenienced by the policies restricting their activity, but between 1918 and 1932, for example, it helped fifty-two carriers with allowances running between $10 and $50 per month.[61]

There is other evidence that health officials provided added services to breadwinners or otherwise treated them with greater lenience than they did those presumed to be without family responsibilities. Health officials helped Tony Labella, who had caused typhoid outbreaks in both New York and New Jersey, to find work outside the food industry. They returned Alphonse Cotils to his family and business. Yet health officers did not offer Mary Mallon similar aid and understanding. In a national study of laws and regulations controlling infectious diseases, researchers noted that "exceptions in favor of breadwinners . . . may be made by local health authorities."[62] Perhaps Mary Mallon did not fit the official definition of a breadwinner because she was a woman or because she had no family.[63]

New York state and city officials, as we have seen, did not isolate most healthy carriers they had located. In this, they followed national public health authorities, notably Milton Rosenau and Charles Chapin, who believed that it was usually not necessary, or desirable, to isolate healthy carriers. In his popular public health textbook, Milton Rosenau offered suggestions for carriers that were significantly less stringent than his proposals for the acutely ill. The textbook first appeared in 1913 and enjoyed seven editions by 1951, becoming the standard for the field and influencing generations of public health workers. The 1935 edition, the last one Rosenau himself wrote, provided this advice:

We cannot lightly imprison persons in good health, especially in the case of breadwinners, even though they be a menace to others. In some infections there are so many carriers that it would require military rule to carry out such a plan. Fortunately in most cases absolute quarantine is not necessary. Sanitary isolation is sufficient. Thus the danger from a typhoid carrier may be neutralized if the person exercises scrupulous and intelligent cleanliness, and is not allowed to handle food intended for others. Such a person might well engage as carpenter, banker, seamstress, etc., without endangering his fellowmen. . . . The price of liberty is "good behavior."[64]

Rosenau's analysis identified the various factors he thought should protect healthy carriers from hospitalization or incarceration: their health; their economic value in the family; their sheer numbers in the population; and their behavior (habits and jobs), which usually could be effectively controlled outside the hospital. Despite obtaining identical laboratory reports for both sick and healthy persons infected with typhoid bacilli, bacteriologically oriented public health officials did not recommend the same regulations for both groups. The sick should be temporarily isolated in homes or hospitals; the healthy carriers could be allowed to walk about on the city streets. The laboratory alone, for these practically oriented public health workers, could not define the full scope of the public health approach.

Rosenau's formula reveals the other factors that entered into determining public health policy about healthy carriers. If carriers had significant financial responsibilities, health officers felt they should not deny them their livelihood. A person's social and economic position as head of a household provided some immunity against the state's authority to intervene. The suspended sentence Alphonse Cotils received when found guilty of violating the health codes reflected this viewpoint. The judge let him go not only because he was healthy but because he was an established businessman.[65] Furthermore, the very numbers of carriers involved precluded their institutionalization. While it might have been physically possible to isolate the growing numbers of healthy carriers, the political and economic restrictions of city health departments already operating on limited budgets made a full-scale isolation policy unrealistic.

Rosenau's precepts for healthy carrier control reflected the common faith of early twentieth-century bacteriologists in the potential for altering human behavior. He assumed that both scrupulous personal cleanliness and cooperating in changing jobs offered workable solutions to public health problems. His optimism was echoed in New York City health officers' statements about the level of cooperation they actually received from most carriers and in the writings of other public health authorities. In his 1910 text, *The Sources and Modes of Infection*, Charles Chapin similarly found the suggestion to isolate healthy carriers impossible, unjust, and ineffectual.[66] Chapin, like Rosenau, advocated retraining carriers to allow them to find jobs outside the food handling occupations instead of indefinite isolation.

The limits of laboratory findings become evident in this differential treatment of sick typhoid fever sufferers and healthy carriers of typhoid fever. Both carried equally virulent and dangerous bacilli in their excreta; both could transmit the bacilli to others. Chapin argued, in fact, that, although both healthy and sick were "equally dangerous potentially," the "well person moving freely about may be more dangerous to the community than the sick person who is confined to the house."[67] Sick people felt too ill to prepare food for others or carry on their normal duties; the healthy continued their usual patterns. The sick presented a recognizable threat, whereas the well hid their invisible dangers. If notions of risk to the community were the measure of public policy, the healthy carrier should be more restrained than those ill with the disease. Yet Chapin, Rosenau, and other public health officials advocated and practiced almost the opposite differential treatment. Public health workers sought control of carriers in ways that acknowledged their health, their place in the community, and the near practical impossibility of constraining them all, considerations well beyond laboratory findings.

The policies developed concerning typhoid fever patients and carriers led to considerable success in typhoid control over the first half of the twentieth century. Water and milk controls earlier had dramatically reduced the number of people suffering from the disease, and further reductions became evident in the years that carriers became closely associated with disease transmission. Authorities often tied the good results to health department activities. Friedman concluded his study of carriers with the observation that the isolation of acute cases in hospitals and at home, and the injunctions against carriers working as food handlers, nurses, and teachers "interrupted the cycle of disease transmission and effected a steep decrease in the yearly number of cases of typhoid fever in New York City."[68] Any evaluation of carrier policy must take this positive finding into account.

Early twentieth-century public health opinion about healthy carriers of typhoid fever did not routinely advise quarantine as it did for typhoid sufferers; for healthy carriers, isolation was a last resort. C. L. Overlander of Boston, for example, thought attempts to follow carriers might be a "will-o'-the-wisp," out of the grasp of local officials' financial and manpower abilities. He concluded that "detention of such persons in quarantine . . . is a proceeding unwarranted viewed from either the standpoint of the patient himself, the health officer or the community."[69] Accepted public health policy emphasized helping carriers survive in the community, not taking them outside of it.[70]

Despite this prevailing opinion, and distinct from their actions as they evolved in other cases, New York health officials' first response to Mary Mallon when she was located in New York City in March, 1907, was isolation. Health officers might have meant her isolation on North Brother Island to be temporary until they determined another course of action, but, if so, they forgot about Mary Mallon and left her alone in the cottage on the grounds of Riverside Hospital. William Park remembered her sixteen months after her initial capture, but did not act to release her. Until she herself initiated a court action seeking her release, health department officials did nothing to return her to society. Yet, according to the theory of the day, Mary Mallon walking the streets of New York would have endangered no one. It was only necessary to separate healthy carriers from the general population if they could not be stopped from carrying out activities, such as cooking, that would actually put others at risk of infection. In 1907, officials did not yet know whether Mallon would successfully take up other work: they chose to isolate her merely on the basis of their prediction that she would not give up cooking.

Health officials outside of New York City, including most significantly Charles Chapin and Milton Rosenau, explicitly objected to the immediate isolation of Mary Mallon. As Rosenau stated during the first meeting at which George Soper revealed Mary Mallon's initial capture and isolation, in April, 1907, "It is not necessary to imprison the bacillus carrier; it is sufficient to restrict the activities of such an individual."[71] Chapin, too, concluded his 1910 analysis of how healthy carriers should be handled with an indictment of New York's incarceration of Mary Mallon: "What result is secured by keeping her in confinement, other than the placing of discredit on public health work, it is difficult to see."[72] Both men believed that isolation was too strong a penalty, as well as an impractical remedy, for healthy carriers in general and for Mary Mallon in particular. For these two prominent public health officials, bacteriology, while emphasizing the importance of germ hosts, did not reduce the solution merely to removing carriers from society or demand that carriers' civil liberties be denied.[73]

Yet New York officials kept Mallon isolated in her island cottage until she brought a law suit seeking release, in July, 1909. Failing in that attempt, she returned to the island. In 1910 a new health commissioner, Ernst J. Lederle, finally decided to let her go. He recognized that such a total isolation as Mallon had been subjected to was not medically indicated for typhoid fever carriers who were dangerous only when they cooked the food that others ate. Also, Mallon's small part in New York City's typhoid saga, in which hundreds of carriers were free and thousands of new cases occurred each year, did not seem to warrant the attention and expense. Lederle told the press, "She has been released because she has been shut up long enough to learn the precautions that she ought to take."[74] The *New York American* quoted him more informally: "For Heaven's sake, can't the poor creature be given a chance to live? An opportunity to make her living, and have her past forgotten? She is to blame for nothing—and look at the life she led!"[75]

Mallon signed an affidavit swearing to give up cooking, and Lederle helped her find employment in a laundry.[76] He told reporters that he was doing this because, "She was incarcerated for the public's good, and now it is up to the public to take care of her."[77] The department tracked her for a while, as they did other carriers under their observation, but in time, Mary Mallon disappeared. Along with many other carriers, she absconded from officials' view and tried to lead her life without close observation.

In early 1915 an outbreak of typhoid fever occurred at the Sloane Maternity Hospital in New York City. Twenty-five doctors, nurses, and hospital staff were stricken, and two died. Investigation of this outbreak uncovered a Mrs. Brown, a new cook who had been employed in the hospital for three months before the outbreak.

Both S. Josephine Baker and George Soper claimed to have played a role in identifying Mrs. Brown as Mary Mallon. Dr. Baker told a newspaper reporter, "I was head of the Child Hygiene Bureau at the time, but I was interested in the Sloane case and went up to make an investigation for that reason. As I walked into the kitchen, the first person I met was Typhoid Mary Mallon. She had been cooking for the hospital under the name of Mrs. Brown."[78] George Soper related a different story. He wrote that Dr. Edward B. Cragin, the chief physician at the Sloane Hospital, "telephoned me asking that I come at once to the hospital to see him about a matter of great importance." Cragin told Soper about the outbreak of typhoid fever in the hospital: "The other servants had jokingly nicknamed the cook "Typhoid Mary." She was out at the moment, but would I recognize her handwriting if she was really that woman? He handed me a letter from which I saw at once that the cook was indeed Mary Mallon, and I also identified her from his description."[79]

Whoever might have helped in the identification of Mrs. Brown as Mary Mallon, officials finally found and trapped her in a Corona, Queens, house and brought her back to North Brother Island.[80] Health Commissioner S. S. Goldwater promised "she would never endanger the public health again."[81]

The resolve of health department officials to isolate Mary Mallon in 1915, when she was found cooking after having agreed not to, is easier to understand than their initial decision to send her to North Brother Island in 1907 before alternative strategies were tried. Their later decision was more in keeping with contemporary thinking that isolation should be used only as a last resort. Soper expressed common sentiment on the subject: "Whatever rights she once possessed as the innocent victim of an infected condition . . . were now lost. She was now a woman who could not claim innocence. She was known wilfully and deliberately to have taken desperate chances with human life. . . . She had abused her privilege; she had broken her parole. She was a dangerous character and must be treated accordingly."[82]

We might understand the officials' reasons for Mary Mallon's second isolation, the one that became lifelong, but even that incarceration presents a puzzle. Other carriers, once relocated, were not necessarily isolated, as the case of Tony Labella indicates, and he had even carried his destructive force across state boundaries, a fact that would seem to argue for stiffer penalties. Was Mary Mallon isolated twice, the second time until her death, because she was the first carrier to be traced or because she was indeed more dangerous than other carriers? Was it to give a message to other carriers to behave themselves or risk similar treatment? Why did officials not choose to retrain her for a job that did not involve food handling and let her go?

The policies developed in New York City, and indeed, around the country, during the years following Mallon's second incarceration certainly allowed for occasional isolation. In Mallon's case, as we will see in the next chapter, Biggs and his associates had judicial sanction and acted within their prerogatives as they understood them. Nonetheless, such isolation was an extreme response to healthy carriers, especially when seen in the context of a public health system that could not locate most of the carriers in the population and that could not control so many of the ones it was able to identify. In the early part of the century—as today—it was rare, if not completely unheard of, to take a healthy person in the prime of life and keep her a virtual prisoner until her death. The existence of a policy that permitted isolation of healthy individuals does not itself explain how and why Mary Mallon became chosen for long-term and indefinite isolation.

What does seem clear from an overview of the health policy of the early twentieth century is that officials chose Mary Mallon as an extreme example of what might happen if health policies were not obeyed. Because she was the first identified carrier, it is reasonable to conclude that officials used her case as an example for others at the same time as they determined policy based on what they learned from her. Science found her to be dangerous; but she then refused to accept the scientific explanation and did not cooperate with authorities. If all carriers responded as she did, any health department control of typhoid fever would be profoundly threatened. Therefore, some health officials, like S. Josephine Baker, were convinced that "the only answer was to keep her in the custody of the Department, out of contact with other people's food." Her own "bad behavior," Baker concluded, "inevitably led to her doom."[83] Mary Mallon's public defiance of authorities during her initial arrest, her continuing refusal to obey proscriptions, and, as we will see, her denials of being a carrier made in court and in interviews with the newspapers provoked health officers to assert their authority and court the public confidence by forcibly keeping her out of the kitchen. She became proof positive that with an effective health department alert and ready, "Public health [was] purchasable."

The health department had determined that Mallon was

dangerous above and beyond other carriers and needed to be isolated from the public as a "menace to the public health."[84] Other carriers remained at large during the years of Mallon's incarceration—in fact, most carriers avoided detection at all—yet such distinctions did not bother New York officials, who continued to believe they acted properly in her case. Mallon provided an example of the extreme, extraordinary power of the state, perhaps even its "arbitrary powers" in Biggs's phrase.

Was it necessary to restrain even one person's individual liberty in order to achieve health? New York public health officials believed so, especially when that individual had achieved public notoriety. Public health officials saw Mary Mallon as a menace to the public's health, and their actions fit their perceptions. Today, as we again weigh the relative importance of public health and individual liberty in discussions about whether to isolate (and for how long) people with tuberculosis or HIV infection, public officials are, in the same tradition, making similar choices and isolating a few in the name of protecting the many. In the next chapter we will look more closely at the laws that applied to Mallon, and in succeeding chapters delve further into the question of why authorities kept her isolated in her island cottage for so many years, explore how the public responded to her isolation, and evaluate the personal cost of such actions to epidemic disease carriers themselves.

"A
Menace
to the
Community"

Law and the Limits of Liberty

CHAPTER THREE

*W*hen health department officials
forced Mary Mallon into the city ambulance and took her against
her will into Willard Parker Hospital and then to her isolation on
North Brother Island in March, 1907, they acted with uncertain
legal authority. The basic question of whether or not health
officials could take away a healthy individual's liberty in the
name of protecting the public's health had not yet been answered
in court. William Park and Hermann Biggs knew that they had
legal authority to isolate, by force if necessary, people sick with
diseases who they believed might transmit those illnesses to others if not confined. They had experience in taking people sick
with smallpox or tuberculosis against their will to isolation hospitals run by the health department. In 1907, for example, the same
year they secluded Mary Mallon on North Brother Island, health
officials removed thirty-five people suffering with pulmonary tuberculosis to Riverside Hospital "by force as being nuisances and
dangerous to those about them."[1] But never before had they attempted to take a healthy person, a person who did not show any
symptoms of suffering from any disease, away from her home
and employment to put her in a city institution in the name of
protecting the city's health.

As we have seen, William Park felt uncertain about the

health department's authority to deprive a healthy Mary Mallon of her liberty "for perhaps her whole life."[2] Newspapers made these official concerns a matter of public debate. Thomas Darlington, commissioner of health when Mallon was taken, admitted to a reporter that there was "considerable doubt as to the legal right of the health officials to detain the germ woman. She had violated no laws." While science knew her to be a menace, he said, her legal status remained uncertain.[3] The *New York American* reported that health officials were going "to appeal to eminent lawyers to determine what action they can take."[4]

In this chapter, I examine the legal perspective on Mary Mallon's situation. While lawyers and judges shared basic viewpoints with scientists and public health officials in defining the menace she posed to healthy New Yorkers, the legal experts put concerns about individual citizens' legal and constitutional rights in the foreground. Their actions generally upheld health department actions, but in the legal arena the courts applied their own particular logic to the problem of how to handle healthy carriers in general and Mary Mallon in particular.

The "extraordinary and even arbitrary" board of health powers that Hermann Biggs touted as he traveled around the country and the world (see chap. 2) rested in part upon sections 1169 and 1170 of the Greater New York Charter. These sections included the following provisions:

The board of health shall use all reasonable means for ascertaining the existence and cause of disease or peril to life or health, and for averting the same, throughout the city. [Section 1169]
Said board may remove or cause to be removed to [a] proper place to be by it designated, any person sick with any contagious, pestilential or infectious disease; shall have exclusive charge and control of the hospitals for the treatment of such cases. [Section 1170][5]

These provisions had been written and in use before any concept of healthy carrier was known. What officials needed to know in 1907, when they first isolated Mary Mallon, and in 1909, when the case came to court, was if these laws applied to this new situation of isolating a person with no physical symptoms but whose body harbored pathogenic organisms.

If health officials indeed consulted with lawyers in 1907 about how to proceed in their actions concerning Mary Mallon, no record of the deliberations remains. Either officials received encouragement from their legal consultants to go ahead with their plans to isolate her or they proceeded on their own to separate Mary Mallon from society and take away her liberty without legal advice. According to the newspaper, city officials not only kept her against her will in a hospital and subjected her to repeated laboratory tests, they also refused to permit Mallon "even by telephone, to converse with her relatives or any one else excepting the surgeons and her guards."[6] After a few weeks the health department removed Mary Mallon from the city hospital to a cottage on North Brother Island, and the issue of the legality of her isolation faded from view.[7]

Officials remained cognizant of their need to keep Mallon's identity private. Soper described the process of discovering a cook who was a healthy carrier of typhoid fever to the Biological Society of Washington in 1907, and Park expanded on her case to an American Medical Association audience in 1908.[8] Neither named the woman at the center of the case. Health department reports for these years merely noted briefly that "a woman who had served as cook in various families" was "examined from week to week."[9] Mary Mallon meanwhile remained in her one-room bungalow—described by one contemporary as a "shack," by another as a "pig sty," and by a third as "a lonely little hut"—accompanied by her fox terrier, alone with her thoughts.[10]

It was not until late June, 1909, two years and three months after her initial arrest, that newspapers revealed her identity because the opportunity came for Mary Mallon to test her banishment in a court of law. At that time she and her lawyer, George Francis O'Neill, filed a writ of habeas corpus, initiating a legal proceeding guaranteed all citizens. Habeas corpus may be used when a person has been arrested or deprived of liberty, as in this case through isolation or quarantine; it requires authorities—in this case, the health department—to bring the person to court for the purpose of obtaining a legal judgment about the detention. The writ is issued as a matter of right, but a release, which Mallon and her lawyer hoped would result from the hearing, does not always follow.[11]

The precipitating events that allowed for Mary Mallon and lawyer George Francis O'Neill to begin habeas corpus proceedings remain somewhat hidden. The *New York American* reporter covering the case believed that "some welathy [*sic*] New Yorkers" supported Mary Mallon in her effort to seek release after reading of her plight in the newspaper's pages on June 20, 1909, in an article that moved them to "pity for the lone woman who has not a relative or a friend to whom she can turn."[12] The reporter did not identify the benefactors. Possibly William Randolph Hearst himself funded the legal proceedings—he had done so for other people whose stories interested his newspaper's readers—but we can only speculate on whether and why he may have helped Mallon.[13] The June 20 story in the *American* was no doubt important to the case and critical to the release of Mallon's actual identity. However, it seems unlikely that it was the sole cause of Mallon's legal suit.

Mary Mallon had been determined to obtain her freedom from the early moments of her detention. She resisted strenuously when she was first arrested in 1907, and she continued during her years on the island to indicate that she did not accept her isolation. Presumably with an eye toward her ultimate freedom, Mallon obtained private laboratory analyses of her feces and urine beginning in July, 1908, a full year before her court appearance. Continuing through August and September of that year, she sent specimens to be analyzed at the Ferguson Laboratory on 42nd Street in Manhattan. It is unlikely she would have bothered to do this if she were not planning some sort of attempt to prove her innocence. After a six-month hiatus, she resumed her quest for private laboratory opinion in April, 1909, sending seven more samples to George Ferguson in that month alone. Mallon then wrote to Ferguson directly seeking information about all of her specimens and received a response that "*none* of the specimens submitted by you, of urine and feces, have shown Typhoid colonies."[14] It appears from this active communication and documentation of a pattern of negative stool samples that Mallon was planning a legal battle at least as early as April, 1909, if not eight months earlier when she had sent her first feces samples to the laboratory. The legal action ultimately materialized a week after publication of the *American* article at the end of June, 1909.

It is possible that Mary Mallon could not, or thought she could not, financially support legal proceedings until the newspaper publicity generated the money. Lawyer O'Neill's connection to her cannot be documented until after June 20 when his services seem to have been made possible through the benefaction of Hearst or the newspaper's readers, as the reporter suggested. If late June was in fact the first time she consulted with legal counsel, Mallon's previous preparations and documentation through the Ferguson Laboratory served her well in bringing the case quickly to the court of justice. The *New York American* article appeared in the Sunday edition, June 20, 1909; eight days later O'Neill filed the habeas corpus petition hoping it would lead to Mary Mallon's release from her North Brother Island detention.[15]

The June 20, 1909, article, which originated public knowledge about Mary Mallon and revealed her identity, contained a short reportorial statement about Mary Mallon's "predicament." She "is a prisoner for life," wrote the reporter, even though "she has committed no crime, has never been accused of an immoral or wicked act, and has never been a prisoner in any court, nor has she been sentenced to imprisonment by any judge." The newspaper added some "curious facts" about typhoid fever and the difficulties of medical detection work.[16] The prose was surprisingly unsensationalistic for a Hearst newspaper, but the alarming illustrations and photographs were certain to grab readers' attention (see fig. 5.2 and chap. 5 for more on this first news account of Mary Mallon).

The story in the newspaper, whose Sunday circulation reached almost 800,000 New Yorkers, did not question the city's legal right to imprison Mallon for life.[17] In fact, the reporter assumed this would be her fate: "Mary Mallon will probably be a prisoner for life on the Quarantine Island in East River." On these pages, William Park, too, seemed to have conquered whatever doubts he had originally felt about the city's right to hold Mallon, concluding, "It is clear that she will be a prisoner on North Brother Island for a long time, perhaps for life."[18] Yet this was not attorney O'Neill's opinion of what the law demanded.

George Francis O'Neill was thirty-four years old when he took on Mary Mallon's case. The young lawyer had been a customs inspector before being admitted to the New York state bar on May 13, 1907, almost two months after Mallon's incarceration. The *New York Times* identified him as a medical-legal expert, although his legal experience was still very new. Six months after Mallon's habeas corpus hearing, the Medico-Legal Society engaged O'Neill as the personal counsel to Albert Patrick when he sought a pardon on the charge of killing Texas millionaire George Marsh Rice. That case, like Mary Mallon's, rested on medical evidence, and the governor ultimately pardoned Patrick. The record does not reveal very much else about George Francis O'Neill's legal practice. He shared office space with other lawyers; he stood twice as the Republican candidate for the state senate from the 22nd district, apparently unsuccessfully. His physicians diagnosed tuberculosis in 1913, after which time O'Neill traveled outside of New York to try to regain his health. Unsuccessful in this attempt, he died on December 23, 1914, at thirty-nine years of age.[19]

Whatever convinced George Francis O'Neill to take Mary Mallon's case, he was active in his pursuit of justice as he saw it. Scribbled in the court records are two notes that reveal his state of mind. In one he wrote, "absurd to take woman on an alleged report in which no name is mentioned—[.]" He must refer here to the city's seizing of Mallon based on Soper's report, although one assumes that Soper did indeed use her name in his communication with health department officials even though he did not reveal it in the public record.[20] O'Neill's designation of the city's behavior as "absurd" showed his confidence that Mallon might be released. In the second note, he scribbled, "Had a right to examine first and then take, not take and then examine," again a seeming reference to the city's initial actions in March, 1907, when Baker and the health department took Mallon against her will to the Willard Parker Hospital and did not release her again.[21] O'Neill admitted here that the city could under its own regulations examine Mary Mallon, but they could not immediately take her. Both the notes emphasize lack of due process, the key point in O'Neill's legal argument at the habeas corpus hearing.

O'Neill petitioned in the writ on behalf of Mallon that she "is imprisoned or restrained in his [sic] liberty in Riverside Hospital, North Brother Island, N.Y.," and that the cause of her restraint was "unknown." He asked that the superintendent of Riverside Hospital be required to "produce said Mary Mallon before . . . a Justice of the Supreme Court."[22]

O'Neill filed this writ of habeas corpus to test the legality of Mallon's detention in a court of law.[23] The health department had no choice but to bring Mary Mallon before the New York Supreme Court, where Judges Mitchell Erlanger and Leonard Giegerich heard the arguments in late June and early July, 1909.

The health department stated for the record that Mary Mallon was confined on North Brother Island "for the reason that she is infected with the bacilli of typhoid, and is undergoing treatment under the care of physicians therein."[24]

From our late-twentieth-century perspective, it is interesting to realize that the legal issues debated in 1909 were Mallon's rights as a carrier and the health department's obligations vis à vis healthy typhoid fever carriers in general. No one at the time, as far as I have been able to determine, worried about the rights of Mary Mallon's "victims" and their families. No family for whom Mary Mallon worked brought suit or entered the debate in any way. The newspapers freely used the names of those who had employed Mallon as a cook, including such socially prominent names as J. Coleman Drayton and Henry Gilsey. The families' rights to privacy were abridged repeatedly, and details of their private lives and the losses they suffered were held up to public scrutiny.[25] As sympathetic as observers might have been to the plight of those who were said to have contracted typhoid fever from Mary Mallon (or died from it), the victims were not the subject of the legal discussions, nor did they seek revenge or enter the debate then as they might try to do today.

Legal historians have documented how judicial interpretations of the law—even of the Constitution—change significantly over time. Whereas late-twentieth-century courts are extremely vigilant of individual rights and due process, early-twentieth-century judges demonstrated a "preference for social control over individual autonomy," a point of view that was evident in these 1909 proceedings. As legal analyst Larry Gostin has demonstrated: "Courts [in the early part of the century] tended to uphold public health statutes as long as the state did not act in 'an arbitrary, unreasonable manner' or go 'beyond what was reasonably required for the safety of the public.' " These early assessments about what was reasonably required increasingly rested on medical opinion and evidence.[26]

Mary Mallon's habeas corpus case can be best understood historically in its proper legal context, following as it did closely on the heels of the 1905 United States Supreme Court decision *Jacobson v. Massachusetts*. That case involved a Massachusetts citizen, Henning Jacobson, who did not want to submit to vaccination against smallpox. The state legislature had empowered the boards of health to require vaccination if an epidemic of smallpox threatened; the Cambridge Board of Health adopted such a regulation when smallpox appeared in the city and ordered all inhabitants to be vaccinated. Jacobson argued that the ruling violated his individual rights. Justice Harlan and six of his colleagues on the Supreme Court thought otherwise:

The liberty secured by the Constitution of the United States to every person within its jurisdiction does not import an absolute right in each person to be, at all times and in all circumstances, wholly freed from restraint. There are manifold restraints to which every person is necessarily subject for the common good.... Real liberty for all could not exist under the operation of the principle which recognizes the right of each individual person to use his own, whether in respect of his person or his property, regardless of the injury that may be done to others.[27]

The most important issue for Justice Harlan, as it was four years later for Judge Erlanger, was the danger to other people posed by individuals or groups who would not cooperate with health officials. Both judges might have also agreed that there were limits to how far the state could go in protecting the public health. Nowhere in the U.S. Supreme Court decision did the justices rule that people could be forcibly vaccinated against their will. As legal expert James Tobey concluded from his analysis of vaccination laws in general and *Jacobson v. Massachusetts* in particular, "Compulsory vaccination means that all persons may be required to submit to vaccination for the common good, and if they refuse ... they may be arrested, fined, imprisoned, quarantined, isolated, or excluded from school ... but they cannot be forcibly vaccinated, desirable as such a procedure might be from the standpoint of public health protection."[28] Individual liberty and public health, thus, could be protected simultaneously under compulsory vaccination provisions, but there were limits on each.

In this tradition, the New York health officials and their lawyers based the city's right to hold Mary Mallon on its obligation to protect the public's health. Under the provision of police powers, resting with the state and in this case delegated to the city and to its board of health, city physicians justified their inspection, quarantine, and health laws of every description. As Chief Justice John Marshall had defined these obligations, they constituted "the acknowledged power of a State to provide for the health of its citizens."[29] Laws aimed at public health protection were subject to limitations, of course, based upon constitutional rights of citizens. The Fourteenth Amendment requires that no state shall deprive a person of life, liberty, or property without due process of law. Mallon's right to a habeas corpus hearing demonstrated that the courts had the power to curb a city's right to isolate one of its citizens. O'Neill's petition for Mallon's release brought up the questions of how far and under what circumstances the New York City Health Department could abridge one citizen's rights in its efforts to protect the health of others.

Corporation Counsel Francis K. Pendleton and George P. Nicholson, counsel to the health department, based their argument during Mary Mallon's habeas corpus hearing on sections 1169 and 1170 of the city code (see above). "It is evident," they wrote, "that sufficient power rests in the Board of Health for the isolation of Mary Mallon"—evident, they believed, because of laboratory results showing her to be "infected with the contagious bacilli of Typhoid in large quantities."[30] In support of this conclusion, the lawyers presented the numerous positive laboratory reports of Mallon's stool samples.

Section 1170 gave the health department authority over "any person *sick* with any contagious, pestilential or infectious disease" (my emphasis). One relevant question was whether a law written to cover "any person sick" applied to a person who was well but who carried bacilli that could make other people sick. Could a healthy person who was shown in laboratory reports to be carrying pathogenic bacilli be, for legal purposes, considered sick under this clause? This was one of the points that O'Neill wanted to question most seriously. Was a medical conclusion based on laboratory evidence—especially in this early-twentieth-century era when bacteriological evidence was new and not yet systematically applied—sufficient to define a person who felt healthy as sick?

In chapter 2 we looked at the New York City Health Department rules, instituted between 1915 and 1921, that were designed to monitor and control typhoid fever cases and carriers. These attempts to broaden the sanitary code's control of people with infectious diseases specifically to include healthy carriers (all of which followed Mary Mallon's second incarceration) indicate that health officials did not believe the earlier laws written about sick people could rightfully be applied to healthy carriers. In 1919, Health Commissioner Royal Copeland wrote, "The one striking and conspicuous improvement now needed is in the formulation of rules and regulations to be adopted by the Board of Health for the control of typhoid carriers."[31] Copeland ultimately got the regulations he requested and in 1921 happily reported, "Perhaps the most important step made by this Bureau [of Preventable Diseases] during the year was the formation of a definite set of regulations, in co-operation with the Counsel of the Department, for control of typhoid fever carriers. *Heretofore,*" Copeland wrote, "*the Department attempted to exercise control from time to time without any well formulated policy and without legal sanction for its requirements*" (my emphasis).[32] By the department's own later admission, then, not until 1921 did the laws allowing for the isolation of the sick rightfully apply to healthy carriers of typhoid fever.[33]

Yet here in 1909 were department officials appearing in a New York court of law claiming that the laws then on the books were sufficient to detain Mary Mallon. The health officials who appeared in the New York Supreme Court at the habeas corpus hearing to defend their isolation of Mary Mallon voiced no doubts about whether the laws designed to control the sick could be applied to the seemingly healthy. They simply presented the sections of the city code as if they applied to Mallon. They assumed without questioning that they already had the authority they needed. Using the language of the new science of bacteriology to define Mallon as effectively sick, laboratory-defined sick because she could spread disease, they masked the ambiguity of the laws and, apparently, the judge allowed this to pass without comment.

With the health department defining Mallon as sick because she harbored pathogenic bacteria, O'Neill was left to insist that Mallon was not sick because she had no physical symptoms and therefore could not be a health menace to the community. O'Neill did not challenge the authority of the health officials over the sick, and he thus lost an opportunity to challenge and have the judge define more precisely the extension of health department authority to healthy individuals who happened to be disease carriers.

O'Neill's key point in his effort to "discharg[e] the said Mary Mallon from the care and custody of the Department of Health of the City of New York" concerned what he saw as the abridgment of her constitutional right to due process. He argued that the health department did not follow due process in its incarceration of Mary Mallon in 1907: "The said Mary Mallon is being confined without commitment or any other order of any Court within the State of New York, or that of any other person or authority having power to restrain her." He insisted that the health department, given this situation, could not legally continue to isolate her indefinitely. Mallon had not had her day in court.[34]

There really was no disputing this point. Soper himself admitted when he later related her story, "She was held without being given a hearing; she was apparently under life sentence; it was contrary to the Constitution of the United States to hold her under the circumstances."[35] When O'Neill petitioned for Mallon's release in the writ of habeas corpus filed before the New York Supreme Court on June 28, 1909, it was the first (and, as it happened, the last) time her case was subject to judicial review.[36] O'Neill was clearly correct in pointing out that no court of law had yet ruled on the legal issues in the case. But his emphasis on due process was not uppermost in the mind of the judge. The Court focused on whether or not the health department had overstepped its authority in keeping Mary Mallon separated from the general population, rather than on the process officials used to do so. The overarching question for the judge was whether public health protection demanded that healthy carriers like Mallon be isolated from the public.

Hermann Biggs's idea of the broad scope of health department powers notwithstanding, O'Neill eloquently insisted that the health department could not legally keep Mary Mallon in confinement for life:

If such an act as this can be done in the case of any person said to be infected with typhoid germs, it can be perpetrated in the cases of thousands of persons in this city who might be said to be infected with tuberculosis and other kindred diseases. If the mere statement that a person is infected with germs is sufficient, then that person can be taken away from his or her home and family and locked up and imprisoned for life on North Brothers [sic] Island. That is what has happened in this case.[37]

The case indeed related to the issue of how much authority medicine and departments of health could have in their efforts to protect the general healthy population, and specifically, how much authority they could wield over healthy citizens. O'Neill wanted to question health officials' authority; were their "mere statements" sufficient grounds for lifelong isolation of an individual? The *New York American* reporter understood this larger issue at stake in the court case: "It is . . . expected to demonstrate just how far the Board of Health powers go—whether this body has the legal right to banish a human being to solitary confinement in the absence of a court commitment."[38]

Looking back on the 1909 case during an interview with a press reporter two years later, O'Neill tried to make light of the issue: "If the Board of Health," he said, "is going to send every cook to jail who happens to come under their designation of 'germ carrier,' it won't be long before we have no cooks left, and the domestic problem will be further complicated."[39] Sarcasm aside, the point he raised was nonetheless extremely important. Would the courts accept the words of "medical men" as sufficient to deprive a citizen of liberty for life? As O'Neill put it (again with two years' hindsight):

It is quite a problem if a municipality can, without legal warrant, or due process of law, clap some one in jail upon the word of some medical man. If the Board of Health can act this way with any one who is alleged to be a germ carrier, yet who never suffered from the disease, then it can put thousands upon thousands of persons who suffered at some time or another from typhoid fever in confinement.[40]

The power of medicine to define who endangered the public's health received considerable public discussion during Mary Mallon's 1909 court hearing. For example, a "New Thought Student" wrote to the *New York Times*:

If one unfortunate woman must be labeled "Typhoid Mary," why not send her other companions? Start a colony on some unpleasant island, call it "Uncle Sam's suspects," there collect Measles Sammy, Tonsillitis Joseph, Scarlet Fever Sally, Mumps Matilda, and Meningitis Matthew. Add Typhoid Mary, request the sterilized prayers of all religionized germ fanatics, and then leave the United States to enjoy the glorious freedom of the American flag under a medical monarchy.[41]

Public power wielded by established scientific experts and experts of all kinds increased significantly in the early twentieth century. The *Jacobson* decision itself gave authority to the medical community to define the value of vaccination, casting aside its more fringe challengers who believed the procedure to be dangerous. Progressive politicians, businessmen, and reformers were winning elections across the country as they tried to bring "good government," which emphasized order and rationality, to American cities and replace the haphazard and often corrupt partisan ward bosses. The use of educated authorities in all fields was central to this movement.[42] Reform was challenged by those whom the reformers sought to replace, people whose point of view supported O'Neill in his questioning of the right of health officials to curtail individual liberty. In New York City reformers frequently replaced Irish politicians, adding an ethnic layer to the clash of viewpoints.

A second issue raised by O'Neill's arguments before the court in 1909, in addition to due process, was whether or not Mary Mallon was the menace to the health of New Yorkers that officials claimed she was. He stated unequivocally that Mary Mallon was healthy, not in need of medical attention, and that therefore she did not endanger any other person's health. He told the judges: "Said Mary Mallon is in perfect physical condition, and has . . . never been obliged to receive the care and attention of a physician or surgeon." He insisted on the basis of Mallon's health that "she is not in any way or any degree a menace to the community or any part thereof." If the department was holding her in order to treat her, O'Neill denied her need of treatment.

On this point, bacteriology itself was on trial. O'Neill did not accept the new bacteriological concept that healthy people could carry disease to others, and that typhoid fever specifically could be transmitted through fecal discharges, via unwashed hands and food ingestion, from a healthy person to another. He denied her sickness: "We absolutely deny that this woman ever suffered or is now suffering from the affliction alleged," he told reporters.[43] He also denied the charge that Mary Mallon had infected the specific people whose illnesses Soper traced to her. To quote O'Neill again:

It may safely be assumed and we have charged that in some of the houses where this woman was employed the conditions were most unsatisfactory, and unsanitary, and the cases of typhoid referred to by the officials of the Health Department may be undoubtedly ascribed to this. This woman has been a victim of unfortunate circumstances in having been employed in houses where typhoid broke out, the disease having been unquestionably the result of conditions with which she had nothing to do.[44]

Admitting typhoid existed in some of the homes in which Mallon cooked, O'Neill insisted there was no convincing evidence that she was to blame for its presence. He instead drew on the more commonly accepted route of typhoid infection—unsanitary conditions and polluted water supplies, or infection outside the home—to explain the disease incidence. Although he did not call attention to the statistics, he could have bolstered his case even more by noting that in 1907 the city reported over 4,400 new cases of typhoid fever and alleged tracing only two of them to Mallon. There were far more dangers menacing the health of New Yorkers than could be accounted for by this one woman. Typhoid fever lurked throughout the city.

The questions O'Neill raised about Mallon's culpability, even though they did not get full airing in court, remain cogent. It is conceivable that, as the investigators before George Soper had themselves concluded, typhoid erupted in those houses from sources extraneous to Mary Mallon and her cooking. The evidence connecting Mary Mallon to the twenty-two specific cases of typhoid fever was indeed incomplete. The court, and we assume the health department, did not ask for or receive information about the full record of Mary Mallon's employment and the families for whom she cooked who did not report any typhoid.

Mallon claimed to have been connected to many such uninfected homes, one of them a friend's home in which she lived repeatedly when she was not employed.[45] She did name one family to reporters: "I was [a] cook for Mr. Stebbins' family and for other families and nobody fell sick while I was there."[46]

Even those who accepted the healthy carrier concept and accepted Mallon's connection to the specific cases might have questioned along with O'Neill the necessity of isolating her from the general population in order to stop her from being a "menace to the community." Mary Mallon had been isolated from the beginning and not as a last resort. This action implied that health officials believed, although they did not argue explicitly before the court, that Mallon was the equivalent of sick, even though she was symptomless, because her body harbored pathogenic bacteria. Certainly the distinction between a person sick with typhoid fever and a person carrying the typhoid bacilli was irrelevant to the people who ate the food into which the bacilli dropped.[47]

But from Mary Mallon's and George O'Neill's point of view, the difference between sickness and health was paramount. She insisted she was not sick and had never been sick with typhoid fever. She used her personal knowledge about her own body to argue that since she had no disease symptoms she could not menace anyone else's health. She did not want to be treated like someone who was sick when she felt healthy and vigorous, and was in fact leading a productive life when she was taken.

If Mallon had based her definition of herself as healthy on her experiences alone, the case would have represented a stark clash between two conflicting worldviews, experiential and scientific. But the situation grew more complicated, for while she adamantly insisted on her own knowledge of her health, Mallon also assessed it in part by procuring laboratory analyses of her own feces and urine which showed that she harbored no pathogenic bacteria. She seemed to condone the health department's definition of health when she herself sought laboratory analyses.

But Mallon's privately acquired laboratory results from the Ferguson Laboratory were all negative, verifying to her satisfaction what she already believed, that she was healthy. The health department laboratory repeatedly (but intermittently) found her feces infected, suggesting to health officials that her health was only skin deep. The court, for reasons that went unexplained, accepted reports from the laboratory that found her infected and rejected reports that claimed her healthy. The files record no evidence of discussion on this point.

The most important public health issue of the 1909 court case concerned isolation.[48] O'Neill filed the writ in order to seek Mary Mallon's release from her forcibly imposed isolation. In this he had the support, although he did not use it, of the major public health authorities of the time. As we have seen, Charles Chapin thought the only purpose served by keeping Mallon locked up was to give public health a bad name. Either O'Neill was not the "medical legal expert" the newspaper had chosen to call him and did not think of using the testimony of public health experts who would have supported him, or he believed the case too compelling on due process grounds alone to need the outside help. In any case, attempts to understand the full context of legal and medical thinking about Mary Mallon are stymied by the fact that public health experts did not get a chance to participate directly in the court debate.

The health department drew a one-to-one relationship between the positive stool samples as tested in its own laboratory and the necessity to isolate Mary Mallon. Lawyer Nicholson claimed that Soper's epidemiological investigation and "the pathological examination conducted in said Department is positive and complete as to the danger of allowing a person infected as the petitioner, to go at large and mingle with the community." He continued, "The Board of Health shows the danger and menace to the public that the petitioner would be if allowed to be at large in the community."[49] The legal precedent cited in defense of this position was the health department authority to forcibly isolate people sick with contagious diseases.

Two parts of the health department argument in court may amaze modern readers. First is the ease with which the health department lawyer assumed that laws written about people sick with infectious disease could be applied to this new category of healthy people who harbored bacilli (especially when faced with evidence upon which two laboratories disagreed) even while they wrote of their uncertainty elsewhere. The judge, seemingly without consideration or question, acquiesced with the assumption that the two groups—people sick with typhoid fever and healthy carriers of typhoid fever—were identical in the eyes of the law. There was no discussion about it in the record.

The second point is even more striking. Health officials argued that if laboratory analysis showed pathogenic typhoid bacilli in fecal discharges, in order safely to protect the community, the person harboring them should not "mingle" with people or go "at large" among healthy people. At the end of the memorandum filed by the department lawyer, the connection was drawn very starkly, and in capital letters:

THE EXAMINATION OF THE STOOLS OF THE PATIENT SHOWS
CLEARLY OF HER INFECTED CONDITION AND THE DANGER TO
THE PUBLIC BY ALLOWING THIS PERSON TO GO AT LARGE UNTIL
SUCH TIME AS SHE IS FREE FROM THE INFECTION OF THE
BACILLI OF TYPHOID.[50]

If the logic of this statement had been followed generally, health officials would have had to isolate all healthy carriers they found. In 1909 they had identified only five healthy carriers in New York City, but the health officials knew that there were hundreds, if not thousands, of others yet to be found. A general application of the principle even to all identifiable carriers did not get discussed in 1909, nor did the court ask health officials to justify locking up one person in the face of thousands, most unidentified, going free. If they had, perhaps the outcome of Mary Mallon's hearings would have been different. The health department budget and ability (or interest) did not extend to locking up thousands of healthy New Yorkers.

The fact that health officials applied the argument of necessary isolation to Mary Mallon and not necessarily to other healthy carriers identified in the department laboratory suggests that they viewed Mary Mallon as different from other healthy carriers. They did not argue for her difference before the court. They knew they had and would continue to have other healthy carriers in the city of New York, who would be permitted to "mingle." They knew, in fact, that typhoid carriers could mingle with the general population and not cause any risk whatsoever. But they wanted Mary Mallon isolated, and they used the simplest and most absolute argument possible—if infected, isolate—before the judge.

Fred S. Westmoreland, the resident physician at Riverside Hospital who received Mary Mallon and who testified on the department's behalf at the hearing, restated the case and made one important addition:

Owing to . . . her occupation as a cook . . . , the Department of Health concluded that the patient would be a dangerous person and a constant menace to the public health to be at large; and, consequently . . . decided . . . to place her in a contagious hospital and isolate her from the general public.[51]

In bringing Mallon's occupation into the picture, Westmoreland narrowed the definition of who the health department might not allow to mingle with the citizenry. Not all carriers need be isolated, only the ones who handled food and thus endangered others. This position was closer to the view of public health experts nationally in that it related to the activity that might encourage bacteria to be transmitted from carriers' excreta to the mouths of susceptible people. But it suggested that isolation would be necessary for all carriers who were food handlers, a policy that also was never developed or even contemplated in New York, or anywhere else in the country.

The judge listened to the arguments and heard the simple message that the health department intended for the court to hear, that people excreting pathogenic bacteria, whether sick or well, could be considered sick because of their ability to transmit disease, thereby fitting the existing laws, and needed to be isolated to protect the public. O'Neill's contention that Mallon was not sick became irrelevant in the face of the positive bacteriological analyses. In mid-July, 1909, Judge Mitchell Erlanger agreed with the health officials and ordered that the writ be dismissed and "that the said petitioner, Mary Mallen [*sic*] be and she hereby is remanded to the custody of the Board of Health of the City of New York."[52]

In considering the meaning of this court decision, it is important to recall once again the circumstances of Mary Mallon's isolation. When she was first located on George Soper's epidemiological evidence in March, 1907, she was immediately taken. Never before had the health department tried to isolate a healthy person. The concept of healthy carrier was in its infancy, and many people had not yet heard about it. When a laboratory test showed Mary Mallon's feces to be positive for typhoid bacilli, she, the first to be labeled a healthy carrier and herself not yet a repeat offender, was placed on North Brother Island in complete isolation, and she was not released. The judge, two years and three months later, in July, 1909, ruled that the health authorities had acted properly and that they could keep her indefinitely in isolation on North Brother Island.

Officials did not allow Mary Mallon a chance to prove whether or not, upon learning of the situation, she would or could change her behavior and cease infecting others. The health department and the court acted to keep her in quarantine when all she had done was to insist she was healthy and to resist what seemed to her to be an unreasonable arrest. The initial action in 1907 and the 1909 court affirmation of it permitted a healthy woman to be indefinitely kept in isolation upon the charge that she might pass on infection to other people. The court and the health department put the protection of society and the public's health as they saw it above the protection of one individual's liberty.

Mary Mallon's legal case brings to light an important question: is it possible to protect the health of the population and at the same time not infringe on individual liberty? This question presupposes that we *want* the protection public health programs provide, and at the same time that we are vigilant of individual freedom. In pitting these two strongly held values and legal positions against each other, a dilemma arises that is at least sometimes, if not often, impossible to resolve. Public health departments limit what disease prevention they can accomplish if they acknowledge, as they must do under our country's laws, a citizen's right to personal liberty. But individual liberty can be legally abridged in the name of protecting the public's health. As much as we all might wish it, no federal, state, or local agency trying to protect the health of citizens will always be able to do that job without threatening and infringing on the freedom of some citizens. Conversely, protecting individual liberty above all else may sometimes put people at risk for exposure to infectious disease. We as a society have decisions to make—over and over again—about which side of the dilemma we value the most.

In the 1909 legal proceedings, the judge ruled that Mary Mallon's liberty, like Henning Jacobson's in 1905, could be taken away in the name of protecting the public's health. He did not point to any limitations on the health department's authority to protect the public in the instance of protecting the liberty of healthy carriers of typhoid fever. Indeed, S. Josephine Baker learned from the case, "what sweeping powers are vested in Public Health authorities. There is very little that a Board of Health cannot do," Baker concluded, "in the way of interfering with personal and property rights for the protection of the public health."[53] Nonetheless, the health department did seem to recognize some limits to its authority. While it forced Mallon to stay on North Brother Island, it did not force her to undergo the surgical removal of her gallbladder (a procedure, as we have seen in chap. 1, often unsuccessful and dangerous in this period, that had the potential for alleviating her condition). The risks to her of surgical complications or even death were so high that officials, while suggesting the operation, did not insist upon it.[54]

We might speculate that if the New York City Health Department had tried to isolate against their will all the known healthy typhoid carriers—over 400 by the 1930s—the judicial rulings might have begun to go in the opposite direction. The court might have put limitations on health department use of its authority with regard to the isolation of large numbers of healthy people. But the judge seemed to have no problem with a single case, perhaps reasoning that because Mary Mallon was the first healthy carrier to be identified, she made a good example to deter potential future offenders. Whatever other reasons might have motivated him—and I will explore some possible ones in later chapters—the judge interpreted an ambiguous law as allowing him to accept the advice of the city physicians and permit long-term isolation.

Part of what Mary Mallon's case reveals is the early-twentieth-century acceptance of the authority of scientific experts and of laboratory tests as legal measurers of truth and determiners of the abridgment of liberty.[55] Significant parts of American society came to trust these new tools based on microscopic examination instead of relying only on experience. Even in a case of conflict, when a person said she was healthy and one laboratory agreed, but another claimed she was not, health policy seemed to rest with the point of view that favored the new science. Health law stood on the shoulders of bacteriological findings.

There is more at work here than the prominence of medical knowledge or the legal acceptance of new medical theories. Let us posit for a moment that all parties in Mallon's case agreed that she carried and disseminated typhoid fever with her cooking. The question still remained about whether or not people who gave disease to others needed to be isolated. Was it not possible to stop Mary Mallon from cooking without placing her in strict isolation in a cottage on an island? After all, officials did not later isolate most other healthy carriers they found. If health officials and judges believed strict isolation was the only way to stop Mary Mallon's potential dangers, why and how did they reach this conclusion? What differentiated her case from others?

The law was not always interpreted in such a way as to demand isolation. Compare the New York Supreme Court ruling in Mallon's 1909 case with a report the following year of an Adirondack guide, Mallon's "brother in affliction," dubbed "Typhoid John" by one newspaper, who was identified as a typhoid fever carrier and the perpetrator of an epidemic among tourists that killed two and infected over thirty-six more (more in both categories than Mallon had been associated with at the time). The state health department in this case determined that "there was no State law by which a human carrier of typhoid bacilli could be kept from spreading contagion and disease," and did not try to detain him, although it did offer him free medical care. The newspaper similarly concluded that "there is no law in this country restraining the movements of these human carriers of typhoid germs, although medical experts estimate that there are probably some 10,000 such afflicted and afflicting persons in the United States."[56] While comparing Mary Mallon to this man, the reporters and health officials did not, significantly, note the anomaly of her isolation.

In Mallon's court case the health department did not bring up arguments to distinguish her from other carriers, in terms of her resistance or of her being the first carrier to be traced. Health officials presented to the court a situation in which a healthy woman needed to be isolated because the presence of pathogenic bacteria in her alimentary tract defined her as a danger to society. The legal proceedings indicate that the judge was convinced that the positive laboratory tests proved Mallon's dangers and that similar laboratory tests in another case would bring the same conclusion. Science and medicine could adequately define a health menace.

Given the universality of the arguments raised in court, what happened to Mary Mallon as a healthy carrier should have been typical and precedent-setting. But we already know that when a similar case of Alphonse Cotils (a repeat healthy carrier, which Mary Mallon was not in 1907 or in 1909) came before the municipal court in 1924, the judge suspended his sentence (see chap. 2). In that case, the judge thought, "The only object in imposing a prison sentence would be to deter other typhoid germ carriers from handling foodstuffs."[57] He clearly did not see the specifics of Mallon's isolation as precedent-setting or generalizable.

The judges in 1909 and in 1924 did not speak about the universal applicability of their rulings; and the health officials, who understood it, chose not to bring it up. They had no intention of isolating all carriers. O'Neill made some effort at generalizing in his sarcastic remarks about locking up all cooks, but did not effectively carry the argument to its conclusion. Mary Mallon's habeas corpus hearing did not lead to a legal precedent about healthy carriers. Her case was not published in the legal journals, and it was not cited as precedent in other cases concerning typhoid carriers.[58]

In the early twentieth century the law spoke with a single voice and a simple guideline: public health authorities had the medical ability and the legal authority to define a public health menace, regardless of due process or the curtailment of an individual's liberty and regardless of consistency. The judges were willing to give health departments the power to discriminate among carriers and decide which healthy people who carried pathogenic bacteria in their bodies were to go free and which were to be detained.

The public health laws that exist today are basically similar to the ones developed at the beginning of the twentieth century. The states' obligation to protect the health of citizens cannot be abridged or obliterated, but that obligation is constantly open to interpretation as to how it should be carried out and whose expertise might be called upon to help. Legal questions like ones posed earlier in the century continue to face public health officials trying to prevent the spread of HIV infection and drug-resistant tuberculosis. There are public health workers who believe that infected people in both instances should be kept separate from the healthy population, possibly on the basis of laboratory screening tests before any symptoms develop, and others who think that while a few individuals may need to be singled out for such isolation, most do not. Evaluation of the danger of disease transmission is one criterion that remains important to the decision, but other factors enter into the equation today as in the past.

Current fears of living in a police state put limits on plans to isolate large numbers of people, even in the face of potential public health dangers. Mass isolation has been used in Cuba, where the state has created a community within the boundaries of which all AIDS sufferers must live, but such authoritarian behavior on the part of the government in the United States would not easily be met with cooperation.[59] Charles Chapin knew, early in the century, that "there certainly would be most energetic opposition on the part of the public" to such policies. Besides, Rosenau had insisted, "It is unnecessary to place bacillus carriers *incommunicado*."[60] But that is just what health authorities did with Mary Mallon in 1907 and what the court reinforced in 1909: they forced one woman to live in isolation in the name of protecting the public's health. From the legal point of view, justice could be served in allowing such abridgment of individual liberty.

"She Walked More Like a Man than a Woman"

Social Expectations and Prejudice

*W*hen the court ruled in July, 1909, that Mary Mallon had to stay on North Brother Island under health department–imposed isolation, many public health professionals sympathized with the healthy woman and were disturbed by her predicament. Charles Chapin, from his distance in Providence, Rhode Island, wrote about the issues that made her case compelling: "It seems a hardship to keep her virtually in prison, to deprive her of her liberty, because she happens to be the type of a class now known to be numerous and well distributed," he suggested. "There is now a good deal of sympathy for her, for she is simply one of thousands, perhaps an extreme case, but at the same time one of a class of which all the other members are still at liberty." Chapin acknowledged that Mary Mallon should not be permitted to cook for other people, for in such a position she would be "in truth a dangerous focus of infection," but, he went on, "there are many occupations in both city and country in which she could do little harm. . . . there are hundreds of occupations in any one of which she might be free, but under a sort of medical probation, and be shorn of her injurious powers."[1]

In the mind of this national expert on public health policy, there were no medical or public health reasons to keep Mary Mallon isolated in a cottage on an island. The judge in Mallon's case may have been convinced by the New York City Health Department that on scientific grounds isolating Mary Mallon was necessary to protect the health of New Yorkers, but many of those people who understood the public health issues best— and Chapin represented this point of view—believed that New Yorkers could be well protected without such extreme measures. Health Commissioner Darlington had voiced "considerable doubt" about whether the health department needed to detain the "germ woman." In 1910, when Ernst J. Lederle took over as health commissioner, he, too, thought her isolation unnecessary and released her from her quarantine.

Despite the single-mindedness of their arguments in court in 1909, New York health officials in other venues did not limit themselves to bacteria counts and laboratory analyses when they described Mary Mallon and her potential dangers. In this chapter I explore some of the social expectations and prejudices shared by New York health officials that contributed to their perception that Mallon was different from other carriers and in turn affected what happened to her. The fact that Mary Mallon was a woman, a domestic servant, single, and Irish-born significantly influenced how health officials and the middle-class public thought about what should be done with her. Looking at Mary Mallon's story from the perspective of the dominant social values of her times— as from the perspectives of medicine, public health, or the law— does not alone nor fully explain why health officials and the courts acted as they did, but this point of view adds an important dimension to her story.[2]

Health officials viewed women carriers of typhoid fever as more dangerous than men in part because cooking, an activity that provided one of the easiest routes of bacilli transmission, was a traditional female activity. Women more than men cooked for their families; women more than men were employed in domestic service; women more than men provided food at public functions like church suppers. The earliest statistics gathered on typhoid carriers revealed that many more women than men were listed on healthy carrier rosters.[3] New York City's own carrier statistics bore out the gender disparity: in 1923, of 106 identified carriers, 82 were women.[4] Being a carrier was a gendered condition, one defined in part by socially sanctioned sex roles. Cultural expectations about who women were and what they did became part of the explanation of why more women seemed to be carriers and part of the response concerning how to control carrier-transmitted typhoid fever.

One striking example of how ideas about gender roles influenced thinking about the dangers of typhoid fever carriers came from George Soper. In a press interview after Mary Mallon's 1915 capture, Soper made use of the opportunity to warn the public in the pages of a Sunday news magazine that, as food handlers, all women cooks were potentially dangerous to the public health, whether they were employed outside the home or within it. "The first lesson to be learned from the case of Mary Mallon," Soper emphasized, "is in the matter of cooks. Who is your cook? Has she ever had typhoid? Has she ever nursed a typhoid patient?" Almost all women, Soper safely assumed, either cooked for their own families or hired other women to cook for them. Women of all classes, then, by virtue of their culturally defined gendered activities, were potentially dangerous in Soper's eyes.

How does a lady engage a cook? She goes to an office, she has an interview with a number of candidates of whom she has never heard before, she is told they have good references as to character and ability, and she employs the one who makes the best personal impression. In five minutes she has satisfied herself concerning the person who is to perform the most important function in the household.

Soper indicted upper-class women who were careless in making important hiring decisions and urged them to make sure that they did not bring danger into their homes. In even stronger language, he targeted middle-class women, with whom "the danger of transmitting typhoid is increased tremendously," because mothers tend sick children and bring germs directly from the sick room to the kitchen when they prepare the family's meals. Mothers, in carrying out their traditional jobs of caring for their children and feeding their families, might carry disease to the ones they love. Most of all, Soper blamed working-class women domestics who entered the homes of others as cooks, spreading germs to unsuspecting people.[5]

While all women thus became suspect for spreading typhoid fever, health officials did not for a moment consider testing all women and locking up all those identified as typhoid carriers. It was not simply her sex that made Mary Mallon a candidate for incarceration. Mary Mallon was not isolated because she was female, but her womanhood was an important factor contributing to what happened to her. The gendered order of society, embodied in cultural expectations about men's and women's behavior and in language, influenced how women in general and Mary Mallon in particular were viewed.

By the 1930s in New York City, such gender considerations had become a stated component of health department rules for controlling typhoid carriers. As Charles Bolduan and Samuel Frant wrote, "A hard and fast rule has been set. Stools on all who prepare food in the family, as well as on *all women over 40 in the household, and any grandmothers or mothers-in-law*, are required, and also on all those giving a history of typhoid fever in the past" (emphasis added).[6] Men (and young women) living in a household which was being investigated for the cause of a typhoid outbreak would be subject to scrutiny only if they gave a history of having handled food or having had the disease; women over the age of forty, regardless of their typhoid status or their stated connection to food preparation, were all required to undergo medical examination. The rules recognized a socially common sexual division of labor at the same time as they reinforced the expectation that even women who claimed no responsibility for food preparation could not be trusted not to cook.

Because Mary Mallon was a woman, middle-class American society had expectations about how she should act and what she should do that helped lead to her condemnation when she did not follow the acceptable norms. The gendered language evident in some tellings of her story reveals that appropriate "womanly" behavior was on the minds of health officials as they considered Mallon's case. As the following discussion suggests, gender was one very important factor in Mary Mallon's situation, and it interacted closely with class and ethnicity, both of which also carried strong cultural expectations that influenced the outcome of Mallon's story. Mallon was not isolated for life because she was a Catholic, Irish-born, single, working woman. The evidence suggests, rather, that for the middle-class professionals with whom she came in contact these social identifiers created a set of social expectations and evoked certain prejudices, which together helped lead to their perception of her as deviant and expendable.[7]

Gender, class, marital status, and foreign birth all help explain how it happened that Mary Mallon was cooking for the Charles Henry Warren family in their rented Long Island summer home in 1906. She was an Irish-born, working-class, single woman. These facts meant that she had few choices in her life. She did not have a family on which to rely for social or financial support. She had to work, and, like many other Irish-born women, she made her living by hiring out her domestic services to wealthy New Yorkers. She found most of her placements through an employment agency, a fact that later helped George Soper trace her typhoid history.[8] Her career pattern was completely ordinary, following the limited opportunities available to single women of her ethnicity and class.[9]

From Soper's identification of the families for whom Mary

Mallon worked who reported cases of typhoid fever, it is possible to trace Mallon's employment history, although she claimed that his list was incomplete. Between September, 1897, the first employment date we know, and March, 1907, when the health officials first apprehended her, Mary Mallon was fully employed 65.5 months, or 57 percent of the time. Mallon admitted that she was not always working. We can safely conclude that her life was not easy, that money was a problem, and that she, like other women of her marital status, occupation group, and ethnic background, sometimes did not have adequate support.

This, then, is the basic outline of Mallon's situation when she became a public ward in 1907. The statements and attitudes of the health officials reflect that they saw her as a person representing a class lower than their own, as uneducated, and as unappealing in her appearance, her choice of a male companion, and her living spaces. Assessing the attitudes that underlay public officials' thinking about Mallon will help us to understand the conscious and unconscious thought that determined how she was viewed and treated, as well as how Mary Mallon herself understood their words and actions.

We know the events of Mary Mallon's initial encounters with health officials mainly because of the writings of George Soper and S. Josephine Baker. As recounted in chapter 2, Mary Mallon rebuffed George Soper when he first called at her place of employment and when he followed her to her home by lunging at him with a fork and screaming epithets to his fleeing back. The day S. Josephine Baker apprehended her, she came out "fighting and swearing," and would not be talked to "sensibly." She was "maniacal," and finally, in the ambulance on the way to the hospital, like "an angry lion."[10] These descriptions give us a hint about how these two individuals, the two most responsible for Mallon initially and upon whose accounts most subsequent ones rested, approached Mary Mallon.

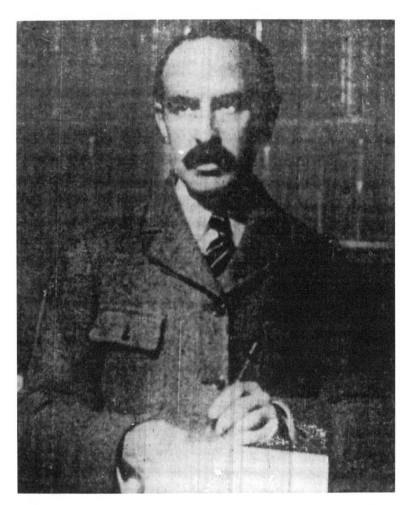

Fig. 4.1. *George Soper, 1915.*

George Soper provided by far the most cited and most comprehensive accounts of Mary Mallon's story.[11] Unfortunately for
historians, he left no private papers to help us flesh out his public
writings and learn more about his personality and motives.[12]
Writer Warren Boroson found in Soper's public persona a man he
described as "intelligent, decisive, authoritarian, cold, ambitious,
and vain." Boroson thought Soper showed no interest in Mary

Mallon as a human being who had thoughts and feelings of her own.[13] (See fig. 4.1.)

Soper's ambition and vanity are evident in two letters he wrote (around the time of Mallon's death) defending his reputation against what he believed had been inadequate recognition in the press.[14] Soper felt that popular accounts of Mary Mallon's discovery, while naming him, "rob me of whatever credit belongs to the discovery of the first typhoid carrier to be found in America.... Suffice it to say," he continued, "I did not stumble upon her in the course of routine duties ... or as a blind disciple of Robert Koch. I was at the time a thoroughly trained and experienced epidemic fighter who had seen service in the laboratory and the field.... It was a difficult investigation."[15] In the second letter, Soper, referring to himself in the third person, insisted that the discovery of Mary Mallon "was the outcome of a scientific field investigation by Dr. Soper, who was a highly trained consulting expert." He claimed that the American Association for the Advancement of Science had recommended him to carry out the investigation, "as the most capable person obtainable to clear up the mystery surrounding an outbreak of typhoid." He felt his discovery "changed the entire outlook of the medical profession upon the management of infectious diseases," and he seemed bitter that his role did not garner him more public acclaim.[16]

Vanity and ambition may partly explain George Soper's approach to Mary Mallon, but other attributes are even more important in interpreting his behavior and writings. What Warren Boroson called "cold" and "authoritarian" may reflect instead a combination of social and cultural attitudes very common to the early twentieth century. Soper belonged to an educated and privileged class of urbanites, mostly Protestant, whose dedication to the truth-telling ability of science put him among an elite group of progressive civic leaders. Urban social activists among whom Soper counted himself attempted in this period to stem social disorder, which they saw everywhere around them in the rapidly expanding cities, with a series of reform proposals for alleviating the worst of urban ills. In the process, they espoused both democratic and elitist goals.[17]

Soper believed that science could be used in the public service. Much of his work on urban sanitation, subway ventilation, and sewer systems reflected his belief that urban problems could be conquered through the application of rational and scientific principles.[18] Mary Mallon's situation, however, provided an example of how what he regarded as nonrational forces might interfere when officials tried to apply scientific advances in the public sphere. At the same time as Soper believed in the rightness of his actions, he acknowledged that they did not produce the desired result. Perhaps the impatience he showed with Mary Mallon was rooted in frustration that the scientific task which should have been straightforward was not.

Soper's ideas about women's roles were similarly in keeping with his time and with his own encounters with working women. Few middle-class married women worked outside the home. A married woman who worked outside her own home usually did so because she was poor or her husband had become sick or lost his job. If a woman was single, the extra income she could earn outside the home could help support her family. Such jobs as were available to women did not often involve positions of public leadership and usually were based in other people's homes or "involved tasks that were an extension of housework—in laundries, canneries, textile and clothing factories."[19] Thus, with the exception of a small number of professional women like S. Josephine Baker, Soper would have encountered women working outside their homes mainly in domestic employment, and the women he would have come into contact with likely would have been immigrant working-class women. Most American-born women of his age and class would not have labored outside their homes. It is fairly safe to predict that, as a result of this experience, Soper would have assumed basic class and ethnic differences with women like Mary Mallon. Viewed through the lens of his own gender and class expectations, Mary Mallon would have seemed a social inferior. His own social orientation, as well as his strong commitment to science, help explain the ways Soper tried to solve the public health dilemma Mary Mallon posed.

Soper and Mallon were about the same age, in their late thirties, at the time that they first met in 1907.[20] For reasons it may be impossible to know with certainty, they did not get along from the very first minutes of their meeting in the Bowen family's Park Avenue kitchen in March, 1907. Soper insisted he was "as diplomatic as possible," but we cannot know the precise words he used to try to explain to Mary Mallon that she was a healthy carrier—a concept not yet known in the lay world and still barely understood in the medical community—and why he wanted her to come downtown for laboratory tests. We can analyze the words Soper used to describe that meeting and two other direct encounters he had with Mary Mallon.[21] In all his descriptions we see the gulf that separated George Soper and Mary Mallon.

Soper used some straightforward words to describe Mary Mallon's appearance: she was an "Irish woman," about forty years old, "tall," "heavy," "single." She was, he admitted, in "perfect health."[22] When he met her, he wrote, she was "at the height of her physical and mental faculties. She was five feet six inches tall, a blond with clear blue eyes, a healthy color and a somewhat determined mouth and jaw. Mary had a good figure and might have been called athletic had she not been a little too heavy."[23] He described Mary Mallon ambivalently. She was blond and blue-eyed, but these conventionally attractive features were offset by her "determined mouth and jaw," a phrase that seems to connote that Soper did not think her pretty or feminine. He similarly negated her healthy athletic appearance in his comment about her weight.

Soper also equivocated in his description of her educational

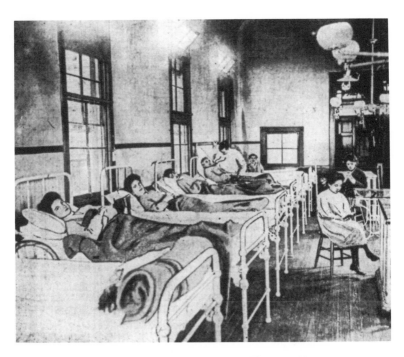

Fig. 4.2. *Mary Mallon in bed in Willard Parker Hospital, 1909.*

level. "She could write an excellent letter," he wrote, "so far as composition and spelling were concerned." He complimented the form but not the content of what she said. "She wrote in a large, clear, bold hand," Soper observed, and with "remarkable uniformity." The bold hand seems positive, although it might compare in Soper's mind to how a man might write and seem to him inappropriate in a woman. The notion "remarkable" seems to indicate Soper's incredulity that she, an Irish working-class woman, could perform so well.[24] He praised her (possibly to showcase his own humanity and compassion); but there were limits to the positive qualities he would attribute to Mary Mallon.[25]

Soper's ambivalence completely fell away with his further description: "Nothing was so distinctive about her as her walk, unless it was her mind. The two had a peculiarity in common," he thought. "Mary walked more like a man than a woman and

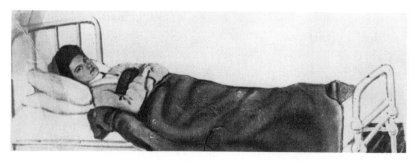

Fig. 4.3. *Close-up of Mary Mallon in bed in Willard Parker Hospital, 1909.*

... her mind had a distinctly masculine character, also."[26] These comments leap off the page as we read them today. In Soper's eyes and, he tells us, in the minds of others who knew her, she was no ordinary woman. Her very appearance, her mind, and the way she walked showed her deviance from acceptable female norms.

Soper never claimed that Mallon's walk or the character of her mind influenced the bacilli lodged in her gallbladder. Yet he could not refrain from calling attention to her ways of walking and thinking, medically irrelevant though he surely knew these traits to be. The *Medical Record*, with similar disregard for relevance, described Mallon as "a perfect Amazon, weighing over 200 pounds." She was set aside in these descriptions as different, deviant, unfeminine. Of course, these characteristics were not relevant to Mallon's public health status; her weight and her femininity were extraneous to the health dangers she potentially posed. Even more startling, the one early photograph I have been able to find of Mary Mallon indicates that the physical description of her was not only immaterial, it was false. In this photograph (and in the following close-up), taken in 1909, Mary Mallon lies in a bed in Willard Parker Hospital. She is the woman in the bed closest to the photographer, a neat, conventionally pretty, distinctly "feminine" woman.[27] (See figs. 4.2 and 4.3.)

The physically imposing masculinized woman seems to have existed only in the eyes of the anxious beholders, in the vision of those like Soper who needed to see in her an aberrant "other" in order to justify their actions against her. His description may also reflect what different worlds the two moved in and the fact that Mary Mallon did not meet George Soper's ideal of womanhood. Whatever it signified to Soper, his description reveals to us that factors other than science entered into his evaluation of his target. Consider his description of her lifestyle:

I found that Mary was in the habit of going, when her work for the day was finished, to a rooming house on Third Avenue below Thirty-third Street, where she was spending the evenings with a disreputable looking man who had a room on the top floor and to whom she was taking food. His headquarters during the day was in a saloon on the corner. I got to be well acquainted with him. He took me to see the room. I should not care to see another like it. It was a place of dirt and disorder. It was not improved by the presence of a large dog of which Mary was said to be very fond.[28]

Soper went beyond anything that might be considered necessary to a scientific investigation in this description. He could conceivably want to know the hygiene of Mallon's living quarters in his consideration of the public health dangers she might pose. But his characterization of her friend, A. Briehof, as "a disreputable looking man" was not necessary to build a sanitary indictment against Mary Mallon. No doubt it contributed to creating social disapproval. Here was a single woman seeming to cohabit with a man who spent his days in a saloon. Soper did not test Briehof (or Breshof) for typhoid, but he and Mary Mallon failed the test of moral and social rectitude Soper did apply.[29]

Soper described Mallon and Briehof's home as "disordered." For people committed to bringing order and rationality to city life, as Soper was, this was strong language. Soper did not want to see another apartment like theirs; he did not think such living spaces should exist. In a statement preceding the quoted paragraph, Soper wrote, "Mary had no home." He said she was "in the habit of going" to this apartment after work, and yet he would not call it her home. Mary Mallon lived under conditions George Soper abhorred, on which he could not refrain from passing judgment. Her out-of-wedlock cohabitation, her perceived disordered life, and even her dog were all relevant to George Soper in his justification for keeping close watch over this particular healthy carrier. He believed Mallon could not care properly for herself in part because she did not meet his social standards.

Soper's investigation of Mary Mallon's activities included looking into her personal hygiene on the job, since she transmitted the typhoid bacilli in large part because she did not keep her hands clean. But the engineer epidemiologist did not limit himself to cleanliness when he observed, "She was careless in her personal habits, but so are most cooks."[30] His class bias came into play when he placed Mary as part of a group which he, and by implication, his social class, denigrated. The stigma attached to healthy carriers could be linked to the inferior status of domestic workers to further justify Mallon's incarceration.[31]

The distance Soper felt between himself and Mary Mallon is evident in his drawing a line between "we" and "them." He wrote, for example, that Mary Mallon's situation "shows how carefully *we* should select our cooks," continuing, "*we* ordinarily know very little about *them*. [The case] confirms the truth of the adage that the more *we* pay the less *we* know about our servants" (emphasis added).[32] Soper saw himself a class apart, and above, the one occupied by Mary Mallon, a hierarchy which helped define some of his suspicions about Mary Mallon. His observations that she was not "particularly clean," which he repeated, fit his characterization of the class. Since Soper had only second-hand knowledge of Mallon's cleanliness on the job, learned from housekeepers and employers whom he interviewed, we cannot be sure how accurately he described her personal habits.[33] Other commentators picked up on Soper's observations, and one, exaggerating Soper's descriptions, said that in one "place where she had been employed she left the kitchen in such a filthy condition that it required the services of a scavenger to cleanse it."[34]

As important as were physical appearance, home, hygiene, and occupation to Soper's analysis of Mary Mallon's problems, he saved his strongest language to describe her behavior and beliefs. When Soper met Mallon at her home to try to bring her into the hospital for laboratory tests, he noted, "Although I recited some well considered speeches committed to memory in advance to make sure she understood what I meant . . . I could do nothing with her."[35] Soper's conversations with Mallon did not go as Soper had anticipated they should, because in his view, Mary Mallon did not behave rationally. "It was impossible," Soper complained, "to deal with her in a reasonable and peaceful way." From the beginning, when he turned over his records to the health department, Soper advised that the officials "be prepared to use force and plenty of it" when dealing with this woman.[36]

Soper's impatience with Mallon spilled out onto the pages of his published accounts. He related that when he visited her in the hospital, a few days after the health department apprehended her, he found a "fearfully angry-looking person [with] a startling appearance." He told her, "You would not be where you are now if you had not been so obstinate. So throw off your wrong-headed idea and be reasonable."[37] These were not words to gain her trust or ease her mind as she lay there alone in the Willard Parker Hospital, following her dramatic arrest.

Mary Mallon responded by not speaking: "Mary looked at me steadily, but neither spoke nor moved. Her eyes gleamed angrily." When Soper explained to her that "you don't keep your hands clean enough," Mallon did not "utter a word." When he offered to write a book about her, hiding her identity but promising her the profits, if she would only talk to him, "Mary rose. She pulled her bathrobe about her and, not taking her eyes off mine, slowly opened the door of her toilet and vanished within. The door slammed."[38]

Soper was at a loss. In his experience people did not act like this; everything about this woman was foreign to him. After their first interaction, he put some of the blame on himself, admitting he needed to figure out ways to say the words more comprehensibly. But after the second time, when he followed her home, he put more of the onus on her. By the third encounter when he met her in the hospital he could hardly contain himself. He concluded that she "possessed a violent temper against which, when fully aroused, few persons had ever been willing to contend." She used her "weapon" against him three times, and during her incarceration threatened to use her temper more often to keep people at bay. Soper related, "Mary knew how to throw herself into a state of what Dr. John A. Cahill, Superintendent of Riverside Hospital, called 'almost pathological anger.' " As Soper told it, Mary was in the driver's seat, able to use her "personal weapon" at will.[39]

How do we interpret this description of Mary Mallon's behavior and temper? Was Soper venting his feelings about the Irish alongside his own frustration at not having events go the way he planned? Were his notions of womanly behavior so totally attacked by this woman that he could not himself respond rationally? Was it coldness and authoritarianism that characterized his reactions? Or was Mary Mallon really acting beyond the bounds of normal human response? Because of our distance and the limited documentation available, we will never be able to answer these questions fully. Nonetheless, it is clear that the feelings Mallon evoked in Soper were powerful, and his telling of their interactions was clearly filtered through the lens of his own frustration, bewilderment, and anger. He may be describing Mallon's temper, but we see his own anger at work in the process. His rational, considered, and socially acceptable notions of how people should behave were deeply challenged by this "stubborn" and "perverse" woman. He thought he approached her with "tact and judgment"; she responded with "indignant and peremptory denials" to his appeals.[40]

The most positive explanation Soper provided for why Mary Mallon behaved the way she did is that she did not understand her unfortunate condition. He blamed this on her refusal to talk with officials about the meaning of being a healthy carrier. Soper suggested, on the one hand, that she did not understand what it meant to be a healthy carrier, that she did not accept "the claims of science and humanity" and thus was "non-communicative." Health officials (including himself) should work harder to find ways to help her understand.[41] On the other hand, he wrote, "It is beyond belief that she has failed to grasp [the scientific facts'] significance."[42]

Soper grew harsher in his evaluation after Mallon was found cooking in 1915, following her three years of incarceration and five years after her release on the promise that she would not handle food. "She did this deliberately and in a hospital where the risk of detection and severe punishment were particularly great," Soper reflected. Her behavior argued "a mental attitude which is difficult to explain." But, Soper continued, "Aside from such behavior as this, Mary Mallon appears to be an unusually intelligent woman. She writes an excellent hand, and the composition of her letters leaves little room for criticism."[43] This is a striking juxtaposition. Soper brought up Mallon's handwriting at the height of his criticism about her behavior and her refusal to accept scientific expertise. He would not have expected that a woman of her class would have good penmanship. The fact that she did indicated she had some education, and she should therefore behave more reasonably. His expectations for her station in life were minimal, but they helped to define her deviance: "Most persons will agree that no amount of dullness, anywhere this side of downright feeble-mindedness, can excuse [her return to cooking], and Mary Mallon is not feeble, either in mind or body. She is an excellent cook and has shown considerable ability in various other ways."[44] If a person is smart enough to write a letter and cook a meal, Soper implies, she should be expected rationally to accept the authority of science.

The idea of intelligence repeatedly emerged in the literature about typhoid carriers, and Soper was not alone in concentrating on it. Only if carriers were considered intelligent could they be released to their homes, for on that basis rested public assurance that they would obey the rules. For example, public health official L. L. Lumsden wrote that "to require a strict isolation or quarantine of [carriers] as a class would be decidedly radical, almost as radical, in fact, as it would be to require the isolation of all cases of incipient pulmonary tuberculosis." Yet Lumsden believed that local officials should keep in quarantine "any typhoid bacillus carrier who will not take or who from lack of intelligence can not be expected to take the necessary precautions prescribed by the health officer."[45] For Lumsden and Soper, only "intelligent and conscientious" carriers could be trusted to take the necessary precautions.

By 1915, Soper threw up his hands and retreated. He acknowledged it was very hard to teach carriers of their dangers. "Mary had ample opportunity to know the danger which she constituted toward those whose food she prepared. . . . She knew that when she cooked she killed people, and yet she deliberately sought employment as a cook."[46] As if in response to Charles Chapin and his belief that typhoid carriers did not need to be locked up, Soper wrote, "To many persons who did not know Mary it seemed that she ought to be given her liberty." But, he believed, those who knew her best knew better than to let her go free. "Mysterious" and "noncommunicative," Mary Mallon was "a character apart, by nature and by circumstance," Soper concluded, "strangely chosen to bear the burden of a great lesson to the world."[47] To him, Mary Mallon's incarcerations were justified in the name of protecting the public from this woman who could not and would not act to protect herself.

S. Josephine Baker's descriptions of Mary Mallon and her detailed accounts of health department activities in the early years of the twentieth century provide another window on officials' attitudes toward the first healthy carrier to be traced by the health department. In her autobiography, Baker provided numerous examples of her attitudes and those of her fellow public health officials about issues that concern us here.[48] She shared the American-born, Protestant, middle-class views about immigrants in general and about the Irish specifically, and, despite her own unusual career choice, she held many traditional views of women's roles as well. When she was a child, her mother had taught her to cook because she believed all women should have this skill. Baker seemed to agree, although she did not enjoy or use the skill as an adult. Because of her training, not her experience, she boasted, "I feel quite confident that I could walk out into my own kitchen tomorrow and bake bread that would be a credit to our old Bridget."[49]

Baker's attitudes toward the Irish were on the whole condescending and negative, although she saw herself as compassionate. Baker was a professional woman who spent her career promoting progressive causes, including child welfare and women's rights. She, like Soper and other urban professionals of the period, worked to increase democratic reforms yet did so from a platform of elitist assumptions and perspectives. Her attitudes toward immigrants reflected this ambivalent progressive stance.[50] We might assume that she thought her own cook diligent and hardworking, but Baker described the Irish more often as "shiftless." After caring in her clinic for an Irish woman who had burned her feet while trying to keep them warm and dry in her oven, Baker decided the best word to describe her was "Numb— that seems to be the right word for all of them."[51]

When Baker began her work as a medical inspector for the health department, she worked in Hell's Kitchen, a neighborhood on the west side of Manhattan peopled at the time mainly by Irish and African Americans. She described her days:

The heat, the smells, the squalor made it something not to be believed. Its residents were largely Irish, incredibly shiftless, altogether charming in their abject helplessness, wholly lacking in any ambition and dirty to an unbelievable degree. . . . Both races lived well below any decent level of subsistence. . . . I climbed stair after stair, knocked on door after door, met drunk after drunk, filthy mother after filthy mother and dying baby after dying baby.[52]

She had chosen to spend her life improving conditions of the urban poor, and in so doing analyzed their poverty as largely situational, but she did not seem to respect the people among whom she toiled.

Baker's descriptions of Mary Mallon largely fit this pattern, although her personal connection led, at least in retrospect, to genuine sympathy. She had not been warned "that Dr. Soper had reasons to suspect that Mary might make trouble" when her supervisor, Walter Bensel, sent her to collect blood, stool, and urine specimens in March of 1907. Baker found Mary to be "a clean, neat, obviously self-respecting Irish-woman with a firm mouth and her hair done in a tight knot at the back of her head." With the exception of "firm mouth," the description was straightforward and positive. But the fact that Baker did find it necessary to note the clean and neat appearance suggests that she did not expect it, given Mary's Irish immigrant status and her occupation. The firm mouth notation indicates that Baker observed some physical evidence of resistance. She, like Soper, described her approach to Mallon as "using as much routine tact as possible," and her initial encounter yielded, again, a set jaw, glinting eyes, and a firm "No." Baker thought, "Obviously here was another case of that blind, panicky distrust of doctors and all their works which crops up so often among the uneducated." Baker did not regard

Mary Mallon as an individual but rather as someone representing a class, the uneducated, who behaved as Baker would expect, irrationally.[53]

Baker found herself in a difficult position. Unlike Soper, she was a department of health employee, and her superior officer instructed her to get the specimens or to bring the cook to the Willard Parker Hospital. Possibly Dr. Bensel had sent Baker thinking that a woman could approach Mallon more successfully than a man, and he expected results. But Mallon greeted Baker with the same kitchen fork she had used against Soper. The two women's worlds collided during the five-hour search for Mallon. The servants (many of whom themselves may have been Irish immigrants) helped Mary Mallon; the police helped S. Josephine Baker. It was, in some respects, a class war. Baker wrote, "The rest of the servants denied knowing anything about her or where she was; even in my distress, I liked that loyalty."[54]

Despite the show of what Baker termed "class solidarity," the physician's resources were greater and she got her woman. When Mallon emerged from her hiding place "fighting and swearing," Baker "made another effort to talk to her sensibly." But Mallon, after five hours in a dark corner contemplating her situation, "was convinced that the law was wantonly persecuting her, when she had done nothing wrong." Baker took the "maniacal" woman into the ambulance, and "literally sat on her all the way to the hospital; it was like being in a cage with an angry lion."[55]

This characterization of Mary Mallon, some of which I repeat from chapter 2, bears closer scrutiny here because it is so stark. The two women represented two opposing groups in America at that moment: educated, privileged, American-born, physician Baker, armed with science, public health expertise, and the police, against working-class, ill-educated, Irish immigrant Mallon, who eked out her living as a domestic servant. How could the two have comprehended each other? Mallon was confused and hostile in the face of Baker's direct onslaught; Baker on the other hand was afraid of possibly having to face Dr. Bensel without having accomplished her duty. The two women each experienced a certain lack of power within her own world; neither had much room for compromise.

Writing after Mallon's death, Baker confided, "I learned to like her and to respect her point of view." As one woman to another, Baker felt some compassion for Mallon. Yet despite the connection of gender, the gulf between these two women was enormous. Mallon evoked Baker's negative feelings about immigrants and the poor that she had voiced repeatedly. In forcing Mary Mallon into the Willard Parker Hospital, Baker was doing her job; she helped bring a public health menace under control. Baker's focus on Mallon's refusal "to listen to reason," on her temper, and on her inability to believe "all this mystery about germs" overtook her sympathy and dominated her perceptions. Believing as she did, she was able to carry out her duties.

Mary Mallon became, as historian Alan Kraut puts it, "synonymous with the health menace posed by the foreign-born."[56] Kraut includes the Mallon story in his account of America's long history of fear of contamination from abroad, a medicalized nativism that he traces from colonial times to the present. Certainly this attitude was present in Baker's anti-immigrant prejudices.

Anti-immigrant sentiment, widespread among health officials, might in this period have been aimed more often against southern and eastern Europeans than it was against the Irish, who, having emigrated earlier, already dominated much of New York's public and political life. Alan Kraut, too, found that by Mary Mallon's time, the Irish Catholics were "increasingly assimilated socially and dispersed geographically" and did not arouse as much open prejudice as did newer central European immigrant groups, and especially Asian and African groups whose physical appearance set them apart from native whites.[57] Nonetheless, Irish people like Mary Mallon, who were not well integrated into middle-class New York City life and did not meet American standards, still felt the stings of officials' disrespect.[58]

Perhaps if Mary Mallon had had a home to shelter her that authorities recognized as safe or a family to take care of her, she might have been released despite her initial refusal to cooperate with health department guidelines. Perhaps if she had been a housewife and not a domestic laborer, no matter how hot her temper, health authorities might have found reason to liberate her. Certainly Alphonse Cotils gained liberty, if we can read meaning into the judge's decision in his case, in part because he had some of these social options in his life: he could promise to carry out his business from his home on the telephone, for example. Perhaps if Mallon had not been Irish, with a stereotypical hot temper, she might have been coerced less. We can never know what would have happened if Mallon had been someone else, if the first healthy carrier followed so carefully in this country had been someone who, even if uncooperative, represented more "respectable" middle-class America. We can know that gender, class, and ethnic biases did much to shape official thinking about Mary Mallon.

Soper's and Baker's descriptions of Mary Mallon's appearance and behavior differed considerably from officials' descriptions of Alphonse Cotils, the Belgian-born New York baker who refused to cooperate with authorities, and of Tony Labella, the uncooperative typhoid carrier who escaped to New Jersey from the health department's surveillance during these years. Officials and the news reporters who covered the stories did not explicitly label these two male carriers in terms of sex, ethnicity, race, or personal habits. Whereas officials almost always referred to Mary Mallon as an "Irish woman," they did not put such identifiers on these two men. Nor did they once describe them as clean or neat, as if they did not expect them to be. Officials did not indicate anything about these carriers' education level or handwriting ability, or remark extensively on their appearance. They did not even write about how either of these men behaved when approached by health authorities. Apparently health officials did not deem the social signifiers necessary in these instances, even though they routinely used them to label and denigrate Mallon. Health officials indicated their own social biases when they omitted labels as much as when they used them.

Cotils and Labella were on the healthy carrier list because they had been found to carry the typhoid bacilli and because they were in the food handling business. Both did not cooperate with restrictions placed on them and continued to prepare food for others. I have already examined the case of Alphonse Cotils, who in 1924 received a suspended sentence from the New York municipal court judge who reviewed his case, and was back in his bakery the following year.[59] Labella needs some further discussion. He disappeared from New York health department view after causing an outbreak of typhoid affecting eighty-seven people and resulting in two deaths. New Jersey health authorities found him after tracing another outbreak to him, one that resulted in thirty-five cases of typhoid fever and three deaths. They isolated him for two weeks and then released him. Rather than incarcerating this healthy carrier for repeated violations and breaking parole when he returned to the city in 1922, the health officials in New York added him to the list of carriers and concluded the case with the remark, "This carrier is now employed in this City as a laborer in building construction work and is required to report to us weekly."[60]

By all public health measures, Labella was as dangerous to the health of others as was Mallon. In fact, he had already been identified with more typhoid fever cases and more deaths than Mallon. He had disobeyed the law in two states with repeated violations, certainly showing a lack of respect for science and refusal to cooperate with the law. Yet health officials continued to allow him his freedom to find construction work and live at liberty. One reading of Labella's story, which unfortunately cannot be followed more closely with extant documentation, is that as a male (even though possibly immigrant and Catholic) wage earner, he was viewed as a family breadwinner and necessary to the family economy. As recalcitrant as he was and as much a menace to the public health as he was proven to be, he was not locked up. Mary Mallon, in parallel circumstances, was denied her freedom and not retrained for a different job.[61]

The cases of Cotils and Labella evoked an official stance very different from the one in Mary Mallon's case; for these two men lifelong isolation was not considered a necessary response to the public health danger posed. The same was true for the Adirondack guide described in chapter 3. A case of a typhoid carrier who had infected ten employees at a New York hospital where he worked as a kitchen helper reveals another way in which health officials perceived Mary Mallon differently from others they identified and tracked. In this 1923 instance, health officials located the unnamed carrier, "a man who for twelve years had been an inmate of an institution for the care of mental cases." The man's duties included slicing bread, which provided ample opportunity for him to transmit typhoid bacilli from his hands to the food of others. The health commissioner, in releasing the information to the press, blamed the "laxity on the part of hospital authorities in the method of engaging employs who may handle their food supply." The carrier himself was released and added to the list of carriers under the observation of the health department.[62] Unfortunately, there is no extant discussion of this case, and we can only speculate about how and why health officials differentiated this man with his long-term history of mental problems from Mary Mallon. In Mallon's case, officials relied on descriptions of her antisocial behavior to help condemn her, yet evidently they did not consider this unnamed carrier's long history of mental health problems to be a factor necessitating his isolation.

Unfortunately the extant records do not permit a very complete search of the people other than Mary Mallon who, as healthy typhoid carriers, found themselves in health department isolation hospitals. One such carrier was Richard Voigt, who went to Riverside Hospital in early 1916 voluntarily seeking treatment for his condition. He was a fifty-six-year-old married man, who earned his living as a waiter in a restaurant. He was discovered to be a carrier after four stool samples tested positive in December, 1915, and he admitted himself to the hospital for therapy on January 10, 1916. He stayed for one month. We cannot follow him further.[63]

Two unnamed women voluntarily accepted hospitalization in the 1920s when health officials identified them as typhoid carriers. According to a news account mentioning them, they had "been in Riverside Hospital two years, but are not forcibly detained. They have no home and have elected to remain in the hospital" indefinitely. From the same source, we learn that an eighteen-year-old female carrier was hospitalized for treatment and released. Those few carriers who were hospitalized seem most often to have followed this pattern of brief hospitalization for observation and treatment and then release.[64]

The case of Frederick Moersch, about whom we can learn a little more, helps us understand that the social factors influencing Mary Mallon's case were not uniformly or predictably applied. Moersch, a German-born confectioner from Brooklyn, was identified as a carrier in 1915, following an outbreak of typhoid affecting fifty-nine people, traced to ice cream that he dispensed.[65] Moersch was not isolated for his role in the outbreak; he was, however, placed in Riverside Hospital following a later 1928 epidemic traced to him.[66]

Moersch was a married man, aged thirty-eight at the time of the 1915 outbreak; he then had four children. The health department described him as "well disposed and quite amenable," and entered him on the roster of carriers, releasing him with instructions to find work that did not involve food handling.[67] He apparently worked for a time as a mechanic's assistant and as a plumber. Beginning in June, 1915, the Brooklyn Bureau of Charities paid his rent.

What little information is available about Moersch indicates that health officials viewed his situation with sympathy and generosity. "The case of Fred Morsch [*sic*] is worthy of special[68] note," wrote G. L. Nicholas, chief of the division of epidemiology, to his director at the Bureau of Infectious Diseases in 1916. "His wife is not in good health and cannot help with earning money. They have four small children and a fifth child, born a few months ago, has since died." Significantly, Nicholas noted, "He is a skilled workman, and . . . he was suddenly excluded from work at his trade." Nicholas used the worthiness of Moersch's case to suggest that the department find ways to subsidize or find employment for needy carriers.[69] "It appears quite probable," agreed Bill Waters, the acting director of the Bureau of Infectious Diseases to the health commissioner, "that this Department will have to provide, through some source, for the maintenance of those dependent upon such persons as are prevented by us from continuing their usual occupation."[70] Moersch was discovered the same year as Mary Mallon's second incarceration, but health officials thought more sympathetically about his case and treated him much more leniently.

In March, 1916, the health department approved Moersch for innovative medical treatment (which they also gave to Mary Mallon) to try to alleviate his carrier state, but unfortunately we cannot follow his course in the extant records. He may have been hospitalized briefly for this treatment.[71] Health officials were convinced in 1916 that Moersch "made no attempt to work at his trade in secret," and were pleased to note that he did find work as a plumber. The health department did not isolate him and continued to list him as a carrier living at his Brooklyn home.[72]

In 1928, when he was out of work, Moersch returned to the confectionery business, this time in partnership with his daughters. Authorities traced as many as sixty cases of typhoid and a few deaths to him when they found him dispensing ice cream on Bleeker Street in Greenwich Village, Manhattan, in October, 1928.[73] Knowing Moersch had a history of typhoid transmission and had been informed of his status as a healthy carrier, the health commissioner sent him to Riverside Hospital. The health official promised to protect the public from this health menace, telling the press: "His isolation will now be made permanent."[74] Another department spokesperson, Dr. Edward L. Creedon, head of the division of communicable diseases, hedged on this promise, telling the press only that Moersch "would be kept [at Riverside Hospital] for prolonged observation."[75]

It seems that Moersch did, in fact, spend many years on North Brother Island, but the records do not reveal whether he was kept voluntarily or forcibly.[76] Emma Sherman, who ran the bacteriology laboratory on North Brother Island beginning in 1929 and who worked with Mary Mallon in that laboratory, insists that Mallon was the only healthy typhoid carrier on the island.[77] The fact that Sherman did not know about Fred Moersch suggests that his presence during those years was significantly more private than was Mallon's. There are a few possible explanations for this: it might have been a voluntary detention, or Moersch's identity might have been known only as a hospital worker, or the passage of time might have made his case seem more ordinary and therefore less memorable. Officials issued few public statements about Moersch, and they did not write about him in their own publications or private writings. This itself seems to indicate that they distinguished between Moersch and Mallon.[78]

Officials distinguished between the two healthy carriers in another important respect. Not only did they not isolate Moersch in 1915, after he had infected more people than Mallon, and instead sympathetically helped him find financial aid, but they also provided him with work shortly after taking him to North Brother Island. The city employed Moersch as a "hospital helper" at Riverside Hospital fifteen months after they brought him there, presumably when they decided his carrier state was intractable. He retained that job until he moved off the island and returned to his Brooklyn home, sometime in 1944. The fact that Moersch was able to leave North Brother Island may mean that he had stayed there as a voluntary employee, a very different status from Mallon's. He remained on the city payroll, with a job at Kingston Avenue Hospital in Brooklyn (giving a home address in Brooklyn), until his death.[79]

Differences in the treatment of Mallon and Moersch by officials cast doubt on any notion that health officials based their decisions about healthy carriers solely on scientific or objective criteria. Clearly, socially constructed views of the two carriers intruded into decisions made about them. The factors that most strongly labeled Mary Mallon and stigmatized her, which officials used repeatedly in their descriptions, were based on views of appropriate gender roles and influenced strongly by prejudices about class and ethnicity. Officials repeatedly used identifiers that connoted stigma and deviance in Mallon's case when they did not do so when referring to other carriers, including Moersch and Tony Labella, whose specific and documented dangers to the public were larger than her own.

It is reasonable to conclude, as Clarence Darrow observed in a different carrier case in Chicago, that the vagueness of the quarantine laws permitted health officials to "discriminate between individuals":

They may permit one carrier complete liberty to go about in his usual manner, transacting his ordinary business, while another may be confined under the strictest quarantine. Or one may be allowed his freedom upon merely giving his word that he would sterilize his discharges and another denied that privilege. . . . At present the Board [of health] assumes the right to arbitrarily discriminate between persons of the same class.[80]

Clearly, there were no strict rules to determine which carriers health officials should isolate, and officials had considerable latitude to decide who would receive the strongest application of the possible regulations.[81]

The definition of the danger Mary Mallon posed was not limited to bacteria counts; it extended to include the social context within which typhoid itself was most often transmitted. The social views of health officials—conscious and unconscious—were potent. They could help determine whether a particular healthy carrier would go free under health department observation or whether a carrier would be isolated. All healthy carriers could potentially endanger the public's health, but only a select few individuals were singled out to pay the price of their freedom in the name of protecting the public health. Expectations and prejudices about Mary Mallon's social position—her Irish immigrant status, her job as a domestic servant, her femaleness—all contributed to defining her as dangerous in the eyes of those who pursued her.

"This
Human
Culture
Tube"

Media and the

Cultural Construction

of "Typhoid Mary"

CHAPTER FIVE

*H*ealth officials labeled Mary Mal-
lon a social undesirable and helped to build a case against her by
setting her up as an example of how carriers should not act. Creating an image of an unnatural woman became an important
part of the case—social stereotyping in the service of protecting
the people's health. But the health department was not alone in
developing a negative connotation to the term *Typhoid Mary*. In
this chapter, I explore the ways in which the media's portrayals of
Mallon even more strongly shaped and reflected public opinion
about healthy carriers, first to challenge and then to reinforce the
health department's representation of Typhoid Mary as a social
pariah. The public viewpoints about Mary Mallon, however, insofar as they are recoverable and reflected in published writing,
retained an emotional connection to the human misfortune represented in her story. Early accounts foregrounded sympathy for
the woman caught by circumstance. The media later combined
this sympathy with a stronger story of the public health menace
she represented to construct a lasting negative imprint. Especially
around the time of her reappearance in 1915, the media, in blaming Mary Mallon for her return to cooking, capped and gave

permanence to this singularly negative construction of *Typhoid Mary.*

The obvious place to begin to explore the construction of cultural meanings of Mary Mallon's story is with the words *Typhoid Mary* themselves which have become a metaphor for a dangerous person who should be reviled and avoided. While the press helped the term gain national notoriety—keeping it alive and in use throughout Mallon's life—reporters did not invent it. As far as I can determine, a national public health expert first publicly used the term in a medical setting. The scene was a joint meeting of the Section on the Practice of Medicine and the Section on Pathology and Physiology at the American Medical Association Annual Meeting in Chicago in June, 1908. William Hallock Park, the head of New York City's bacteriology laboratory, presented a paper on typhoid bacilli carriers in which he related the first sixteen months' experience with "a cook" found to be a healthy typhoid carrier. Park did not name Mary Mallon, nor did he use any descriptor to identify her except for "cook" and "woman." Park was not present at the discussion of his paper, and his colleague Milton J. Rosenau of Washington, D.C., responded to a comment by a physician from Tennessee who suggested that carriers undergo a surgical operation to cure their condition: "I can not take Dr. Park's place," said Rosenau, "but [I] feel sure that if he were here he would say that 'typhoid Mary' refuses to submit to surgical interference."[1]

This first public use of the term appeared in print when Park's paper was published in the *Journal of the American Medical Association* on September 19, 1908. Using the small "t," the editor emphasized the descriptive nature of the term. In the same year biologist George Whipple published a textbook about typhoid fever, and in it he reported on the new phenomenon of healthy typhoid carriers. "One of the best known," carriers, he wrote, is " 'Typhoid Mary,' a cook in New York City, who . . . left a trail of at least twenty-eight [*sic*] cases in the houses where she had served." Whipple's almost casual use of the phrase seems to indicate it had already become common parlance in the medical community.[2]

It is possible that neither Rosenau nor Whipple knew Mary Mallon's name in 1908. They may have used the term merely out of convenience; we should not assume that *Typhoid Mary*, now pejorative, carried a negative connotation when it was first coined. During the period before Mary Mallon's real identity was publicly known—before June 20, 1909—anyone needing to refer to the New York City carrier may have used the term to describe and yet protect the identity of the real person.

Typhoid Mary was not the first substitution for Mary Mallon's name to appear in print. Reporters learning about Mallon's arrest in 1907 (two years before her habeas corpus hearing when her name became known) did not use the phrase. They used the pseudonym "Mary Ilverson"—either a name they made up or one the health officials themselves had used as a cover to reporters. The name did not have a very long life, however, and it never developed the cultural significance associated with *Typhoid Mary*.

On March 13, 1907, William Randolph Hearst's *New York American* reported the new medical discovery of healthy carriers of typhoid fever. In a story called "Germs of Typhoid Carried for Life," a reporter discussed a New York Academy of Medicine meeting at which Charles Harrington of the Massachusetts State Board of Health presented a paper on these carriers, who he said represented about 4 percent of recovering typhoid fever patients.[3] The newspaper did not know that Soper was then on the trail of New York's own healthy carrier, who would be apprehended less than a week later.

But reporters soon learned of Mary Mallon's capture, and on April 2, about two weeks after her arrest, the *American* revealed the "Human Typhoid Germ" held in the city's hospital. "Presence kept a Secret," the newspaper screamed. "A case hedged about with more safeguards against publicity and attended by more mysterious circumstances than any which has been recorded," the reporter wrote, congratulating himself for breaking the Board of Health's publicity barrier and discovering that " 'Mary Ilverson,' a cook, has been a prisoner in the institution for some time."[4]

"The startling fact was revealed," boasted the reporter, "that this woman . . . has caused thirty-eight [*sic*] persons for whom she worked to contract typhoid fever. It was also disclosed that she is practically a human vehicle for typhoid fever germs." There was more:

It was admitted to an *American* reporter last night by a well-known member of the Board of Health that this human culture tube has worked for prominent families in this city and communicated the disease to some of its members. . . . "Mary" is an Irish girl. . . . she constantly makes attempts to escape. . . . "Mary" is rosy of cheek and buxom of form. Her spirits are always at concert pitch, and the only thing in life that worries her is the restraint.

The reporter went on to quote Walter Bensel (S. Josephine Baker's superior officer) as saying, "This woman is a great menace to health, a danger to the community, and she has been made a prisoner on that account. In her wake are many cases of typhoid fever," which she caused when she "unwittingly disseminated—or, as we might say, sprinkled—germs in various households."[5]

Here was a story worth breaking, but it was not followed in the press. As far as I have been able to learn, only one other newspaper ran the story. Joseph Pulitzer's *New York World*—the *American*'s biggest rival—wrote about Mary Ilverson, using no quotation marks. Reporters in that newspaper depicted a "walking typhoid fever factory," but also "a buxom woman, a cook, in perfect health."[6] Nothing more followed in either newspaper, indicating perhaps that health officials successfully reimposed a veil of secrecy.

In this first public telling, the description of "Mary Ilverson" revealed attitudes that later reemerged attached to "Typhoid Mary." The language of the 1907 reports began a process of dehumanizing Mary Mallon. She became a "germ," "vehicle," "factory," and "culture tube." In articulating the connection between "typhoid carrier" and "menace," the articles indicated an acceptance of Mary Mallon as "prisoner." They reported that she, a cook, had infected members of "prominent" families, suggesting she was a threat not only to public health but to social hierarchy as well. Yet, even though much in these early accounts reduced Mary Mallon to a social evil, they still evoked some sympathy for her. She had acted "unwittingly" and "unconsciously," they reported, and they remarked on her Irish heritage in a fairly positive, if patronizing, manner.

The health department might have chosen to turn the *American*'s and *World*'s revelations of Mary Mallon's capture into a lesson for public education. Health officials had come to understand that they needed social as well as medical arguments to help shape public opinion and discourse about healthy carriers. The articles and quotations from officials created an image of a social undesirable, a frightening and dangerous person, which officials could have used directly to educate the public about this new danger to their health. In 1907, however, New York health officials did not yet themselves understand the full dimensions of the situation they had on their hands, and they did not consider turning the media interest to public use. They were more interested in keeping the story to themselves while they figured out how to handle it. The suppression of news about Mary Mallon's detention indicates the health department retained control of information dissemination.

But in 1909, when the popular media and the medical press no longer needed a pseudonym like Mary Ilverson for a woman whose real identity was finally publicly known because of her habeas corpus hearing, the health officials could no longer contain public interest. The public, cultural construction of Mary Mallon's story and of "Typhoid Mary," separate from the woman and from official definition, began to emerge. It was not until 1915, upon Mary Mallon's second incarceration, that it took full form.

Media scholars now recognize the extent to which news reports are not merely accounts of what happened, but stories "with characters, action, plot, point of view, dramatic closure."[7] The dramatic qualities of news reporting are possibly no better exemplified than in William Randolph Hearst's newspapers at the turn of the century, and the telling of Mary Mallon's story epitomizes the genre.

Hearst believed daily newspapers should grab their readers' attention with bold statements and dramatic stories. His biographer wrote of him that any story "that did not cause its reader to rise out of his chair and cry, 'Great God!' was counted a failure." Hearst worked to "convulse his readers with excitement," and in the process helped to change the standards of American journalism. In the 1890s, Hearst set out to compete with New York's highest circulation daily, Joseph Pulitzer's *New York World*. As a young reporter, he had worked for Pulitzer and learned his technique of mixing sensationalism with democratic idealism. Now, with his *Morning Journal*, which changed its name to the *New York American* in 1901, Hearst proved himself the master of the new journalism. He shamelessly courted readers with crime and scandal stories alongside some anti-establishment rhetoric and support for public reforms. In the words of his biographer,

In the strict sense, the Hearst papers were not newspapers at all. They were printed entertainment and excitement—the equivalent in newsprint of bombs exploding, bands blaring, firecrackers popping, victims screaming, flags waving, cannons roaring, houris dancing, and smoke rising from the singed flesh of executed criminals.[8]

The June 20, 1909, story in the *American* that identified Mary Mallon for the first time for the American public was a masterful example of Hearst's brand of journalism. The layout design alone told a story of death and disease certain to alarm any reader. Framing the two-page spread and dominating its announcement of a new public health danger was a full-page drawing of a buxom cook, a woman breaking human skulls like eggs into a skillet (see fig. 5.1). Here was an aproned woman, hair carefully coiffed, arched eyebrows: an ordinary woman. But look closer. Her mouth is set, she has a double chin. The shading indicates—perhaps—a degree of masculine hairiness on her face and arms. Her ordinary occupation of cooking is perverted by the clear reference to the demonic. This hairy, heavy-set, determined woman is one who rolls up her sleeves to cook humans: a killer. Mary Mallon is transformed into Typhoid Mary: a real woman made into a caricature.

The picture is more powerful than the text that accompanies it. Certainly the image is hard to dispel, even today, and just like today its contemporary viewers kept this image before them and referred back to it repeatedly. The characterization of Mary Mallon as inhuman, a devil in the shape of a woman, was powerful. It made people uneasy: who would want to eat in her kitchen? Mary Mallon, an immigrant woman domestic, has turned the ordinary task of cooking into a death-producing act.

The *American*'s readers faced this headline on opening the Sunday magazine section: " 'Typhoid Mary' Most Harmless and Yet the Most Dangerous Woman in America." The paradox in the headline captured Mallon's situation. Its bold use of the phrase *Typhoid Mary* set the person Mary Mallon apart from the new public health concept she represented. The reporter noted that "she has committed no crime, has never been accused of an immoral or wicked act, and has never been a prisoner in any court, nor has she been sentenced to imprisonment by any judge." Yet, he concluded, "It is probable that Mary Mallon is a prisoner for life."[9]

From the time this article was first published to the present

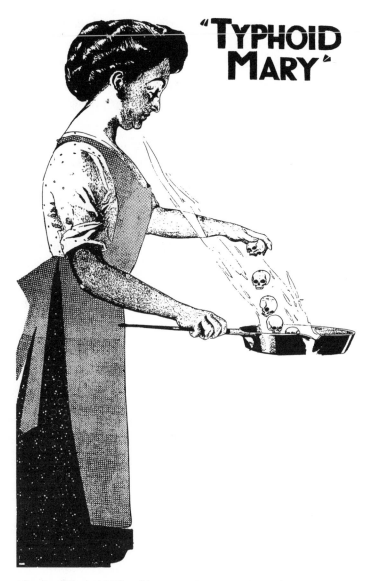

Fig. 5.1. *"Typhoid Mary" breaking skulls into skillet, 1909.*

day, it is possible to see two distinct parts to Mary Mallon's story: the woman, who was caught in a dilemma over which she had little control, and the symbol, which represented meanings imposed on her story that changed over time and reached far beyond her specific case. Our present-day use of the epithet *Typhoid Mary*, instead of the name Mary Mallon, not only in discussions of public health problems but also in our general language, is clear evidence of how potent the term is. The woman herself has receded in historical memory.

The language of the June 20, 1909, *American* news report evoked sympathy, as its author no doubt intended. Here was a woman who could not help herself, who could not stop being dangerous; she was doomed to sit "forever" in her island prison. "Through no fault of hers, Mary Mallon is a living, walking incubator of typhoid fever germs." The reporter revealed about Mallon herself that "she has served in the kitchens of many New York millionaires with entire satisfaction for many years."

The sympathetic report about Mary Mallon's "extraordinary predicament" accompanied a short statement by William Park revealing that the New York carrier was one among fifty healthy typhoid carriers so far discovered in the country. Park stated that Mallon was "remarkable" among all carriers because of the large number of cases associated with her, by which he may have meant that Soper's tracing of her typhoid-transmitting history was the most complete. Like other health officials, the bacteriologist described Mary Mallon as "a large, healthy looking woman, a typical cook, and there is nothing in her outward appearance to indicate that she is other than normal." Park also told the press, curiously (since it was not the case), that "she is, of course, segregated with the typhoid patients." North Brother Island sheltered tuberculosis sufferers, and department reports indicated no typhoid patients there at all. Park probably intended to reassure the public that health authorities had the situation well under control.

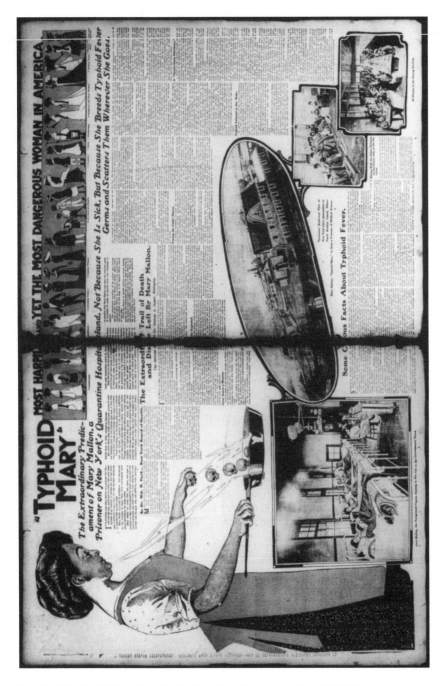

Fig. 5.2. *"Typhoid Mary" article in* New York American, *June 20, 1909.*

Park's statement, the reporter's coverage, the third section of the article (a reprint of George Soper's 1907 paper describing his tracing of Mallon's employment and carrier history), and the final section, a description of some "curious facts" about typhoid fever, all presented with sympathy the dilemma of a healthy person locked up possibly for life, but nowhere is much attention paid to the individual involved. We learn surprisingly little about Mary Mallon herself in these pages.

Whatever sympathy the story might have evoked for Mary Mallon was counter-balanced by the combined effect of the illustrations and photographs that framed it (see fig. 5.2). Readers confronted not only the large drawing of the demonic cook but also silhouettes of her victims marching silently across the top of the two-page spread: "4 Laundresses, [3 Grounds]keepers, 1 Gentleman Visitor, 3 Society Women, 6 of a Lawyer's Family, 1 Footman, 1 Nurse, 1 Workwoman, 2 Daughters and Their Mother, 1 Trained Nurse, 1 Parlor Maid, 1 Negro Servant Girl." The grouping served as a warning: all sorts of people were at risk from people like Mary Mallon.

Four photographs also accompanied the story, scattered across the two-page spread. One shows Mary Mallon in bed, "resting in her cot" at Willard Parker Hospital (see chap. 4, fig. 4.2) looking vulnerable and alone even though her bed is in a ward full of other patients and staff. The reader saw a young woman the newspaper story said was healthy, prone, in a room full of sick people. The second is a photograph of buildings on North Brother Island, among which the mind's eye could envision a lonely Mary wandering. The caption to this "panoramic bird's-eye view" of the island says it is where Mary Mallon is "held a prisoner of medical science" (see fig. 5.3). The third photograph shows a group of patients sitting in the sun outside one of the island's buildings, one of whom is said to be Mary Mallon (see fig. 5.4). Apparently the *American* saw no problem in publishing this photograph even though the story describes Mary as living alone on

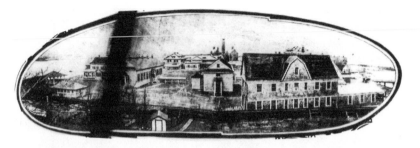

Fig. 5.3. *"Panoramic Bird's-eye View of ... North Brother Island."*

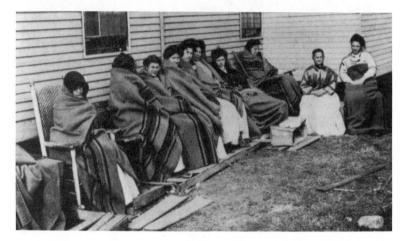

Fig. 5.4. *Group of patients on North Brother Island; Mary Mallon is probably fourth from the right, but she could be the woman with her back to the camera.*

the island and as a prisoner. The fourth photograph shows "dinner in the dining pavilion," again implying that Mallon ate with others in a common dining room, although later reports insist Mary always ate alone in her own bungalow (see fig. 5.5). Readers could come away from the story wondering how a healthy woman in the prime of life could survive this daily regimen designed for sick patients, possibly for the rest of her life. But this article would give them no cause to question the medical science that held Mary captive or to wonder if her imprisonment were necessary. It was simply sad.[10]

The *American*'s June 20 story made one very telling point,

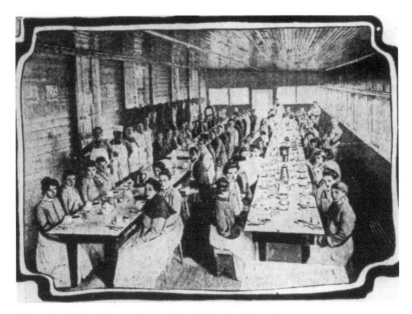

Fig. 5.5. *Patient Dining Room, North Brother Island.*

which must not have eluded Mallon herself. Referring to the other contagious disease patients on the island, the reporter wrote, "While Mary sees these unfortunate victims of various diseases come on the hospital boat and, in due time, return to their homes and friends—Mary stays on forever." Isolation on the island when one was sick and expected to recover in time was difficult; but the reporter wanted his readers to ponder something much more devastating: life-long isolation when one was healthy.

All New York newspapers picked up the story of Mary Mallon and her lawyer George Francis O'Neill who in June of 1909 were in court seeking her release from her isolation on North Brother Island. The *American*, ten days after first scooping the story of her isolation, again offered the most drama when it covered the habeas corpus hearing. "Why Should I Be Banished Like a Leper?" ran a three-column header on page one on June 30. The analogy to people infected with leprosy was itself very powerful. Three illustrations accompanied the article, all of which depicted a more appealing woman than the cook breaking skulls into the frying pan. The shift might indicate the *American* was responding to a sympathetic public and making an intentional play for readership. It completely challenged the health department view of Mallon as a social "menace," the view department officials presented during the court hearings.

In these *American* renditions, and in the accompanying text, Mary Mallon became more a victim than an aggressor. A portrait of her dominates the page, a drawing which seems to be taken from a photograph. In it, a serious but attractive young woman, whose hairdo and dress fit the fashion of the day, gazes directly from the page (fig. 5.6). She does not look like a woman who could be guilty of bringing death to others by her cooking. If it were not for the accompanying text, we might take her for the daughter of a prominent New Yorker, perhaps on her way to a party.

Two cartoon-like drawings are set directly under the portrait. The one on the left, a cook preparing a deadly stew, intrudes onto the formal portrait with—again—skulls steaming out of the cooking pot. But this drawing, despite its depiction of death, is milder than its predecessor. The skulls float from the pot on their own; in the previous version, the cook dropped them into the skillet. In this picture, too, the cook is more feminine, even a bit jaunty, thinner, more at ease. Her face, although not drawn in detail, is innocent. If she is cooking up destruction, she does not seem to be aware of it. The caption reads, "Worked as a cook and was supposed to have spread typhoid germs." *Supposed to have*: the text follows the illustrator and is not sure of her guilt.

The injustice of the situation and Mallon's innocence in the artist's eyes is further portrayed in the right-hand drawing under the portrait. Here Mary Mallon is being dragged into an ambulance by four men. She is giving them a hard time; on her face is her hurt and her outrage. But her lack of cooperation is sympathetically shown—she is not a devil who needs to be seized, but

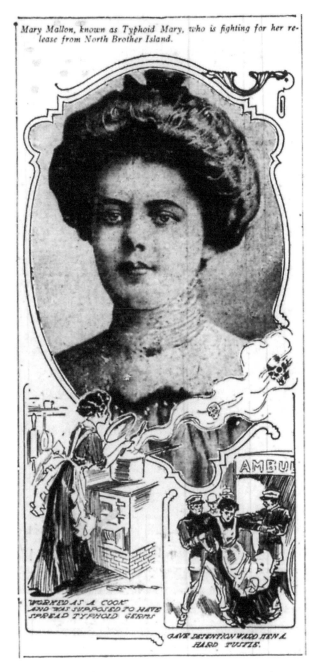

Mary Mallon, known as Typhoid Mary, who is fighting for her release from North Brother Island.

WORKED AS A COOK AND WAS SUPPOSED TO HAVE SPREAD TYPHOID GERMS.

GAVE DETENTION WARD MEN A HARD TUSSLE.

Fig. 5.6 *Mary Mallon portrait with two accompanying cartoons, 1909.*

rather a woman, still in her apron, who may not deserve to go. The two officers' faces are not gentle or kind. They are not monsters, either, but they are doing their job with a certain lack of sympathy. The bowler-hatted health officer behind them (even though Mary Mallon was taken by a woman health officer) is solemn; her arrest is serious business. There are no demons in this tripartite grouping; but there is a heroine with whom viewers can identify and sympathize. The newspaper's illustrator emphasized the human aspects of the story that connected Mary Mallon to the newspaper's readers.

American reporters interviewed Mallon on her way to the New York Supreme Court hearing and presented to their one million morning and evening readers a human interest portrayal of the woman, who, "Never Ill, Begs Freedom."[11] The story focused on the sad facts of a woman about to turn forty whose life was ruined through no fault of her own. "No stranger who saw Mary Mallon yesterday," the reporter wrote, "would have suspected the danger the Health Board alleges it finds in this young woman. She has a clear, healthy complexion, regular features, bright eyes and white teeth." The news reporter treated health officials with some skepticism here, which had not been the case ten days earlier, when, possibly, the newness of the revelations brought more respect to the medical side of the story. The reporter went on, in questioning Mary Mallon's situation, to notice, "Strangely enough, the Island is now a retreat for only tuberculosis patients." The text questioned both whether Mallon really carried the germs attributed to her and the wisdom of putting her in an institution catering to another disease.

During the early twentieth century, the press generally covered new advances in medicine and science in a positive and sympathetic way. Samuel Hopkins Adams in *McClure's* (as Paul De Kruif later on) helped spread promising news of scientific triumphs, and, as historian Terra Ziporyn has shown, newspapers and journals around the country increased coverage when new vaccines were developed or other breakthroughs occurred.[12] The Hearst newspapers capitalized on the public's interest in science but also, still in the cause of capturing readers' attention, emphasized the human and emotional aspects of their stories. The Typhoid Mary story was intriguing both because it exemplified the latest scientific discoveries and at the same time it allowed reporters to write about an individual caught by circumstance.

After the judge ruled that Mary Mallon had to return to North Brother Island, the *World*, too, carried an emotional and sympathetic story. " 'I'm Persecuted!' Is Plaintive Plea of 'Typhoid Mary,' " ran the headline to an article about a "stout, jovial cook who was loved by the children in every family in which she was employed." The reporter quoted Mary Mallon: "As there is a God in Heaven, I will get justice, somehow, sometime," she insisted. " 'Typhoid Mary,' " the newspaper wrote, "as the Health Department has christened her, is a large, fairhaired woman of forty. Her face indicates character." The reporter distanced himself from the negative meaning implied by his use of the term Typhoid Mary by blaming that on the health department, and he portrayed Mallon as a woman caught in a situation beyond her control.[13]

Although they acknowledged the health officials' claims that Mary Mallon transmitted typhoid fever to people for whom she cooked, the newspapers filled space with sympathetic human interest about the woman herself. Such personal appeal peaked with the *American*'s story of Mallon's marriage proposal from a Michigan farmer, Reuben Gray, quoted in a letter to the health department: "If Miss Mallon is not over ten years older [than his 28] and has nothing other than what you have found to bar her from the society of the world, and you will pardon her and get her into Michigan and see that the authorities of Michigan are not wise that she is here, and she will agree to become my wife, I will agree to become her husband." But, Gray warned, "One thing she should be made aware of before the tie is bound and that is that I have (the 'have' is underscored three times) been insane, but it was over three years ago, and I was pronounced cured then and never had a return of the disease." Apparently some Michigan neighbors or the health department dissented, and nothing further came of the proposal.[14]

Other New York newspapers, less sensationalist or with smaller circulations than the *American* or the *World*, also became interested in the Mary Mallon saga. The *New York Tribune* carried the story about the "unfortunate woman" only after the judge remanded her back to the island.[15] The *New York Times* editorialized that her stigma and notoriety would follow her until "her unique propensity is dispelled" through medical treatment, indicating considerable faith in science to be able to cure her.[16] The *Evening Sun* limited itself to reporting the events in court, except when describing Mary Mallon: "She was the picture of a healthy and well-fed cook. She is about 40 years old, with a mass of light-colored hair, florid complexion, and weighs about 200 pounds." This physical portrayal echoes what became the standard view of Mallon's bodily proportions, although, again, such size is not reflected in her photograph.[17]

The *New York Herald* repeated the story available in all the other newspapers. However, its reporters described a smaller Mallon as "about forty years old, weighs perhaps 160 pounds and is medium in stature. Her cheeks were slightly colored and her blue eyes seemed clear and sparkling."[18] The socialist *New York Call* portrayed the story as a "fight for freedom," but did not add any new dimensions in its descriptions.[19]

One significant discrepancy emerged in the various June and July, 1909, news stories about Mary Mallon. The *American* presented a rendition of Mallon living alone on North Brother Island, seeing virtually no one, and having only "a dog for a companion," which was repeated in all newspapers except the *World*. That newspaper conducted its own interview with the cook and came away with a more social version of her life on the island. Pulitzer's

World, then with a daily circulation over 700,000 and a Sunday readership numbering almost 450,000, insisted Mary Mallon mingled freely with patients and staff. "Mary Mallon is permitted the freedom of the island," the reporter wrote, "and the doctors are glad to have her nurse the children who are there with every kind of contagious disease."[20] These different versions of Mary Mallon's North Brother Island life will be explored in the next chapter; for the moment, we can see that both images served to evoke public sympathy for Mary Mallon's personal story.

The sympathy voiced in the press in 1909 seemed to portray public sentiment at the same time as it worked to shape it. Mary Mallon was a woman caught by circumstances, not a woman to blame. The news stories revealed a certain ambivalence toward her, as the illustration of the cook breaking skulls in the skillet suggests, but any negative view that the health officials may have wished to promote did not capture the public imagination at the time of the habeas corpus hearings, insofar as we can judge it from the popular press. Although health officials believed Mallon a sufficient threat to the public's health to hold her in isolation on North Brother Island, they did not successfully communicate to the public how dangerous they believed Mallon was. To the news readers, the human misfortune spoke louder than the potential danger, perhaps in part because the public still had trouble understanding the concept of a healthy person transmitting disease through invisible organisms lodged in the gallbladder.

The divergence between sympathetic public opinion and the health department's portrayal of a menacing healthy carrier in 1909 may have prevented the officials, once they secured Mallon back on the island following the habeas corpus hearing, from launching a visible campaign to protect the public from the danger carriers posed. Knowing that carriers lived throughout the city and that many of them prepared food for others, officials could have used the opportunity of overcoming the legal challenge in court to launch a widescale attack on the problem. Instead, perhaps in response to the loud sympathy for Mallon voiced in the press, they remained silent.

Health Commissioner Lederle himself may have been affected by the public sympathy toward Mallon's situation when he decided to release her from North Brother Island in February, 1910. Interestingly, this action evoked only a little press attention. Those newspapers that carried the story seemed to support release from "the torture of solitary confinement" for the unfortunate woman.[21] The *New York Times* agreed with the health commissioner that she had paid long enough for her situation, especially given that "there might be other persons quite as dangerous to their neighbors as 'Typhoid Mary,'" and that "she should [not] be any longer singled out for confinement."[22] The media consensus was that Mary Mallon deserved help, not isolation.

The *Times* mentioned in this story that there were possibly large numbers of typhoid carriers. Newspapers had barely noticed this fact in the reports they published during Mary Mallon's habeas corpus hearing in 1909, but the information made more of an impact elsewhere. Medical writers especially emphasized that Mary Mallon had a lot of company in her condition as a healthy carrier. For example, the *Boston Medical and Surgical Journal* wrote: "There is reason to believe that there are other persons now at large who may be quite as dangerous to the community as regards the spread of typhoid as this woman," continuing, "and this was one reason why it was thought that she should no longer be singled out for confinement."[23] Health authorities and lay observers around the country agreed that Mary Mallon was one of many—perhaps tens of thousands—healthy typhoid carriers in the country. "The young woman is not a scientific wonder . . . in spite of the sensation she creates in the newspaper," wrote one author. "Individuals who are chronic spreaders of typhoid fever are not rarities at all."[24]

Despite clear medical unanimity on this point, Mary Mallon

remained the best known among typhoid carriers, and many people continued to think she was "unique in the annals of medical history," as the *American* put it.[25] Maintaining this singular view of Mary Mallon (especially when opinion about her turned in a decidedly negative direction in 1915) helped promote public interest in her story and sold newspapers. The emphasis on her uniqueness represents one way in which media perspectives differed from other points of view and indicates how the press helped to shape events. In the popular portrayals of her uniqueness we can begin to understand the particular burden she carried and why her story resonated so strongly in the public's perceptions.

A novel published in 1910, the year Mary Mallon was released, offers a different but revealing popular representation of her story.[26] Arthur Reeve, who had made a name for himself as a columnist for *The Survey*, a magazine of social work and reform, wrote his first fiction to promote the use of science to solve crimes. His hero was chemist Craig Kennedy (an American Sherlock Holmes), who, aided by his sidekick, old college chum and reporter Walter Jameson (Dr. Watson), solves society's crimes by using the most up-to-date scientific methods.[27] Kennedy wants to run "the criminal himself down, scientifically, relentlessly." He tells his friend, "I am going to apply science to the detection of crime, the same sort of methods by which you trace out the presence of a chemical, or run an unknown germ to earth." In a series of episodes, erudite and suave Kennedy does just that.

One of his first challenges involves investigating the death of oil magnate Jim Bisbee at the request of Bisbee's ward, the beautiful Eveline. The rich man had died from typhoid fever, and around him servants similarly fell prey to the disease. Eveline suspects foul play, and, fearing for her own life, consults the modern science sleuth. Kennedy proves her suspicions correct using the latest bacteriological, fingerprinting, and handwriting analyses. Kennedy's efforts demonstrate that Bisbee's lawyer, and heir under his latest will (to be revealed as a forgery), had hired Bridget Fallon (notice only one letter and a substitution of a different popular Irish name separates her from Mary Mallon), referred to as "Typhoid Bridget," to cook for the old man, knowing she was a carrier. The lawyer carefully immunized himself before dining with Bisbee. (This is a very advanced use of typhoid immunization, since the procedure was adopted by the military in 1911 and in public use only after that: Reeve had done his homework.) Reeve does not present the cook in a positive light. While she claims her innocence, she is characterized as a drunk and an abusive person. She is nonetheless not a villain but instead the pawn of a villain; she is an instrument of someone else's evil. This perspective on Mary Mallon's story adds a new dimension to the range of public thinking about her meaning. A carrier was someone to be feared, someone to sympathize with, someone dangerous to others, and now someone whose dangers might be manipulated for specific gain or malice.

Another early literary rendition of Typhoid Mary is a satiric poem, "The Germ-Carrier," written by "O. S.," and published in the British humor magazine *Punch*.[28]

> *In U.S.A. (across the brook)*
> *There lives, unless the papers err,*
> *A very curious Irish cook*
> *In whom the strangest things occur:*
> *Beneath her outside's healthy gloze*
> *Masses of microbes seethe and wallow*
> *And everywhere that MARY goes*
> *Infernal epidemics follow.*

The poem recounts the story of her cooking for unsuspecting families, who "bite the dust" in her wake, while she, after two years of life in isolation, "is just as germy as the day / On which she went in quarantine." O. S., perhaps with typical British sensibility toward those whom he considers the inferior Irish, seems to approve her ultimate fate of lifelong quarantine and concludes the poem wishing similar treatment of the germ carrier's political analogue (to the poet's mind), Chancellor of the Exchequer Lloyd George.

> *And yet she's not the only one*
> *That flings destruction far and wide,*
> *And still contrives somehow to shun*
> *The horrid poison housed inside.*

O. S. draws the analogy to the liberal member of parliament whose government had recently raised taxes on wealthy Britons with his "People's Budget." The poet writes,

> *Yet where he goes the microbes spread;*
> *You mark, though* he *is never ailing,*
> *Horror that vainly scoots ahead,*
> *And pestilence behind him trailing.*

O. S. would have George ("the one who bears about / These germs of Socialistic rot"), like Mallon, "clapped in quarantine, / There to abide the country's pleasure." The poem, accepting Mallon's danger at face value, expropriates her story as a tool for political commentary.

There are three representations of Mary Mallon in these earliest public productions of her character and life. The first, the social deviant cognizant of her own evil and insistently continuing her dangerous behavior, is the most powerful image, but it was not yet very common at the time of her release in 1910. This image, represented most strongly by the drawing of the cook who kills, puts the blame squarely on the carrier and absolves her captors from any guilt. The second, the innocent who unknowingly or unwittingly causes harm, is similarly compelling and as resonant today as it was in Mallon's time. A basically humane stance, it excuses the person of conscious complicity and guilt—she was an inadvertent menace—but still admits that sanctions may be brought and remedies applied. The third depiction, of a person who has no say in how her dangers will be used and is a mere instrument in the hands of evil, is significantly less appealing in

American culture today when human agency and will are such valued attributes. But it, too, has not disappeared, and remnants of "Typhoid Bridget" can be recognized in our present-day efforts to find villains and assign blame for our own epidemic woes.

In these early-twentieth-century portrayals there is a range of responses to Mary Mallon that continued throughout her life. We recognize a level of comfort sought by the healthy and established in stigmatizing an identifiable enemy, an enemy determined by science but also recognizable by specific social markers. Mary Mallon, in all of her various levels of culpability, represents pollution—pollution of food, pollution of healthy unsuspecting bodies, pollution of womanhood and the home. She is a deviant, a threat to the very core of society through the germs that grow in her body and spew out to infect others. She must be shunned. She may stir the pot innocently, but the ultimate result is sickness and death for those who come into contact with her. Mallon herself remains healthy, perhaps the final proof of her guilt and her power to harm. No matter what she brings upon others, she remains unscathed. She gets away with it.

When Mary Mallon resurfaced in 1915 after five years out of the news and was found to have violated the agreement she made with the health department not to cook again, the tide of public sympathy as depicted in the popular press turned sharply against her. The news reports of her capture, although still very dramatic, this time lacked compassion for her situation. The (New York) *Sun*, for example, published a gripping account:

A squad of sanitary police who had been immunized against typhoid climbed into a department automobile and surrounded the house. . . . Down a side street lurked another automobile in which sat waiting Dr. Westmoreland of the Health Department and more policemen. When all was ready Sergt. Coneally rang the door bell. There was silence. He rang again and again, but no sound came from the house.

Having thus captured readers' attention, the report continued: "A ladder was then found and Coneally climbed to a window at the second floor." When Coneally "poked his head into a semi-dark room," a dog "snarl[ed] from the shadows," and another dog joined the chorus. "Down the ladder came the sergeant discreetly and procured some pieces of meat."

The peace offering allowed the officers to enter the house by the second floor window. They heard the "muffled sound of a slamming door in a room beyond."

And so the officers last Friday were expectant of trouble. As they went from room to room the muffled door slamming was always just a room ahead of them. At last they pushed open the door of a bathroom and found a woman crouching there. She told them finally, they say, that she was Mary Mallon.[29]

Cornered. The editor showed no "cheap sympathy" with Mary Mallon this time. "What would have been done in the case of a man with hysterical homicidal tendencies who had been convicted of murder and had fought detention by every legal and other quibble?" he asked, immediately answering his own question, "Surely he would not have been discharged under parole." And neither should Mary Mallon have been given a second chance to harm people. This "wretch who disregarded the plain warning of the health authorities and deliberately went forth on her mission of death and misery" should be kept in "real isolation." And other carriers too, the editor continued, should not receive any "sentimental sympathy on account of innocence and misfortune." He called for laws to protect the people against such menaces to the public's health.[30]

Other newspapers added vivid details to the story. The *New York World* revealed that the woman had been "well veiled and apparently very anxious to escape attention," but that an officer was convinced it was Mary Mallon "since he remembered peculiarities of her walk from having had a part in her apprehension eight years before"—an assessment that hearkens back to

George Soper's description of Mallon's walk (and her mind) as "masculine."[31]

The *New York Tribune* put the common media view about Mallon starkly the second time around: "The sympathy which would naturally be granted to Mary Mallon is largely modified for this reason," wrote the editors. "The chance was given to her five years ago to live in freedom, and . . . she deliberately elected to throw it away." Thus, "it is impossible to feel much commiseration for her."

Doubtless there are others no wiser—there were many, and they were very noisy, when her case first came to public notice—who think it an outrage that her liberty should be interfered with. But the plain and obvious fact is that we have no way of dealing with these unlucky persons except by keeping them where they cannot do harm to others. Many epidemic outbreaks of typhoid fever have been traced indisputably to carriers. These may involve hundreds of people and cause many deaths. Are such sacrifices to be made on the score of individual liberty where we have to deal with persons that do not know how to make a reasonable use of their liberty?[32]

Mallon's use of an alias, "Mrs. Brown," at the Sloane Hospital where she was caught cooking in 1915 particularly angered public commentators. Using a pseudonym more than implied—it seemed to demonstrate—that Mallon was aware that she should not be in the kitchen. She had been deliberately deceptive. As George Soper told the *New York Times*, which now seemed to agree, given these conditions, "liberty is an impossible privilege to allow her."[33]

The 1915 popular reports on Mary Mallon helped turn public opinion from sympathy and curiosity to anger and fear and gave support to her long-term isolation. Her high profile, as well as the strong negative judgment that dominated the media, made it easier for health officials to isolate Mary Mallon once again. Officials acted in the wake of loudly voiced public approval. She was now

Typhoid Mary, a villain who could not be trusted, who had to be locked away in order to protect innocent people.

Although commentators continued to see personal misfortune in the situation after 1915, few lamented it anymore. Mary Mallon could now be blamed outright; this time she had consciously done wrong. Newspapers supported and advertized Soper's views: "She has long been confronted with the facts and yet, she has had the assurance to go to a hospital, and of all places, a maternity hospital, to cook and possibly pollute the food of some 300 people."[34] This was unforgivable. This was evil. By 1915, the negativism voiced first in 1907 about potential danger and pollution from healthy carriers now dominated the media's perception of Typhoid Mary. The human qualities and personal tragedy of Mary Mallon fell away to be replaced by an inhuman monster who would deliberately use her body to inflict harm on others.

Scientific American united all the negative qualities assigned to Typhoid Mary in a single editorial and indicated how closely the popular media and the scientific community interacted by 1915 when Mallon reemerged as a cook:

The great trouble with Typhoid Mary has been her perversity, exceeding even that which obtains in her most temperamental of callings. She has never conceded herself a menace; she has not obeyed the sanitary directions given her; she would not wash and disinfect her hands as required; she will not change her occupation for one in which she will not endanger the lives of others; under an assumed name she had competed with the Wandering Jew in scattering destruction in her path.[35]

The litany identified the areas of Mary Mallon's culpability: she refused to accept official authority, she persisted in cooking, an occupation itself without virtue, and she consciously deceived. The analogy to the "Wandering Jew" emphasized an ethnic component to Mallon's perceived guilt and made it clear how her story evoked deep-seated social prejudices and powerful emotions.

The passion evident against Mary Mallon in this period of her second, and now to be life-long, incarceration was stronger than any attached to other healthy carriers who also disobeyed health department regulations and continued to cook after being informed about their danger. Just as health officials did not usually label and stigmatize men like Alphonse Cotils, Tony Labella, and Frederick Moersch as to their ethnicity, sex, or personal appearance, the news media remained nonjudgmental and unemotional about the culpability of these other recalcitrant carriers, people who returned to cooking after being informed they endangered others. In their lopsided coverage, the editors showed themselves to be players and shapers, and not just reflectors, in the events.

The *New York Times* articles about Tony Labella, for example, called him an "alleged" typhoid carrier even though both the New York and New Jersey health officials had determined this to be his status. The reporter concluded a matter-of-fact story about him (with no personal description) with, "He persists in handling food, although he has been warned repeatedly by the State Board not to do so, it is alleged."[36] Labella, who had been traced to more cases and deaths from typhoid fever than Mary Mallon and had disobeyed health regulations repeatedly, was only very briefly isolated by the health department (in New Jersey) and never received an emotional condemnation by the press.[37]

Personal details about Alphonse Cotils are also scarce in the news stories informing the public that this bakery owner, "despite warnings from the Health Department, ... had been discovered preparing a strawberry shortcake."[38] The judge's suspended sentence that permitted Cotils to return home, and possibly to his surreptitious cooking, received no disapproving judgment in the press. The *Tribune* revealed that "the Health Department at various times ... had tried to keep Cotils away from food handling, but was unsuccessful until his recent arrest." Identifying the accused as a "Belgian baker," with no other social identifiers, the reporter added, "He was frequently warned ... but did not heed the warnings."[39] When the health department "asked him to sign a pledge never to engage in business having to do with foodstuffs," and "Cotils refused, declaring his physician ... had found him in a perfectly healthy condition," the court released him anyway and the newspaper still did not find fault with this judgment.[40] Similarly, the *World* reported that Cotils may have "obtained the [food-handling] certificate under false pretenses," and yet did not question whether or not he could be trusted when "Cotils said he would leave his wife and two children, for a while at least, [and] take a residence in the country."[41] Apparently, his defiance of authorities after being informed of his dangerous carrier state did not cause authorities or the press to distrust him.

The *American*, true to form, headlined a lengthy story on Cotils, "Health Board Bars Robust Baker, Typhoid Carrier." This rendition was the only news story to give a physical description of Cotils, noticing his "ruddy cheeks and broad shoulders." The image presented of a robust man in the prime of health was positive, whereas nearly identical words were used to describe Mary Mallon negatively. "I am a well man," Cotils told Gene Fowler, the *American* reporter. "Do I look sick? ... You say I am a menace. I am not a menace, for all I do is mind my own business and work hard."[42]

One of the reasons health officials did not trust Mary Mallon was that she claimed not to accept the medical finding that she was a dangerous carrier. Alphonse Cotils, too, told reporters, "I am a healthy, normal person." Cotils continued, "To-day we asked our regular customers if they had any typhoid fever in their families. They all said no."[43] His skepticism seemed as genuine as Mallon's, although the fact that he was informed of his carrier state seventeen years after Mary Mallon's initial capture and nine years after her rearrest had familiarized the public with the carrier phenomenon should have made his excuse somewhat less convincing. Yet the popular press, like the judge, accepted his promise that this time he would stay out of his bakery. Perhaps influenced by the same class-, ethnicity-, and gender-based perceptions that affected the health officials, the media seemed content with Cotils's suspended sentence and did not voice a desire to isolate him from his fellow New Yorkers either by words or in fact.

News reporters got a little more excited when Frederick Moersch reappeared in 1928 as a healthy carrier who knowingly continued to prepare food for other people. The dramatic quality of their stories almost equalled those about Mary Mallon. But the coverage was, for the most part, nonjudgmental regarding Moersch himself. Only one newspaper made reference to "Typhoid Freddie," and the term was not used elsewhere. Moersch was not stigmatized in the reporting, and writers noted no public anger directed against him. On the other hand, reporters remembered Typhoid Mary in all articles about these other typhoid fever carriers, and set her aside as the example of the ultimate in potential health danger.[44]

Writing about the fifty-one-year-old Moersch, the *World* bemoaned that he was "fated to spread disease and death in his path." Yet the focus of their news story was on the scene at his ice cream parlor: "Crowds, aroused by rumors of the case, surged about it all yesterday afternoon. Children, unaware of all the aspects of the tragedy, darted in to throw insults and curses upon Moersch's oldest daughter." The twenty-eight-year-old "blond and strikingly pretty" woman particularly concerned the reporter, who noted sympathetically, "She perhaps will suffer more than many other innocent victims of her father's germ-spreading influence. . . . She already has experienced more than the average share of misfortune." The woman's husband had died four months before this event, and she had given birth to her second child only weeks following his death. "Now the store, her only means of livelihood, is doomed to certain failure."

"What's going to happen to me and my children?" Fredericka Kraus sobbed to the reporter: "It's not our savings alone that's invested in this store. It's our insurance, every penny we have. . . . And the way people are treating us! Don't they realize it isn't our fault?"[45] The health department closed the store, destroyed the ice cream that Moersch had made, sterilized the display cases, and then allowed the ice cream parlor to reopen.

As a result of the excitement over Moersch's case in Greenwich Village, Will F. Clarke of the *World* studied the phenomenon of healthy carriers of typhoid fever and reported his findings to the public in "City Watches 208 Typhoid Carriers." Clark wrote about all the healthy people "walking about the streets of New York almost every day" who could cause typhoid epidemics. "Just so long as they exercise such judgment [not to prepare food] they are permitted their liberty," he wrote. Realizing that Moersch had returned to confectionery work knowing he was a carrier, Clarke wondered "whether this was done unthinkingly or willfully." The press had not posed such a generous question about Mary Mallon's 1915 return to cooking. Clarke did not mention Tony Labella or Alphonse Cotils here, but he wrote the outline of Mary Mallon's story, finding that after "the better part of twenty-one years in isolation . . . she is near sixty, has her own little cottage and seems resigned."[46]

Over the years Mary Mallon lived on North Brother Island, occasional stories about her appeared in the public press. For example, in 1933, the Sunday magazine section of the *New York Daily Mirror* printed, "I Wonder What's Become of—'Typhoid Mary.' "[47] Both the text and visuals of this article are softer than the earlier hostility toward Mary Mallon. Reprinting the original and much used 1909 photograph of Mallon in bed at Willard Parker Hospital following her initial detention, the article featured a sketch of a kindly older woman, a contemporary rendition of the aging Mallon (see fig. 5.7). Bespectacled and grandmotherly, the portrait looks directly from the page with honesty and

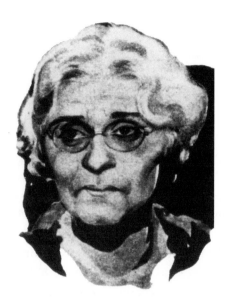

Fig. 5.7 *Mary Mallon, drawing, 1933.*

innocence. The woman here is again the innocent vehicle, one who is shown to be motherly and kind. The only "menace" on this page is in a third illustration, a separate drawing of the "germs, greatly enlarged by microscope," that Mallon's body carries. The difference between this and earlier benevolent depictions is that the blame is more clearly shifted away from the human carrier to the germs she carried.

Interestingly, the reporter who traveled out to North Brother Island to do his research on Mallon did not mention the other healthy carrier who then still lived and worked on the island, Frederick Moersch.[48] As discussed previously (see chap. 4), Moersch was a carrier who had broken parole and had endangered about three times as many New Yorkers as did Mary Mallon, but he had never attracted an emotional response from the public media.

In 1935, three years before Mallon's death, Stanley Walker wrote an extended narrative on "Typhoid Carrier No. 36" for the *New Yorker* magazine.[49] George Soper found Walker's article "flippant" and the "source of much of the misinformation" about Mary Mallon, but, in fact, it contained no more distortion than others.[50] Relying heavily on Soper's own published work, Walker characterized Mallon as "defiant, sly, and difficult to capture or control," again repeating and accepting some of the social prejudices that earlier characterized stories about Mallon. Perry Barlow's drawing that accompanied the story depicted a cook, a woman without a face, hard at her work (see fig. 5.8). No skulls floated out of her cooking pot, but the large shadow lurking behind the cook is more than a suggestion that all is not right.

Walker's visit to Mary Mallon on North Brother Island convinced him that in her later years Catholicism provided "some of the consolation which was denied to her during a lifetime as a pariah—unwanted and untouchable."[51] Walker did not question the health department's decision to hold Mallon on North Brother Island, and he painted the picture of a health department in control of the difficult problem of healthy carriers. He acknowledged that for Mary Mallon "life has been pretty tough," and he noted that "the jolly girl who went out to cook when McKinley was President turned out to be that symbol of pestilence known as Typhoid Mary."[52]

In the telling and the retelling of Mary Mallon's story, news reporters and other writers sometimes confused the facts, changing the dates of her incarceration and the number of people she supposedly infected.[53] But more important in analyzing the meaning of the news stories is to understand the characterizations and representations of Mary Mallon and the evolution of the concept of Typhoid Mary. Perhaps because she was the first carrier to be traced and publicized, perhaps because of her social class, or perhaps because the media had already made her story a symbol for something much larger, Mary Mallon continued to fascinate newspaper readers. Her story reached deep into America's cultural imagination, provoking curiosity, fear, and hostility.

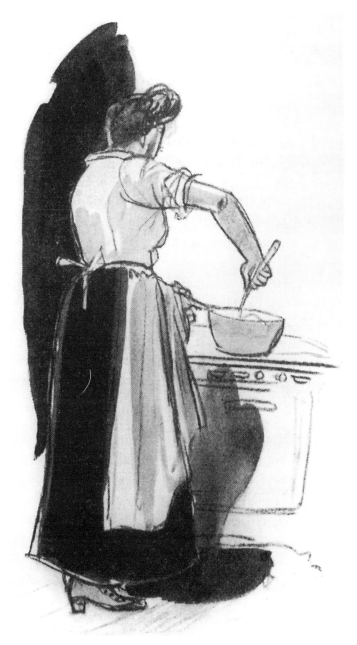

Fig. 5.8. *Mary Mallon at stove, drawing, 1935.*

Even today the phrase *Typhoid Mary* echoes around the world as a rallying cry for the need for protection against individuals who threaten the public's health.

In 1938, when reporters covered Mary Mallon's death, as earlier, they continued to use the dehumanizing terms "human culture tube" and "veritable peripatetic breeding ground" and continued to imply that her situation was anomalous.[54] The *New York World-Telegram* guessed that as many as 200,000 typhoid carriers lived in the United States and noted that 237 were under the New York City Health Department's observation. Nonetheless, their writers believed that " 'Typhoid Mary' was distinct by [being] what psychologists call 'uncooperative.' " Hearkening to gender expectations, the newspaper reflected, "She was not imbued with that sweet reasonableness which would have allowed her to listen to the explanations of learned men about her peculiar case."[55] The implication was that had Mary Mallon been reasonable and sweet—more traditionally feminine—she might not have become Typhoid Mary, a conclusion that continued to single her out while ignoring the numerous other reported uncooperative carriers.[56]

Mary Mallon suffered a series of small strokes, and late in 1932 a major one paralyzed her and left her bedridden until her death on November 11, 1938.[57] The newspapers covered her funeral at St. Luke's Roman Catholic Church in the Bronx. "Nine Mysterious Mourners" attended it, but refused to speak with reporters or identify themselves.[58] She was "alone in death as she had been in life," wrote her advocate, the *New York American*. "In later years Mary lost some of her bitterness after she became interested in the Roman Catholic Faith. But it was a gray, leaden existence at best."[59] More than half of her adult life had been spent in her island confinement.

Over the years of Mallon's life, the popular media did more than report on the first woman in America to be labeled and traced as a healthy carrier of typhoid fever. From the beginning, led by William Randolph Hearst and followed by his competitors for the New York newspaper market, the press presented Mallon's story to the public in a stylized form. Newspaper writers and editors (and their publishing colleagues) shaped and reshaped the message, through positive and negative representations, through omissions, through an emphasis on her uniqueness, through efforts to arouse emotions, and through language that negated Mallon's humanity. In these ways they created and presented their own perspective on why Mary Mallon's story was significant. In so doing, they influenced public opinion and official actions and underscored a potent construction of Typhoid Mary as a woman polluted, a social pariah to be feared and shunned.

"Banished
Like a
Leper"

Loss of Liberty
and Personal Misfortune

*W*hen health officials apprehended Alphonse Cotils in 1924 for violating the health code and preparing food in his restaurant even though he was a known typhoid fever carrier, Cotils protested to the authorities, "I am not a Typhoid Mary.... I always wear a white coat and a white hat and white working pants. I am a clean man."[1] With these words, Cotils set himself apart from Mary Mallon, though both were healthy people accused of knowingly carrying and disseminating pathogenic bacteria through their cooking. His case was different, Cotils thought, because his personal hygiene habits were superior. Cotils refused to ally himself with the notorious woman then isolated on North Brother Island.

Herein lies Mary Mallon's particular tragedy. Not even her fellow carriers would claim her as their own. People accused of transmitting disease to others in the same ways that Mallon did thought themselves innocent, but believed the worst about her. She was dirty; they were clean. She was evil; they were good. She was deviant; they were normal. Alienated even from those who carried the same disease she did, Mary Mallon stood truly alone.

If the world insisted in keeping her at arms' length, Mallon responded by building her own armor to keep the world at bay. Her defenses were very strong and her instincts very private; thus her inner thoughts and her full motivations will never be known. But we can examine and begin to piece together an understanding of how she experienced her role as America's first monitored healthy carrier. We can understand how the early caricature of her as a social evil influenced much of what happened to her. We can see, beyond the caricature, a real woman, of flesh and blood, who stood necessarily in defiance against her public definition.

If Alphonse Cotils could have known Mary Mallon, perhaps he might have recognized a certain kinship in adversity with a woman who believed as he did that she was not a menace to society, and who believed herself to be, as he did, a person misjudged, a person who should be allowed to earn her living doing what she knew best. "I'm Persecuted!" Mallon shouted in the newspaper headline when her story broke. "Before God and in the eyes of decent men my name is Mary Mallon. I was christened and baptized Mary Mallon. I lived a decent, upright life under the name of Mary Mallon until I was seized," she said. Then, she pointed out, in a statement that indicates her understanding of the full power of symbols, "[I was] locked up in a pest-house and rechristened 'Typhoid Mary,' the name by which the world has ever since known me."[2]

Mary Mallon was born on September 23, 1869, in Cookstown, County Tyrone, Ireland. Her parents were John Mallon and Catherine Igo Mallon.[3] She told friends that she had come to the United States in 1883, at the age of about fifteen, and had lived for a while with her aunt and uncle.[4] She told officials that she had lived in New York City since her emigration.[5] As an adult she spoke with a "lilting brogue."[6]

Her employment record before 1897, when she began her three-year engagement as a cook for the New York family that summered in Mamaroneck, is not recoverable. However, in the fourteen years between 1883, when she arrived in the United States and may have first worked out of her relatives' home, and 1897, when Soper picked up her record, it is probable that Mary

Mallon, like legions of other Irish-American young single women, followed a typical work pattern of domestic labor in the homes of relatively well-to-do native-born New Yorkers.

More than any other ethnic group, Irish-born young single women frequently came to the United States alone.[7] The large majority of these women found work as domestic laborers throughout the last half of the nineteenth century and into the twentieth: by 1920 still "81 percent of those employed worked as domestic servants."[8] In the words of one historian, "Irish girls [who came to America] accepted servanthood as a fact of life."[9] Irish-born men and women who settled in America found themselves mired in jobs with minimal occupational mobility, although their children often moved more rapidly up the occupational ladder, the sons often through the church and politics, and the daughters in teaching or trade.[10]

The Irish in America suffered poor health often related to their limited employment opportunities and concentration in congested urban areas. Irish women, particularly, fell prey to tuberculosis, and the rate of infant mortality among the Irish remained high. One historian has concluded, "In the early 20th century the Irish were the only immigrant group in the United States whose [general] mortality rate was higher than in the homeland."[11]

We know from labor and immigration historians that the conditions of Mallon's life as a domestic servant at the turn of the century were undoubtedly grim. Domestic servants worked long and strenuous hours. They were usually single women who lived in the homes of their employers, and (except sometimes for a half-day off) they were always on call. A typical day began at 6:00 A.M. and did not end until after-dinner cleaning, well into the evening hours. Usually the women were on their feet the entire day, except when they took their own meals, which were often leftovers from the family table.[12] A telling rendition of a new immigrant's experiences with domestic labor comes from a labor

journalist who wrote at the turn of the century a graphic fiction-
alized account of the "greenhorns" she had studied. Imitating
what she thought was an uneducated immigrant's dialect, Mary
Heaton Vorse wrote, "I come to this cuntry when I was 15. . . . I
was a tall girl for my age and had fat red cheeks and lookt strong
and helthy."

Fokes dont no how strange things is I usto cry and cry most all the
night just from homesickness and discuragment. . . . nobody showed
me ennything, I was willin an I am no duller than the next one and I
think with a little showin I might have done fine . . . I was just fri-
tened clear through all the time I was in that place they thought I
was sullen . . . green girls is awfull bashfull and don't know how to
speak up for themselvs any more than children.[13]

Historians have well documented the vulnerability of the young,
single, immigrant women who had to make their own way in the
labor market in the period in which Mary Mallon carved her own
niche in New York City's kitchens. The status of domestic work,
never very high, fell by the end of the century, even though most
employed women continued to work in other's homes. Working
women objected to the lack of freedom that domestic work entailed and also to the uniforms that represented their servitude.[14]
Irish women particularly (along with African-American women)
felt the added stings of discrimination. Historian Susan Strasser
has concluded, "The feeling that domestic service implied social
inferiority was 'practically universal.'" Strasser quotes a "shop
girl" from the period who said, "Young men think and say, 'Oh,
she can't be much if she hasn't got brains enough to make her living outside a kitchen.' You're just down, once for all, if you go into
one."[15] A shirtmaker put it even more starkly, "My objection to
housework is that in many places a hired girl is much less than
a dog."[16]

According to historian David Katzman, Irish domestic workers particularly felt unwelcome in their employers' homes. "Most
were Roman Catholic and from rural Ireland, so their religion

and outlook contrasted sharply with those of their employers."
Katzman has demonstrated that the "No Irish need apply" attitude of the pre–Civil War period had declined in American cities
by the end of the nineteenth century, but that "the difference between the religion of the kitchen and that of the parlor" continued to characterize domestic relations. The differences were a
special concern to the "mistresses" who hired the family's help
and who tried to maintain a "Calvinistic or evangelical Protestant mood in their household."[17]

A 1904 study of employment agencies provides further insight into the conditions of domestic employment in the period.
Frances A. Kellor, supported by the Woman's Municipal League
of New York and aided by eight fellow investigators, visited 834
licensed agencies in four cities, including 522 in New York.[18]
Three-fifths of the agencies supplied household workers, and
three-fifths of all household workers found their employment
through such agencies. Mary Mallon, we know, found most of her
jobs through two employment agencies. Kellor described the mis-
erable conditions in run-down rooms where unemployed women
met the "ladies" who looked them over like animals. She wrote,
"In some of these [agencies] girls are actually herded and treated
like cattle. . . . The means of maintaining order in some of the
crowded offices is not only insulting, but brutal."[19]

Kellor's study found that not only were conditions appalling
within the agencies helping people find work, but working conditions were worse. Women domestics frequently changed jobs
seeking better conditions. Kellor revealed that workers "receive
such poor food, and not enough of that," or labored under "defec-
tive sanitation and heat," or found "the over-crowding is in many
instances serious, and certainly girls can have no privacy." Kellor
heard complaints of unwanted sexual advances, poor bathing
facilities, dirty bed clothing, and very long work days with little
time off. She noted, "One employer complained to us that her last
girl was not neat and clean . . . and then showed us [her] room,

which was partitioned off from the coal-bin and could not have been kept clean under any conditions!"[20]

By the turn of the twentieth century, domestic service, in contrast to alternative positions in factories and retail stores, "lack[ed] both protection and dignity in the eyes of girls seeking occupations." The "loss of personal independence" was a particular grievance that Kellor heard as she conducted interviews for her study.[21] Young women may have felt they had no choice but to labor in the homes of others, but most understood the confines of their work.[22]

Mary Mallon's could not have been an exception to the common experiences of her peers. New York domestic labor at the end of the nineteenth century, almost by definition, entailed alienating class, ethnic, religious, and gendered divisions as women from one cultural milieu came to work and live in the homes of families from another. Even when relationships between employer and employee were relatively good, servants' positions were precarious. We can safely assume that Mary Mallon's experiences between 1883 and her 1907 encounter with health officials led her to understand the social, economic, religious, and cultural differences between herself and her native-born employers. She must surely have become aware of the pervasive hierarchy of urban America and been sensitized to her place within it.

Domestic work that included living in others' homes—not all of it did—severely restricted women's social mobility. Many women in domestic service complained to Kellor that they had very few opportunities to meet respectable men, which they felt limited their potential for marriage, the road out of servile employment. Furthermore, their dependence on employers for housing meant that they had nowhere to live in between jobs.[23] We can infer that some of Mary Mallon's jobs did not demand living in the homes of her employers (perhaps cooks had more flexibility than those in general domestic service) because we know that she sometimes lived with Briehof (as when Soper found her in 1907) and sometimes with another family. Even so, it appears from reading between the lines of the Mallon story that she often boarded with her employer families and had few people she could call friends and no known relatives once her aunt died. Indeed, a nurse who befriended Mallon at Riverside Hospital said Mallon told her "on numerous occasions" that "she had no living relations" and "no brothers or sisters, nieces, nephews, grandnieces or grandnephews and that she was the last survivor of her family."[24]

One of the more positive legends to be linked to Mary Mallon through her ordeal was that she became particularly attached to the children in the homes in which she worked. As one newspaper wrote at the time of her habeas corpus court hearing, she was a "stout, jovial cook who was loved by the children in every family in which she was employed."[25] Mallon may, in fact, have been a good companion to the children in the homes in which she cooked, though she may have also fantasized such attachments, or reporters could have exaggerated the relationships. We do know that at one of the homes to which Soper traced her, J. Coleman Drayton's, her employer testified to Mallon's caring warmly for family members when she nursed them through their illnesses with typhoid fever.[26]

No matter how positive Mallon's relations sometimes were with her employers and their families, however, her life was one of struggle and vulnerability. Like the others of her status and occupation, she remained expendable throughout her working career. She could have been replaced without any notice. She experienced periods of unemployment. She understood hardship and deprivation, the vagaries of the domestic marketplace, and probably saw herself—even before any of her dealings with the health department—alone in a sometimes hostile world. She undoubtedly had to learn to pick herself up and get another job when things did not go well, protecting herself against the realities of domestic work. The strong defenses she demonstrated to Soper and the other officials who tried to communicate with her were honed in the harsh world of servitude she had long inhabited.

Soper seemed to think that Mallon's numerous job changes (he traced eight jobs over a ten-year period) indicated something negative about her. "Mary appeared to be a person who moved about a good deal," he wrote. "She did not remain long in any situation."[27] Perhaps he thought her employers were dissatisfied with her work, although there was no evidence for that conclusion. He more than implied that she subconsciously understood her role in transmitting typhoid, and left before she could be blamed for it, claiming once, "It must have looked as though [typhoid fever] was pursuing her."[28] Although Soper suggested that Mallon left her employment when typhoid fever developed in the families for whom she worked, this was not substantiated in his own evidence. Soper traced Mallon to Dark Harbor in the years 1901 to 1902, for example, to a family for whom she worked for eleven months. A laundress developed typhoid fever one month after Mallon arrived; she stayed ten months afterwards.[29] Other commentators nonetheless have continued to suggest such prescience on Mallon's part. "[S]he sensed that something was wrong," wrote Stanley Walker in the *New Yorker*, "and she would go to another job as soon as she saw typhoid developing around her."[30]

In the years during which she carried out her cooking career, Mary Mallon could not possibly have understood that she, a healthy woman, might have caused someone in a family for whom she worked to contract typhoid fever. The best of the world's scientists were themselves only beginning to understand the existence of healthy carriers by the end of the nineteenth century. Typhoid fever was rampant in New York and around the country at the time and was often connected to summer vacations when people left their familiar habitat and wandered to new places, exposing themselves to disease.[31] Even after Soper informed her of the possibility of a healthy person transmitting the disease, Mallon denied her culpability: "She had never had [typhoid] nor produced it. There had been no more typhoid where she was than anywhere else. There was typhoid fever everywhere."[32] Most people believed, as did Mallon, that typhoid was either transmitted by exposure to people sick with the disease or through polluted water and milk supplies. Before cities filtered their water, these were the most common sources of the disease. As Soper himself wrote, "It will be remembered that in those days typhoid fever was far more common than it is today and that the knowledge of its transmission was less complete."[33] At the turn of the century, then, to blame a healthy person with no symptoms for transmitting typhoid fever would have seemed beyond the realm of thoughtful possibility.

It is conceivable that Mallon was fired from some of her jobs, although it is more likely, since there is no record of any dissatisfaction with her cooking and significant record of satisfaction, that she left for her own reasons. Sometimes Mallon was hired only for the summer, and thus had some short-term employment. Soper portrayed her as uncommunicative, claiming that "she did not get on well with other servants and wanted to be moving about."[34] His observation is challenged by the story of her capture in March, 1907, when the other servants helped Mallon hide when authorities came to take her away. Her culinary expertise was appreciated in the homes in which she worked, and even the Warrens, whose home Mallon worked in when she was located by Soper, described their favorite dishes that she prepared. Mallon could make good wages: $45 per month at her Oyster Bay job, which was double the average domestic worker's wage.[35]

There are a few other possible explanations for Mallon's varied job history, which seem to fit more with the time and the situation. The first is that Mary Mallon may have left jobs soon after someone in the family came down with typhoid fever in order not to catch the disease herself. This would not have been a foolish response, but one point against this explanation is that when members of the Drayton household contracted typhoid, Mallon stayed to help nurse them in their illness. In this instance, however, Drayton offered her a bonus for her sick-room help, which may have convinced her to stay. The second possibility is that Mary Mallon perceived some danger to her own employment future when a household became disrupted from disease and "epidemic fighters" began their investigations. Maybe she worried that staff reductions would necessarily follow sickness or death; maybe she did not like the idea of being questioned. She may have wanted to leave before being caught up in a situation that might end her job anyway. We know she left some employment because its term was expired; this was true for those times when she contracted to accompany a family to their summer residence.

As she matured in the New York servant world (by 1897 she was twenty-eight years old) Mallon must have become wise to the ups and downs of her profession. She would have been on the lookout for better jobs, and she might have left abruptly when she found one. She would have developed some protective behaviors that allowed her continued success. One of these may have been not allowing herself to get too emotionally close with the other servants; another may have been a few well-timed exits.

With this historical background, we can return to the story of Mary Mallon's capture and incarceration with a broader understanding of how she may have perceived these events. Through the eyes of a mid-career immigrant woman, thirty-seven years old when Soper first approached her, without family, but with an understanding of how the world divided the haves and the have nots, Mary Mallon saw circumstances very differently than did George Soper or S. Josephine Baker.

George Soper became frustrated when Mary Mallon did not see things as he did: "Reason, at least in the forms in which I was acquainted with it," he wrote, "proved unavailing. My point of view was not acceptable [to Mary Mallon] and the claims of science and humanity were unavailing." Soper complained, "I never felt more helpless."[36] We can see through Mary Mallon's eyes that she, too, felt helpless in this 1907 encounter, and that she, too, found reason in her position.

When George Soper walked up the steps of the Park Avenue brownstone in which Mary Mallon was working in March, 1907, and accused her (albeit, in his terms, diplomatically) of making people sick with her cooking, he initiated a new public health encounter. Investigators previously had looked into other home- and community-based typhoid epidemics. They had come to examine the water supply, the food, and the disease histories of the people in the household.[37] But never before, in Mallon's experience or anyone else's, had an epidemic investigation led to an accusation that a specific healthy individual was causing typhoid in others. Soper himself admitted that "such a thing had never been heard of."[38]

Because of her life experiences in the American urban workplace and her awareness of the low esteem in which Irish women domestics were held, Mallon was probably on her guard when the authorities came to call. Just as the other servants who tried to protect her from S. Josephine Baker's search, Mallon would have seen the attention she received from Soper and then from the health department and police officers as unwanted attention, even persecution, as she put it to the press. What would government officials want with her except to bring trouble? Soper might have assured her that he thought her "innocent" of causing disease in the sense that she did not do it on purpose or knowingly; Baker might have assured her she "only wanted the specimens and that then she could go back home."[39] But by the time Baker approached her with the full authority of the health department and police behind her, Mallon "was convinced that the law was wantonly persecuting her, when she had done nothing wrong."[40] Mallon did not trust her accusers, especially when they appeared with uniformed police officers. What she understood best was her vulnerability in the face of an attack from powerful officials.[41] When at Willard Parker Hospital, the surgeons suggested removing her gallbladder, Baker noted, Mallon "was convinced afresh that this was a pretext for killing her."[42]

Soper approached Mallon with at least two assumptions, both of which were unshared: "I expected to find a person who would be as desirous as I was for an explanation of the way in which the typhoid had followed her," Soper wrote. "Certainly she could not have failed to be impressed by the strange fatality with which the disease had broken out wherever she went."[43] Mallon, however, had not spent the previous months, as had Soper, searching for an explanation of the Oyster Bay outbreak of typhoid fever; she may not have given the occurrence any thought since leaving that job. Moreover, she would not have perceived herself to be at the forefront of a trail of disease. She was a healthy woman doing her job; no more, no less. "She would not allow anybody to accuse her," Soper realized.[44]

What was Mary Mallon supposed to make of this man who seemed intent on blaming her for spreading typhoid fever? Soper found her in her Park Avenue kitchen, he followed her home, he interrogated her friend: why was he harassing her? In the face of his seemingly unreasonable accusations, Mallon tried to defend herself. She might not have even listened to his long explanations about the possible role she played in transmitting disease; if she heard his words, she was surely confused by them. What was clear to her was that her future was in jeopardy, and Mary Mallon reacted understandably to that, by fighting back, by trying to run, by resisting.

Mallon's responses to Soper's uninvited appearance at her employer's home on Park Avenue and the apartment she shared with Briehof on Third Avenue near 33rd Street demonstrated her incomprehension and resistance to the words Soper uttered about her being the cause of outbreaks of typhoid fever, but they also revealed the personal anguish the visits caused her. Soper literally invaded her space. Furthermore, he befriended Briehof in the process, an intrusion that revealed a degree of fickleness on the part of Mallon's "best friend, a man whose name she often went by."[45] Although Soper described Briehof as "a disreputable looking man," he nonetheless "got to be well acquainted with him." Briehof "took me to see the room," Soper divulged, and he "made an arrangement with Mary's friend to meet her in this room." But Briehof did not warn Mallon to expect a visitor, and she was "angry at the unexpected sight" of Soper.[46] She also must have been upset that Briehof had betrayed her to authorities.

Mary Mallon's behavior in these initial encounters with health authorities demonstrates her feelings of being attacked, unjustly accused, alone, and helpless in the face of authority. She felt caged, literally and figuratively, by forces larger than life, uncontrollable. Her responses speak of her vulnerability. She lashed out at what she did not understand, at people who threatened to take away her livelihood. They expected her to listen to their explanations, to comprehend that a healthy person could cause disease in others, and to accept that she had killed a person. But the words of the health officials were unfathomable, not because she was dim-witted, but because she came to those initial encounters from such a different starting place. However well intentioned Soper and Baker believed themselves to be, Mallon could not respond to them in ways they would consider reasonable: they threatened everything she knew. She had to resist.

One response produced another. The more Mary Mallon resisted and refused to communicate with the health officers with whom she came in contact—in her place of employment, her home, and in the hospital—the more they labeled her as uncooperative and saw the impossibility of releasing her. The more they treated her as a pariah, the more she acted like one. This standoff might have been avoided if either side could have stopped long enough to realize what was happening. But this was a new situation. Health officials were feeling their way toward a policy for dealing with the newly identified phenomenon of healthy carriers. In a very different way than Mallon, they too felt vulnerable in the face of a new force they did not yet fully understand but with which they had to contend. In their own excitement and confusion, they were not in a position to negotiate. Neither Mallon nor her captors showed flexibility during those weeks in the spring of 1907.

The initial confrontations between Mary Mallon and health officials defined their respective positions, which became entrenched over time. To the officials, the exciting new medical explanations, especially as they were repeatedly confirmed in the professional literature, remained of primary significance. Mary Mallon's capture represented the triumph of bacteriology, the promise that science could actually solve the urgent disease problems facing the country. While the practical responses to the newly understood phenomenon of healthy carriers were yet to be developed, public health officers were eager to move forward. The fact that a healthy Mallon carried disease in the inner recesses of her body was vital; and it was exciting at the time to learn the new directions bacteriological thinking might take.

On the other hand, Mallon's position that as a healthy woman she did not threaten anyone else's health reflected the predominant understanding of how diseases were transmitted. Even eighteen years after Mallon's identification as a healthy carrier, one health officer concluded that the concept still "seems incredible to many people. If germs cause disease, they reason, how can one be inhabited by 'millions of germs' and yet not become ill with the disease." Furthermore, this New Jersey health officer realized from his own experience that most people could not fathom how such germs lodged in the gallbladder could find their way into the mouths of other people. "The thought is so repulsive that the act itself seems impossible." Even "the microscopic size of all bacteria cannot be imagined by most persons."[47] Mallon, too, found a theory that argued for such strange events incredible and unbelievable. Her own beliefs, experiences, and feelings are

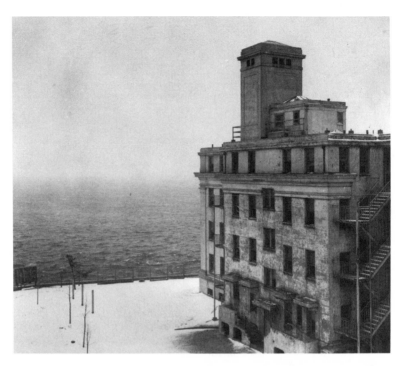

Fig. 6.1. *One of the concrete buildings of Riverside Hospital, North Brother Island, date unknown.*

important determinants in her story, and recognizing them provides a historical perspective that still resonates today. Health officials who encountered Mary Mallon discounted her beliefs, (especially during this "golden age" of bacteriology's promise) which increased their difficulty in controlling her behavior and the health problems she posed. Such a situation could easily repeat itself today if the beliefs of public health officials about a new disease entity were not commonly shared—were literally not even comprehended—by people required to follow policies based on them.

Let us return to North Brother Island, where health officials moved a resistant, scared, and angry Mary Mallon weeks after seizing her in March, 1907. North Brother Island is one of a pair of small land masses in the East River (the other is South Brother

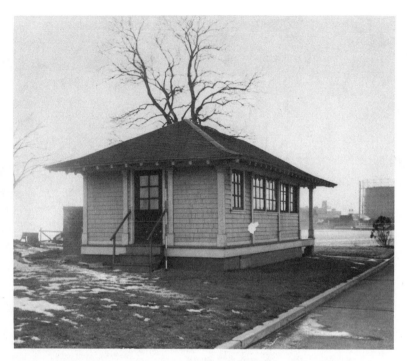

Fig. 6.2. *Mary Mallon's cottage, North Brother Island, date unknown.*

Island), between the Bronx and Riker's Island. A ferry connected
the island with the mainland at 132nd Street in the Bronx, and it
shuttled doctors, nurses, hospital staff, and patients back and
forth across the water. In those years, Riverside Hospital, a city
hospital that catered to tuberculosis patients, dominated the island (see fig. 6.1).[48] Mercifully for her, the health department did
not put Mallon inside the main hospital or in any of its various
concrete satellites, where she would have been exposed to the res-
piratory ailment, but instead let her live in a one-room frame
bungalow on the grounds, where she could contemplate her fate
alone (see fig. 6.2).

When Mary Mallon arrived, there were sixteen buildings on
the island, which ultimately doubled to thirty-two (see fig. 6.3).
Half of the buildings were already aging in 1907, having been
built around the time the island saw its first contagious disease

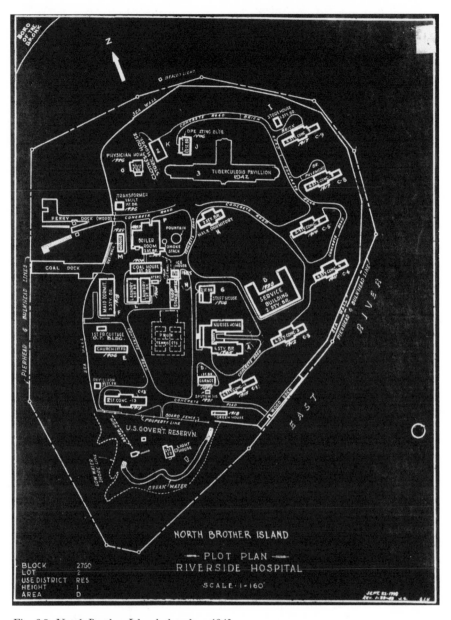

Fig. 6.3. *North Brother Island plot plan, 1943.*

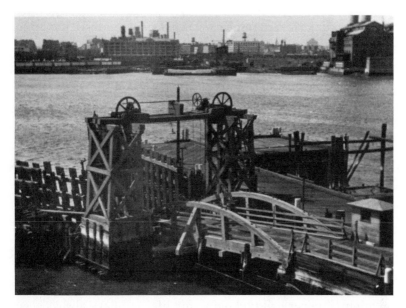

Fig. 6.4. *View from North Brother Island showing the Bronx and the East River, date unknown.*

patients in 1885, and the rest had been built in the past three years.[49] Mary Mallon may have lived in two different buildings during her first confinement, the main one of which was a small building near the chapel.[50] Her view, if she looked off the island toward the docks, was of the Bronx looming across the river (see fig. 6.4). She later told an associate that before she moved there, she knew the island, as did most New Yorkers of the period, as the site of the disastrous sinking of the *General Slocum* steamboat, during a fiery accident in June, 1904, in which over one thousand German-born New Yorkers on a pleasure outing had drowned.[51]

The only extant health department records of Mary Mallon's early years on North Brother Island indicate that her stools underwent repeated and frequent analysis (see chap. 1). There is no evidence beyond Soper's account of his own attempts to explain the situation to Mary Mallon that officials tried to implement for her a program of education or rehabilitation. Given Mallon's strong resistance to being held at Willard Parker Hospital and her determined resolve to keep her own counsel, it is probable that officials initially wanted to study the laboratory reports and meanwhile give Mallon time to cool off. If they had plans beyond this, they left no records of them, nor did they implement any efforts to try to return Mary Mallon to the community.

At the time of her habeas corpus hearing in 1909, the media spread the story that Mary Mallon had been confined alone during her early years on North Brother Island. "She says she has been kept like a leper for the last two years, with only a dog for company," wrote the reporter for the (New York) *Sun*: "She says that her food has been shoved through the door three times a day by a nurse, who immediately ran away."[52] The *New York American*, especially, portrayed the injustice of an attractive and healthy woman, at mid-career, living out her days in complete isolation. "I never had typhoid in my life, and have always been healthy," the reporter quoted from his interview with Mary Mallon. "Why should I be banished like a leper and compelled to live in solitary confinement with only a dog for a companion?" The reporter believed that her appearance in court was "the first time in two years she had been released from the cabin on North Brother Island." The reporter quoted Mallon as saying:

This contention that I am a perpetual menace in the spread of typhoid germs is not true. My own doctors say I have no typhoid germs. I am an innocent human being. I have committed no crime and I am treated like an outcast—a criminal. It is unjust, outrageous, uncivilized. It seems incredible that in a Christian community a defenseless woman can be treated in this manner.

The *American* reporter insisted that on the island "a keeper, three times each day, brings food to her door and then flees as if from a pestilence." The news account claimed that Mallon's "chief fear" during her years on the island was that doctors would "etherize her and perform a surgical operation to prove their theory."[53]

We recognize in this account the voice of a woman who perceived herself to be alone in a hostile world in which she could trust no one and in which she had no allies. The *American* reporter gave her, for the first time in twenty-six months, a sympathetic audience. She could hope that with a lawyer speaking for her and an eager media ready to believe her it might be possible to return to the life she had been forced abruptly to abandon. If she exaggerated her situation in describing the degree of her isolation, it was in the cause of producing sympathy for her attempt to gain her freedom.

Although alone in her cottage, Mary Mallon probably had more opportunities to mingle with nurses, physicians, and possibly tuberculosis patients on the island than these accounts indicate, though unfortunately, there is no logbook record of daily activities on North Brother Island for these early isolation years, either inside or outside of Riverside Hospital.[54] The photographs published in the *American* themselves belied the text, in purporting to show Mary Mallon sitting in the sun with other patients or eating in the common dining room (see chap. 5). Furthermore, there would have been no medical or public health reason to keep Mary Mallon from wandering around the island and seeking companionship.

It is probable that in the early days, weeks, and even months of her stay on North Brother Island that Mallon was in no mood to seek social encounters or graciously receive approaches of friendship. It is also possible that word of her dangers had seeped into island gossip, and that many people went out of their way to avoid her. But there is also some evidence to suggest that, despite such possible barriers, Mallon made friends during the years of her first incarceration and that she interacted socially with at least a few others on the island.

In an interview with a reporter from the *New York World*, Mallon depicted her days as including social interactions. The reporter sympathized with Mallon's "imprisonment which would drive most people insane," but portrayed a less onerous imprisonment than the other newspapers:

Mary Mallon is permitted the freedom of the island, and the doctors are glad to have her nurse the children who are there with every kind of contagious disease. . . . Not only does she nurse them but she prepares their meals. She is allowed to mingle freely with all the other patients on the island and she is employed by both doctors and nurses to do their finer pieces of laundry for them. Doctors and nurses on the Island frequently go to her room and eat the good things she has cooked.[55]

It is hard to believe this description. Just as the *American* portrayal of a woman totally isolated from all human contact seems overdrawn, this one suggesting Mallon often prepared food for others is also suspect. Food preparation was the specific known way that Mallon was said to have transmitted typhoid fever. Her days on the island probably fall somewhere between the two accounts. She described her daily routine to the *World* reporter in these terms: "I get up in the morning, fix my room, eat my breakfast, and then wait until it is time to go to bed again. Often I help nurse the other patients on the Island and often the children will have no one else take care of them when they are very sick."[56] This part of her story, which includes no food preparation, seems believable, especially when compared to descriptions of the years of her second incarceration (see below).

A nurse later confirmed that her acquaintance and ultimate friendship with Mary Mallon began in these months immediately following Mallon's 1907 arrival on the island, clear evidence that Mallon did not live completely unconnected to others. Adelaide Jane Offspring, a registered nurse employed at Riverside Hospital, wrote that she "met Mary Mallon . . . at the said Riverside Hospital in 1907," and that she was "in constant and intimate association" with her during all the years the two were on

the island together, 1907 to 1910, and 1915 until Offspring's retirement in 1935. Offspring returned to the island in 1938 to
nurse Mallon through her final illness. The nurse wrote that
Mallon "was freely permitted to have visitors."[57]

Mary Mallon claimed only a few friends when she wrote her
will in 1933, and Offspring seemed to be closest to her. Mallon
made Offspring the executor of the will, and, after designating a
few small gifts to others, bequeathed everything to her. Mallon
left her money and valuables to her friend, "in appreciation of the
many courtesies and kindnesses which she has extended to me
during the association of twenty-six years."[58] The sullen temper
Mallon showed to health authorities obviously did not extend to
all of her social encounters.

During the years from March, 1907, until her February,
1910, release, Mallon did not have any formal employment on
North Brother Island, or any formal demands placed on her. She
had considerable time to think about her situation, which seemed
merely to harden her resistance to the health department. She
told reporters in 1909 that she felt there were "two kinds of justice in America." The kind meted out to her did not give the benefit of reasonable doubt that even "murderers" were permitted,
but rather she was "flung into prison without a fair trial, denied
the privilege of seeing her lawyer and given no chance to clear
herself." From this, Mallon concluded, "All the water in the
ocean wouldn't clear me from this charge, in the eyes of the
Health Department. They want to make a showing; they want to
get credit for protecting the rich, and I am the victim."[59]

Most who observed and commented on Mallon's situation
and on that of other healthy carriers did not mention the possibility of class biases in any way affecting their treatment as Mallon voiced here. One exception was the socialist newspaper, the
New York Call, and a second was the antivivisectionists' magazine, *The Starry Cross*. The latter wrote: "There is one common

characteristic of carriers, it never varies; they are always plain people in humble circumstances; those with more money and influence who could fight back are never pronounced dangerous."[60]

In addition to the clear class antagonism evident in Mallon's words, she voiced particular animosity toward Soper, whose report on the seven families in which she had allegedly spread typhoid seemed to her to be completely unfair. "He did not see fit to mention the family I always lived with in the Bronx when I was out of work, and where I slept with the children without ever giving them typhoid," she told the *World* reporter. "Will I submit quietly to staying here a prisoner all my life?" Mallon asked rhetorically. "No! As there is a God in Heaven I will get justice, somehow, sometime."[61]

In these 1909 statements, Mallon revealed that "every time the Health Department examines me I send specimens by a friend to a specialist in New York." The friend in this case was A. Briehof, the man Mallon had been living with when Soper located her in March, 1907. Mallon used the Ferguson laboratory to build her own case, wisely choosing a laboratory operated by a professor at the respected New York College of Pharmacy.[62] She was triumphant about Ferguson's findings: "The Health Department report always comes back stating that the typhus [*sic*] bacilli have been found. From the same specimens my own specialist, who is at the head of his profession, reports that he had found none."[63] In 1909, as in 1907, Mary Mallon had continuing reason to doubt the medical evidence behind her forcible incarceration.

For both medical and personal reasons, then, Mallon refused to accept the authority of science purporting to explain her situation and necessitate her isolation. She continued to protest her banishment. She may have found it useful to refer to herself as a victim of discrimination and unjust government forces amassed against her, but most of her language and behavior in 1909 belied passive victimhood. Although captive to the greater force of the state, Mallon behaved as a feisty and still disbelieving and angry woman actively trying to change her fate. She understood her position in opposition to the health department, and she found logic, reason, and even science on her side.

It occurred to Mary Mallon that authorities should have tried to rehabilitate her to return her to society. In her July, 1909, letter, one first intended for the editor of the *New York American* to respond to the June 20 story, but which she redirected to her lawyer, and which remains today with the court record, she wrote, "There was never any effort by the Board authority to do anything for me excepting to cast me on the Island & keep me a prisoner." Because this letter remains one of the very few instances of Mallon's own words and handwriting to survive, it is worth close examination.[64]

Mallon wrote, "When I first came here I was so nervous & almost prostrated with grief & trouble my eyes began to twitch & the left eye did become Paralized & would not move remained in that condition for Six Months[.]" Mallon recognized her poor mental state immediately following her capture, and she had certain expectations that her hospitalization would at least provide access to some needed medical care. While she did not feel she needed medical attention for her carrier state, she did seek it for other ailments that developed. "[T]here was an eye Specialist visited the Island 3 & 4 times a week he was never asked to visit me[.] I did not even get a cover for my eye had to hold my hand on it whilst going about & at night tie a bandage on it." The eye continued to bother her. In December, 1907, a new physician, Dr. Wilson, "took charge."[65] Mallon wrote, "I told him about it he said that was news to him & that he would send me his Electrick battery *but he never sent* [it.]" Her frustration about this problem abated when "my eye got better thanks to the *Almighty God* In spite of the medical staff[.]"

From Mallon's account, physicians did attend to her typhoid infectivity. They tried various remedies, including treating her unsuccessfully with urotropin (see chap. 1), and then considered releasing her. "When in January [1908] they were about to discharge me when the resident Physician came to me & asked me where was I going when I got out of here naturally I said to N.Y. so there was a stop put to my getting out of here then the Supervising Nurse told me I was a hopeless case & if Id write to [health commissioner] Dr. Darlington & tell him Id go to my Sisters in Connecticut." Mallon refused to state what was not true: "Now I have no Sister in that state or any other in the U.S."[66]

Instead of being released, Mallon got a bureaucratic runaround. "Then in April [1908] a friend of mine went to Dr. Darlington & asked him when [I] was to get away he replied that woman is all right now & she is a very expensive woman but I cannot let her go my self the Board has to sit." The friend was Briehof, who was told, Mallon said, to "come around Saturday[.] When he did Dr. Darlington told this man Ive nothing more to do with this woman go to Dr. Studiford [sic] [.][67] He went to that Doctor," Mallon continued, "& he said I cannot let that woman go & all the people that she gave the typhoid to & so many deaths occurred in the families she was with."[68]

The only chance Studdiford provided for Mallon to be released, according to Mallon's account, was "to have an Operation performed to have her Gall Bladder removed." The physician asked Briehof to convince Mallon to undergo the surgery. (As we have seen, most physicians at the time regarded such surgery as risky and not likely to relieve the carrier condition.) He told Briehof, according to Mallon,

She'll have the best Surgeon in town to do the Cutting. I said no[.] no Knife will be put on me I've nothing the matter with my gall bladder. Dr. Wilson asked me the very same question I also told him no then he replied it might not do you any good also the Supervising nurse asked me to have an operation performed. I also told her no & she made the remark would it not be better for you to have it done than remain here I told her no.[69]

Mallon continued to refuse surgery, seeing it as part of a plot against her. She wanted to be freed, but not at such a risk. Obviously, she valued her life, even within its severe restraints.

Then, in October, 1908, another physician visited Mallon on North Brother Island. "[H]e did take quite an interest in me he really thought I liked it here that I did not care for my freedom." Although Mallon set him straight on that issue, she did promise him to try some more medicine. But she was tired of the experiments. She wrote, "I have been in fact a peep show for Every body even the Internes had to come to see me & ask about the facts alredy Known to the whole wide World[.]" She did not like being exhibited: "the Tuberculosis men would say there she is the Kidnapped woman[.]" She resented William Park's lecture describing her situation to the American Medical Association in Chicago: "Dr Parks has had me Illustrated in Chicago I wonder how the Said Dr Wm H. Park would like to be insulted and put in the Journal & call him or his wife Typhoid William Park" (see fig. 6.5).

Mallon's July, 1909, letter and her public statements to reporters reveal a woman still confused and upset by the events that took over her life two years earlier. She had a fairly sophisticated understanding of how the term Typhoid Mary had obscured her individuality, and she was aware that she did not have the full attention of health officials to her plight. They thoroughly examined her feces and urged her to undergo a surgical procedure, but they did not give careful consideration to her other physical complaints or to the adversity of her constrained life as a prisoner on the island. In the letter, Mallon sounds cynical and defeated, attitudes that seem to have overtaken her initial anger and resistance. These sentiments must have been strengthened in July, 1909, when the judge sent her back to the island, this time with little hope of release.

Seven months later, though, in February, 1910, Health Com-

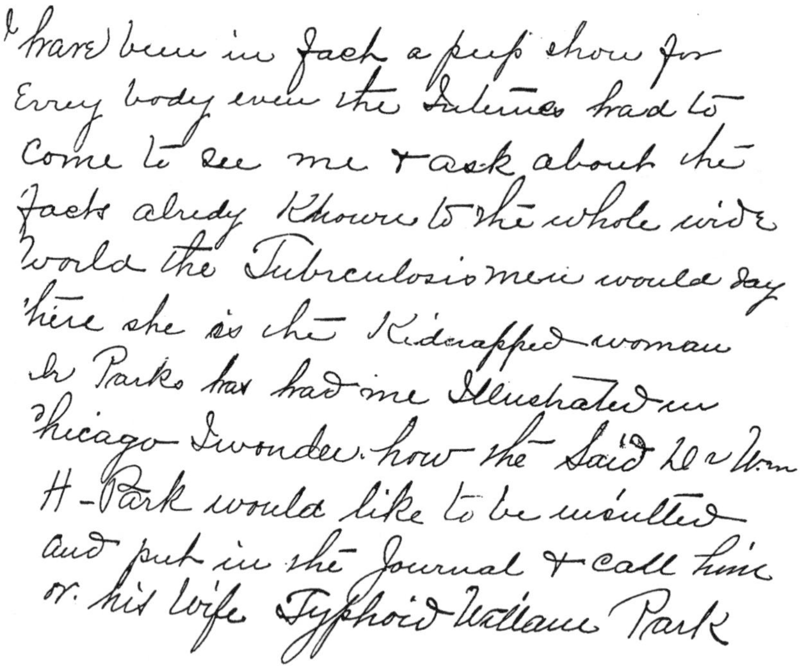

I have been in fact a peep show for Every body even the Internes had to come to see me & ask about the facts alredy Known to the whole wide world the Tubreulosis men would say here she is the Kidnapped woman Dr Parks has had me Illustrated in Chicago I wonder how the Said Dr Wm H.-Park would like to be insulted and put in the Journal & call him or his wife Typhoid William Park

Fig. 6.5. *Excerpt from Mary Mallon letter, 1909.*

missioner Ernst J. Lederle, with the approval of the board of health, did release Mary Mallon and allow her to return to Manhattan and to those parts of her former life that did not involve cooking. George Francis O'Neill, Mallon's lawyer, precipitated the release when he wrote the new commissioner immediately after his appointment in January to call his attention to Mallon's incarceration. The conditions of her release, which she agreed to, were that she "is prepared to change her occupation (that of cook), and will give assurance by affidavit that she will upon her release take such hygienic precautions as will protect those with whom she comes in contact, from infection." In signing the agreement on February 19, 1910, Mary Mallon swore, "I have read and considered the said [board of health] resolution and am willing to abide by the provisions thereof." Her statement promised, "I shall change said occupation upon being released from

Riverside Hospital." While agreeing to "take measures to protect any and all persons with whom I may come in contact from any infection," Mallon's statement added the phrase, "which it is possible I may cause."[70]

Aware of her previous denial that she had transmitted typhoid fever to anyone, the added phrase resonates loudly. Even as she capitulated in a sworn statement that she would not again cook for other people, Mallon equivocated. She was not yet convinced of her culpability.

We do not know what Mallon was thinking at the time she signed the legal document binding her to change her career. Newspapers reported her release from the island, but no reporter interviewed her. Lederle issued a statement to the press about his sympathy for her: "I have taken a personal interest in her case and I am doing what I can for her," he told the *New York Times*. "She is a good cook and until her detention had always made a comfortable living. Now she is debarred from it, and I really do not know what she can do." Lederle said he knew where she was, but he did not divulge that information.[71] Commissioner Lederle told an *American* reporter, "She was incarcerated for the public's good, and now it is up to the public to take care of her."[72]

It is not possible for us to answer with certainty why Mary Mallon agreed to the conditions set forth by the health authorities if she still had doubts about her guilt in spreading disease. Perhaps, after refusing a year before to say that she would go to live with a sister in Connecticut, she overcame such reluctance to stretch the truth, and she signed the statement realizing it was an overstatement of what she intended. A lie seemed a smaller risk than surgery. Or perhaps Lederle had convinced her that she could find employment and adequate income without returning to cooking. Whatever her reasoning, she did convince Lederle that she would desist from cooking in return for her freedom. But as Lederle realized, what was she to do? And where was she to do it?

Apparently, Mallon found ways to comply with the agreement for a few years and prepared no food from her release in February, 1910, through December, 1911, almost two years, and probably through September, 1912.[73] But she claimed at the end of 1911 that since her release in February, 1910, "she ha[d] been unable to follow her trade of cooking, and her chances of making a living have been greatly reduced." Because of her lost wages and status in the labor market, she brought a damage suit for false imprisonment against the city and the board of health again with the help of lawyer George Francis O'Neill.[74] The suit was dropped, for reasons we cannot recover, and Mallon went on struggling to find gainful employment outside her area of expertise. Despite Lederle's compassionate support and his immediate help with finding a job in a laundry, he did not provide continuing practical help over time.[75]

Soper misrepresented Mallon's behavior in this period when he wrote, "On her release Mary promptly disappeared. She violated every detail of the pledge she had given to the Department of Health."[76] But it was not until November, 1914, that the health department admitted that Mallon, like many other typhoid carriers it traced, "ha[d] now been lost sight of."[77] Sometime between September, 1912, when health officials voiced confidence that they had acted wisely in releasing her from detention, and November, 1914, when they first made public that they no longer knew where she was, Mallon, probably finding it impossible to make a living by any other means, returned to cooking. Soper claimed that Mallon had cooked for a private family in Newfoundland, New Jersey, sometime in 1913 and worked in a sanatorium in the same town in 1914. The health department added that she may have worked in an inn in New Jersey in 1913 and 1914. Soper also thought he located her cooking for a small family in New York City in 1914. He said that six cases of typhoid fever resulted from these employments, but he provided no details or evidence that Mary Mallon was indeed the culprit. He also did not add these cases into his own totals for the cases traced to Mary Mallon.[78] We cannot independently confirm Mallon's return to cooking until October, 1914, when the Sloane Maternity Hospital in Manhattan hired a Mrs. Brown as a new cook. The hospital suffered an outbreak of twenty-five cases of typhoid fever in January and February of 1915, which officials subsequently traced to the cook, whom they identified as Mary Mallon.[79] Health officials located her in March, 1915, and returned her to the same cottage she had previously occupied on North Brother Island.[80]

What led Mary Mallon back into the kitchen in 1914? For one thing, sometime during this period her companion Briehof died.[81] Although he may have betrayed her to Soper in 1907, he had stood by her throughout her incarceration and had acted as her laboratory specimen courier. His death added to her financial and emotional vulnerability. Perhaps more significant, she was repeatedly unsuccessful in finding satisfying and rewarding work, as she had already indicated, and she must have felt she had no choice but to return to the work at which she knew she could make a good living. It is possible that she tried cooking for others, and when no one got sick she was reassured and felt safe taking a job at a maternity hospital. It is more likely, though, given the attitude she later expressed, that she continued to deny, to herself and to others, that she ever transmitted typhoid fever. Whatever Mallon's reasons, we know that these years following her 1910 release were not easy for her, and she moved around seeking work. She would not have been inclined, given her previous experiences, to ask the health department to help her. It is probable, however, that once the sympathetic Lederle stepped down at the end of 1913, officials would not have been inclined to offer such help, since in these years no policy of subsidizing or systematically helping carriers was yet in place.

There is no evidence that Mallon returned to cooking willfully knowing she would infect and probably kill people. Such a conclusion would not fit what we know about her life before or after her isolation. She may have been sullen and moody in her responses to health officials, she may have been hot tempered and greatly angered by her isolation, she may have refused to believe her carrier condition, she may have been desperate for work, but there is nothing to suggest that she was a purposeful destroyer of life.[82]

Mallon's use of the pseudonym "Mrs. Brown" at the Sloane Hospital was a seemingly deliberate deception, one that convinced Soper and others that she knew what she was doing and that she deserved to be detained. She certainly knew that the health authorities believed that she should not be working in people's kitchens. But there is no reason to think that she herself had come to agree with the view of herself as dangerous to the public's health, especially if she had, as was likely during the years of her freedom, cooked for people who did not get sick and die. In using a pseudonym she may not have been showing a disregard for public safety but rather her contempt for and disbelief in the new science.[83]

After her return in March, 1915, Mary Mallon's life on North Brother Island eased somewhat. Five new four-and-one-half-story concrete buildings, housing 240 patients, had been added to the facilities, and building continued apace.[84] She resumed her friendship with Adelaide Offspring, and she interacted with others. Whatever question existed about her social interactions between 1907 and 1910, it is clear that after 1915 Mary Mallon had the freedom to leave her one-room bungalow and walk around the island. She started a cottage industry of making and selling goods to hospital employees. George Edington, who grew up on the island and was the son of Edmund Edington, an engineer on the ambulance boat that shuttled between the Bronx and the island, and Edmund's wife, a waitress in the doctor's dining room, recalled that "Mrs. Mallon baked cakes which she sold to the other women who worked on the island." It seems incredible that health officials might have permitted this, but Edington was very clear: "My mother explained that the City provided nothing but her room and board, and that she was a cook by profession." Edington also remembered a safer occupation: "Mrs. Mallon also did bead work and for a long time my mother had a choker of tiny blue beads that she had made."[85]

There were other people with whom Mallon interacted in these years. Adele Leadley, who called herself "a friend and correspondent of Mary's for more than thirty-eight years," shared an interest in the "many hundreds of letters [Mallon] received from all over the world regarding her unusual case."[86] Mallon continued to write threatening letters to Hermann Biggs and S. Josephine Baker, both of whom she blamed for her isolation. Although the letters no longer exist, Biggs's biographer, C.-E. A. Winslow, who had access to Biggs's papers, which have since disappeared, wrote that Mallon "wrote Dr. Biggs the most violently threatening letters." Baker wrote in her autobiography that "she had threatened to kill me if she could get out." Both statements give insight into Mallon's frame of mind during her years of isolation, but bear no relationship to her actions during the years she was free.[87] She kept in contact with the Lempe family of Woodside, Long Island: Mary Lempe, "my friend" to whom Mallon bequeathed "all my clothing and personal effects now located in the bungalow where I reside on North Brother Island," and Willie Lempe, her son, upon whom Mallon bestowed $200. The Lempes may have been the family that Mallon stayed with when she was not employed.[88] One of the porters on the island was Tom Cane, "a charming middle-aged man with an Irish accent," who frequently stopped by to "chat" with Mallon.[89]

Two things changed most drastically for Mary Mallon during the years of her second isolation. In 1918, Mallon began gainful employment in the hospital as a domestic worker. In 1922, her title changed to "nurse," and later to "hospital helper." Sometime around 1925 she began to assist in the hospital laboratory.[90] Also in 1918, authorities began to permit Mallon to take "time off for shopping" with day trips off the island. This gendered comment about reasons for Mallon to temporarily leave the island indicated increasing trust that she would return, and her cooperation justified continuing the practice.[91]

We do not know Mallon's actual duties as a worker in the hospital, or how they changed with the title changes. We do know that her employment did not drastically alter her attitude toward health authorities. In January, 1919, Mallon "refused to Submit stool specimens for examination." A clerk in the division of epidemiology sought advice about this situation, saying "Mary Malon [sic] is loath to give any speciments [sic] of her stools claiming she does not see any improvement in her case and thinks it is useless." The health commissioner penned in the margin, "use persuasive methods."[92] Mallon resumed giving stool samples, but she never accepted her role in transmitting disease.[93]

Mallon's employment and off-island visits provided opportunities for friendships to blossom. Her relationship with the Lempe family continued during these years, and she probably visited them on some of her day trips.[94] Another friendship that was particularly important to her was with a resident physician, Dr. Alexandra Plavska, who interned at Riverside Hospital in the middle of the 1920s and who hired Mallon as her laboratory assistant. Dr. Plavska was a 1917 graduate of the University of Moscow school of medicine. She immigrated to the United States and worked in the bacteriology laboratory beginning (it seems) in 1925, and, in 1927, when she was licensed to practice medicine in New York, opened a private gynecology practice in Manhattan.[95] Mallon appreciated her laboratory job and remembered Plavska in her will, in which she bequeathed her $200 in memory of their association in the laboratory. She described Plavska as a "beautiful person" who was always very kind and who "believed in her."[96] According to Plavska's daughter, the two became "close friends." Mallon visited their home when she was able to leave the island on day trips, and the Plavskas returned the visits once

Mallon was confined to the hospital by her stroke. Plavska and her daughter attended Mallon's funeral.[97]

In 1929, two years after Plavska left Riverside Hospital, a young Hunter College graduate, Emma Rose Goldberg (soon to be Sherman), took a job as laboratory technician and bacteriologist at North Brother Island.[98] She set up a laboratory on the second floor of the old chapel, and Mary Mallon worked with her from then until her stroke almost four years later. According to Sherman, Mallon did general cleaning up, bottle washing, and assisted with sputum smears and urine analysis, as she had done in the laboratory previously when she worked with Plavska. Sherman felt that Mallon's work was not very reliable (in fact, she called it "slipshod"), and she repeated most of the tests herself. But Sherman understood that the laboratory work was very important to Mallon who thought she was making a contribution. The two got along well, despite the great differences in their age, education, and experiences. Sherman said that Mallon was not forthcoming with information about her life. Sherman observed Mallon walking around the hospital grounds and talking with a nurse friend, probably Offspring, further confirmation of her continuing social interactions.

As long as typhoid fever was not a topic of conversation, Sherman disclosed, Mallon was pleasant to be with. But she would not talk about typhoid and continued to show anger and distrust of health department officials. Sherman revealed that the doctors and nurses, out of Mallon's presence, referred to her as Typhoid Mary but never would do so to her face. If they had, Sherman believed, Mallon "would have become physically violent."[99] As Soper had noted, "Nobody ever talked to her about anything she did not want to talk about."[100] Emma Sherman, feeling the same unease, let Mary Mallon choose the topics they would talk about. Sherman remembered that Mallon remained "hostile" when she referred to health authorities and to her isolation on the island. After a day trip off the island, Mallon sometimes presented Sherman with a shiny apple as a friend might, but Sherman knew her colleague was a carrier of typhoid fever, and put it away without eating it.[101]

One day sometime in 1931 or 1932, Sherman and Mallon had their photograph taken (see fig. 6.6). The photograph reveals two women in white laboratory coats: petite and young Emma Sherman and Mary Mallon, showing her age, weight gain, and the possible effects of minor strokes that preceded her massive one. Mallon's smile was distorted, Sherman says, by the loss of teeth as well as possible nerve damage. Sherman tried to get Mallon to see a dentist, but she always refused. She did not seek medical attention, and indicated she did not trust it.

Because of all the media commentary on Mallon's large physical size, I want to examine this photograph closely. It is hard to see in this photograph the Mary Mallon of the 1909 photograph. Sherman was short, under five feet; Mallon is one and one-half bricks taller, approximately five feet four inches in the photo, perhaps down a few inches from, but confirming, what Soper said was five feet six inches when he first met her in 1907. The average height of women in this period was five feet four and one-half inches, indicating that Mallon in her prime was only one and one-half inches taller than average.[102] The photograph shows the elderly Mallon as a heavy-set woman, but even so she does not appear to be a 200-pound "Amazon," as reporters described her in 1907 and 1909, when she likely would have weighed less. One suspects they must have exaggerated her physical appearance as huge in light of their perceptions of her personality.

Sherman said that on the days when Mary Mallon left the island to visit friends, she dressed up and looked "quite stunning, and she returned in good spirits." She described Mallon as a steady worker in the sense of always being on time and dependable in her habits. Each morning she would climb the stairs to the laboratory, where she had her own desk and work area. Other observers of Mallon during these later years agreed that "she has

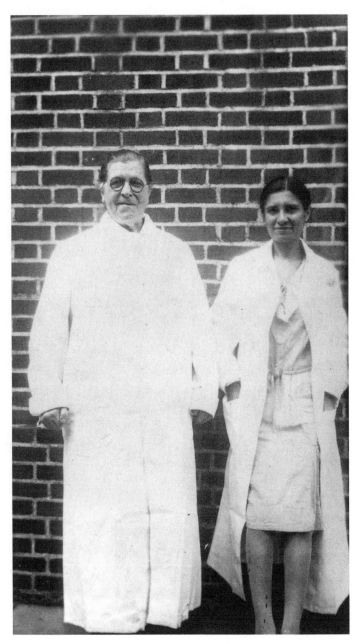

Fig. 6.6 *Emma Sherman (right) and Mary Mallon, North Brother Island, 1931 or 1932.*

apparently been satisfied with her life at Riverside Hospital."[103] From the time she began her laboratory work, Mallon seems to have settled down to the routine of her life on the island, and found some personal satisfaction.[104]

Stanley Walker visited Mallon's cottage in 1935 (after Mallon no longer lived in it), and provided a description: "A plot of lawn surrounds the cottage. There is an elm in front. The cottage is about twenty feet by twenty, a one-story affair with green-shingled walls, which are decorated with white trimmings around the windows and doors." He revealed, "Mary lived in the one large room, where she could entertain friends. There was a large oak table in the centre, old-fashioned rocking chairs with cane seats and backs, old colored prints on the walls, and a cot at the south side of the room, where Mary slept." The back of the house contained a bathroom and small kitchen. Walker made it sound almost cozy, and he concluded, "This was better than freedom." There is no evidence that Mallon shared his sentiment.[105]

According to Sherman, Mallon never became convinced that she transmitted typhoid fever. Sherman said, "She said [the health officials] didn't know what they were talking about and that they picked on her and that there was nothing wrong with her. That's the way she put it, that they picked on her and she was healthy and how could she make people sick when she's healthy." Whatever efforts officials might have made earlier to convince her of her public health danger, toward the end of her life these stopped. Sherman thought the doctors on the island "were completely indifferent to her. They let her alone. . . . No doctor that I know of ever went to visit her and discuss anything with her." Mallon thought the health department took advantage of her and blamed her for things that were never "my fault." Officials "stuck her away for a reason she couldn't accept." To the end of her life Mallon denied her role in making others sick; as Sherman said, "She denied it to her teeth."[106]

One day, probably December 4, 1932, Mallon did not come to

work on time.[107] Sherman, knowing her work record, became worried, and went over to the bungalow, into which she had ventured only briefly before. She found Mallon lying on the floor, having suffered a stroke. She later reported that the cottage had not been well cared for, and that it smelled badly. Mallon was then removed to a bed in the children's ward in the hospital. From that hospital bed, "considering the uncertainty of this life," Mallon dictated her will to an attorney, on July 14, 1933.[108] She remained bedridden and hospitalized the rest of her life. Adelaide Offspring returned to Riverside to attend Mallon during her last week. Mary Mallon died on November 11, 1938.[109]

Some of Mary Mallon's friends attended her funeral, indicating that her associations with them continued into her final years. The people at the funeral mass at St. Luke's Church in the Bronx, who refused to identify themselves to reporters, were identified by Adelaide Jane Offspring as herself, Mary Lempe, Willie Lempe, Joseph Lempe (another son of Mary Lempe's) and his wife, Alexandra Plavska, and Plavska's daughter. Although the newspaper indicated nine people attended, Offspring mentioned only these seven. Four of them (Offspring, Mary and Willie Lempe, and Alexandra Plavska) were Mallon's beneficiaries, along with the Catholic Charities of the Archdiocese of New York and Father Michael Lucy, who had regularly visited Mallon once she was bedridden.[110]

Mary Mallon, whose own estate paid for the gravestone that read "Jesus Mercy" (see fig. 6.7), ultimately became resigned to her life on North Brother Island, and left positive memories with the people who knew her during her final years. But she never came to terms with her status as a healthy carrier, and she railed against the label Typhoid Mary.[111]

Mary Mallon denied throughout her life that she transmitted typhoid fever to people for whom she cooked. Despite working for seven or eight years in a bacteriology laboratory preparing sputum slides for physicians to use in the medical diagnoses of tuber-

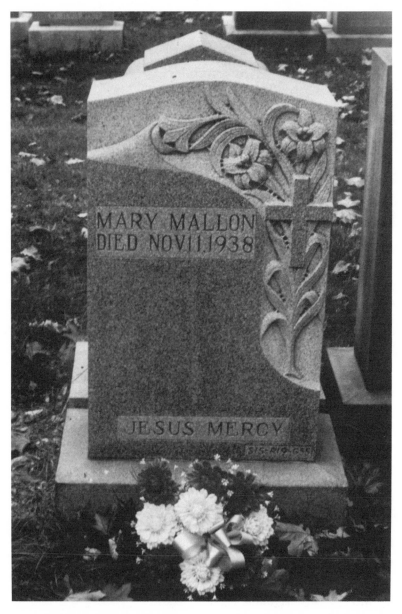

Fig. 6.7. *Mary Mallon's tombstone, St. Raymond's Cemetery, the Bronx.*

culosis, she never came to understand the connection between the sputum that carried tuberculosis bacilli and her own gallbladder that carried typhoid bacilli. She did not accept that she was dangerous to others. It may be hard for us today to see her resistance, at least by 1915 and thereafter, as anything other than a stubborn refusal to admit what she must have come to know was true. But the vehemence of her temper about the subject of typhoid fever and her lifelong refusal to engage in discussions about it indicate that her obstinacy was not a sham; it is very likely she continued until her death to believe she was not a carrier.

Mary Mallon felt deeply and, I think, honestly that she was not what the label "Typhoid Mary" signified. She never believed that the attributes associated with the label applied to her. She was not dirty or shiftless; her life had been, before health officials interfered, an example of hard work and skilled achievement. Furthermore, until her stroke, she was always in excellent health, which the Ferguson laboratory tests confirmed by finding no typhoid infection. In rejecting the stigma that Typhoid Mary represented, as well as the concept of healthy carrier that accompanied it, Mary Mallon refused to acquiesce or consent to her loss of freedom. She took comfort in her few friends and kept her distance from the rest of the world, secure in her beliefs.

Health authorities saw Typhoid Mary as someone who was a threat to their efforts to preserve the public's health; Mary Mallon saw health officials as persecutors who unfairly took away her identity, her independence, and her ability to earn a living. Neither view is entirely right; both, nonetheless, had a point.

"Mis-
begotten   *The Stories Continue*
Mary"

*M*ary Mallon's story has, over time, struck a sensitive chord with Americans, evoking strong and long-lasting impressions. The term Typhoid Mary has entered the English language as a phrase independent of Mary Mallon herself. The range of meanings applied to the person and the phrase, created and used throughout her life, has continued to resonate since her death in 1938. Soper's story of tracing and finding North America's first identified typhoid fever carrier and Mary Mallon's 1907 capture and 1915 recapture have been often repeated in medical literature and the popular media. As with reports made during her lifetime, small misrepresentations in these later accounts alter and dramatize her story. But these modern stories are more interesting for their perpetuation of the concept of Typhoid Mary and the threat of contagion and pollution the term has come to evoke than for adding any details to our understanding of Mallon's life. Their perspective is the final one examined in this book, the cultural persistence and long-term tenacity of Mary Mallon. Her life ended in 1938; her story and its meanings live on.

The post-1938 representations of Typhoid Mary can be usefully divided into two chronological groups. Those written before the time when HIV and other newly emerging viruses became known examined Mallon's story out of curiosity or human interest and frequently used it to teach an audience how much science had contributed to improving the quality of modern life. The attention given to Mary Mallon after the first cases of AIDS were publicized focus instead on the risks people can still pose to one another and try to find practical messages in her story. These accounts also examine the key dilemma her story poses, how to protect the public's health and at the same time maintain the rights and freedoms of individuals. Throughout both periods the phrase Typhoid Mary continues to refer to a person to be feared and shunned, someone who carries contagion inside her body and uses it to harm people around her. Even the most recent portrayals, again following the trends of their times, which strive to find strength and some agency in the individual woman herself, have to come to terms with the deadly meaning of the metaphor.

Fourteen years after Mallon's death, *New Yorker* medical writer Berton Roueché in his popular "Annals of Medicine" series of medical detection tales chronicled a 1946 typhoid fever epidemic in New York City.[1] His epidemiological adventure revealed how the epidemic was finally traced to a healthy carrier. Roueché's articles typically championed medical successes, and this one fit his pattern of highlighting the effective work of New York City's Bureau of Preventable Diseases. In teaching his readers about typhoid carriers, Roueché wrote, "Typhoid Mary Mallon, a housemaid and cook who was the stubborn cause of a total of fifty-three [*sic*] cases in and around New York City a generation ago, is, of course, the most celebrated of these hapless menaces."[2] Three parts of this sentence are significant. One, Roueché combined Typhoid Mary and Mary Mallon as if they were one name. The epithet and the woman merge and are indistinguishable. Two, he referred to Mallon as the "stubborn cause" of transmitting typhoid fever. He found her culpable. Yet, and this is the third observation, he also described carriers—generally—as "hapless menaces." They were dangerous but blameless.

Roueché's observations echoed common usages. He saw Mallon as part-concept, part-human, and in his merging of phrase and name he continued the dehumanization that had begun immediately following her 1907 incarceration. In the same vein, he found Mallon guilty of actions that caused harm to others while he acknowledged that most carriers were cooperative and would not purposely harm others. He, like many writers before and since, set Mary Mallon apart from other carriers and used her story to illustrate the benefits of modern science.[3]

Also during the 1950s, Madelyn Carlisle reminded *Coronet* readers of "the strange story of the innocent killer." The author emphasized the march of medical progress as she recounted Mallon's story mainly in terms of George Soper's heroism. She described Soper as a "health expert" who had a "burning hatred of typhoid fever" and through whose "patient investigation" the bizarre tale unfolded and was solved. Carlisle concluded that, "though the case was strange and the action regrettable, it was right that a public menace be imprisoned." Mary Mallon, the author thought, rightfully spent the remainder of her life in "penance" for the lives she had endangered.[4]

The illustration accompanying Carlisle's article underscored the title's "strange" and added a furrowed brow of guilt. Here a distressed and anxious woman looks up from her cooking, worried perhaps about the harmful effects she causes (see fig. 7.1). She might not be purposeful in her actions, yet she clearly has something to worry about. In this drawing readers saw their own anxiety projected onto the face of the cook.

A few years later, M. F. King, writing in the *American Mercury*, depicted a more clearly guilty "Irish Pariah" whose "bacillus ridden body proved to be a major breakthrough for modern preventive medicine." King told Mallon's story in a way that emphasized the cook's confusion and deception and ended in her personal defeat. When Mallon was returned to North Brother Island in 1915, King wrote, she was "now terrified by the awful knowledge of her guilt." Through her ordeal, he claimed, "the basic secret of typhoid fever germs was made known to medical

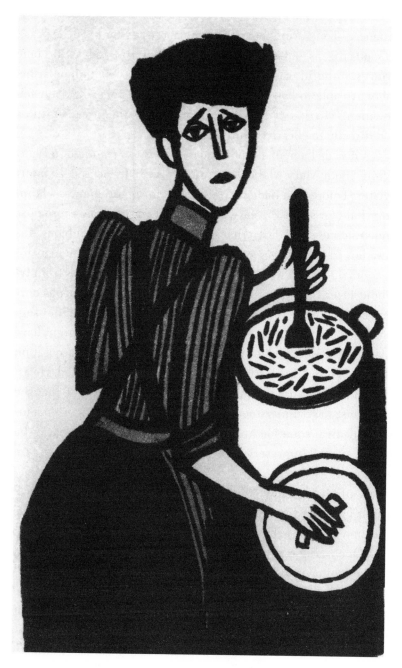

Fig. 7.1 *Mary Mallon, "Innocent Killer," drawing, 1957.*

science." King trumpeted the new successes built on her case: "Good citizens and whole-heartedly cooperative, today's Typhoid Marys, mindful of the dreadful potential of their unique affliction, are able to live useful lives without endangering their fellowmen."[5] In this writer's perceptions, Mary Mallon's misfortune led directly to effective controls.

A decade later, in a 1966 article in *Today's Health*, John Lentz wrote about Mary Mallon's "strange case." He focused, as many writers before him had, on Mallon's seeming uniqueness, claiming that "for some 15 years, this woman was the sole cause of so much sickness and death that she gained a lasting, if dubious, distinction in the history of medicine." Lentz did not inform his readers that Mary Mallon caused fewer cases and deaths from typhoid fever than other identified carriers nor that she was only one among many thousands of typhoid carriers. He did not suggest the possibility that Mary Mallon's pioneer status might have made it difficult for her to understand or accept the accusation that she caused the deaths of people for whom she worked. He assumed that because we now understand the carrier state that she also must have understood the concept. He depicted an uncommon medical situation and a singularly evil person. She was, he wrote, "a walking reservoir . . . lacking in regard for the welfare of others."[6]

A dramatic tinted illustration accompanied Lentz's article and underscored the theme of intent and blame. Four servants are shown on the full-page drawing, three women and a man (fig. 7.2). One young woman is depicted as feeling faint and in need of the help offered by the older woman and the man. In the foreground, not helping and understood to be in fact the cause of the problem, is Mary Mallon. She is busy with the coffee mill, but looking up with powerful emotions. In her face are fear and anxiety, with a considerable dose of malice. Readers may see reason to feel some sympathy for her, but, once again, the artist powerfully points the finger of blame.

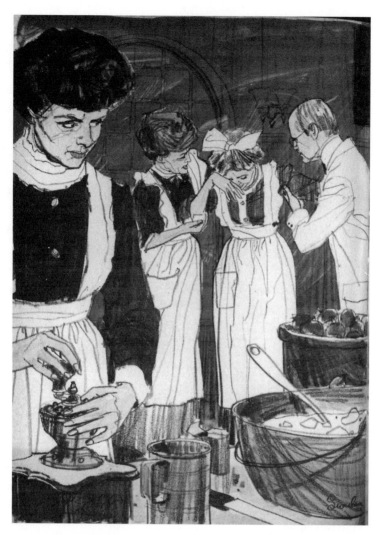

Fig. 7.2. *Mary Mallon in kitchen, drawing, 1966.*

The following year, in 1967, medical historian and physician Gordon W. Jones wrote a survey article on "The Scourge of Typhoid" for the popular *American History Illustrated.*[7] In a small section on Mary Mallon, Jones wrote about the "most famous" healthy carrier that "she had a great tendency to change jobs." By picking up on a previously voiced suspicion that she must therefore have realized her culpability, Jones underscored prevailing negative views. He attributed to her the 1903 epidemic in Ithaca, New York, in which 1,300 people contracted the disease, relying on sources before him that had confused Soper's investigation of that epidemic with Mallon's guilt in causing it.[8] At the same time as he attributed considerable blame to Mallon, however, Jones commiserated with her plight: "No leper of the Middle Ages ever felt the hostile attention of the authorities more strongly."[9]

Three years later, in 1970, writer Mark Sufrin produced "The Case of the Disappearing Cook" for *American Heritage.*[10] Illustrated by Lawrence DiFiori and following closely upon Soper's published work, the article presented Mallon's story at its most dramatic. Sufrin wrote an action-packed rendition of Soper's pursuit of Mallon, her forcible arrest, her release, her return to cooking, and her recapture, and in so doing he furthered the, by then, common understanding of Mary Mallon's negative qualities. She was an "elusive creature"; she denied her guilt. When found hiding in 1907, she "sprang from a crouch and came out fighting and cursing. . . . A big, strong woman, Mary put up a bitter struggle for her freedom." She was "silent and grim" when Soper tried to talk with her, and she refused to cooperate with authorities. Sufrin repeated many of Soper's earlier observations, including that when she was released in 1910 she immediately "vanished." She was, Sufrin concluded, "dangerous, an incorrigible." The story, befitting a magazine that tries to make history popular with its general readership, successfully emphasized the dramatic aspects of Mallon's story.

DiFiori's accompanying illustrations carried the readers' interest one step further. Most telling was the full-page drawing of Mallon wielding her carving fork against an intimidated Soper (fig. 7.3). In a domestic setting, with a table on one side, a rug on the floor, and pots and pans stacked neatly on shelves behind, a buxom, young, and angry Mallon advances with fist clenched and weapon raised upon Soper, who, hat in hand, is ready and eager to retreat. The caption read, "Easily enraged, Mary seized a

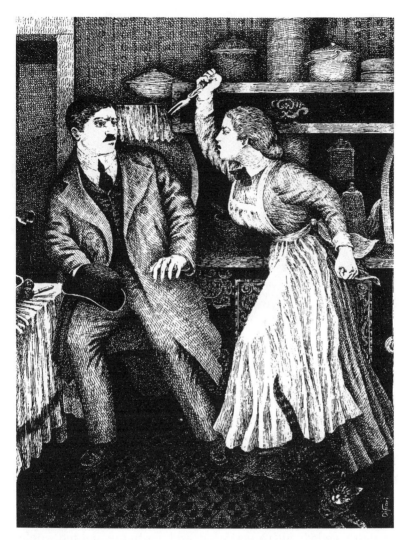

Fig. 7.3. *Mary Mallon advances on George Soper, drawing, 1970.*

carving fork and frightened off Soper when he first told her that she was probably a typhoid carrier."[11]

In another drawing, DiFiori depicted an aproned Mallon, screaming and flailing her arms against the five uniformed officers who surround her (fig. 7.4). The picture captures some of Mallon's outrage and confusion in a sympathetic way, but its caption reminds readers, "Kicking and screaming, she was rushed off

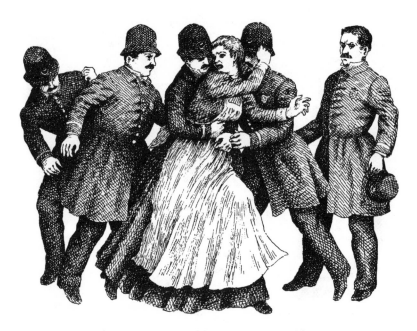

Fig. 7.4. *Police officers arrest Mary Mallon, drawing, 1970.*

to a hospital, where tests proved that she was 'a living culture' of typhoid bacilli."

Revealing in a different sense was DiFiori's third illustration, a rendering of Mallon's 1915 recapture (fig. 7.5). Here two bowler-hatted and serious health officers, called "detectives" in the caption, study a veiled woman as she walks down a street. Mallon, except perhaps for the shading that encompasses them all, is shown in a positive manner, as the essence of a lady. She is modestly veiled, with a perky hat, and her figure, not too ample, is maturely robed in the latest fashion. She carries a modest purse and looks—almost demurely—away from the men's gaze. Were it not for the accompanying story, readers would not suspect her as a public health menace. The full measure of the illustrations plus the story, then, asserts her guilt but also evokes some sympathy.

A 1979 illustration of "Typhoid Mary" by Gary Viskupic takes Sufrin's story in a different direction.[12] Accompanying the

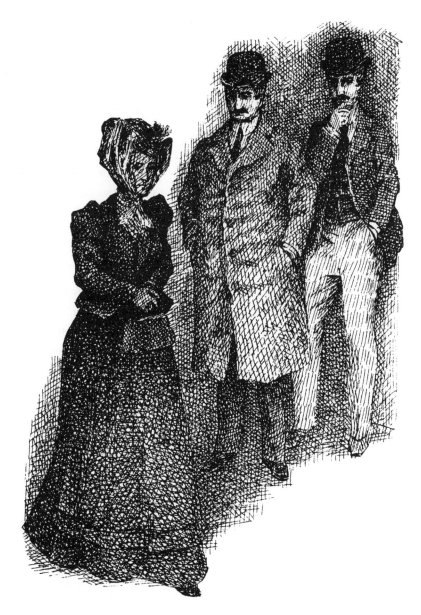

Fig. 7.5. *Mary Mallon followed by health officers, drawing, 1970.*

printing of a revised version of Sufrin's 1970 *American Heritage* article almost a decade later in *Newsday*, the popular Long Island newspaper, the artist presents an attractive, sexualized young woman ladling food onto a platter, adding skulls and bones to the mix (fig. 7.6). This Mary Mallon knows what she is doing. She is not put off by the destruction she wields; in fact, she looks satisfied with it all. Her shirt is unbuttoned far enough to reveal some cleavage, and her apron/jumper shows the curves of her body. Except for the rough, peasant hand holding the spoon, the image would be completely feminine and extremely evil, a witch hidden in modern dress. In this instance of conscious death-dealing associated with an attractive woman, we know who to hold responsible.

In 1979, the same year that Long Island's *Newsday* reprinted Sufrin's article, Long Island physician Mary C. McLaughlin published her version of Mallon's story in the American Irish Historical Society's journal, *The Recorder*.[13] McLaughlin concluded that Mallon had "consciously refused to face the fact that she was a source of illness and death," and wondered if her "nights were filled with guilt and dread seeing the faces of those who became ill." But she softened her judgment by acknowledging that Mallon might have had "a blind spot, which prevented her from recognizing her potential for harm to others."[14]

McLaughlin added a new dimension to Mallon's story, unfortunately one that cannot be corroborated by extant documents. When doing her research, McLaughlin spoke with a friend of her husband's, who "said his family had hired Typhoid Mary." The informant told McLaughlin that Mary Mallon had worked for his grandparents in Marblehead, Massachusetts, and that she "was closely tied into the Irish Movement in America, raising money to support the Irish cause." In fact, McLaughlin's source claimed, Mallon's cause was championed by Countess Markiewicz (the poet Yeats' friend) who "waged a campaign through the American-Irish press to get signatures for a petition to the au-

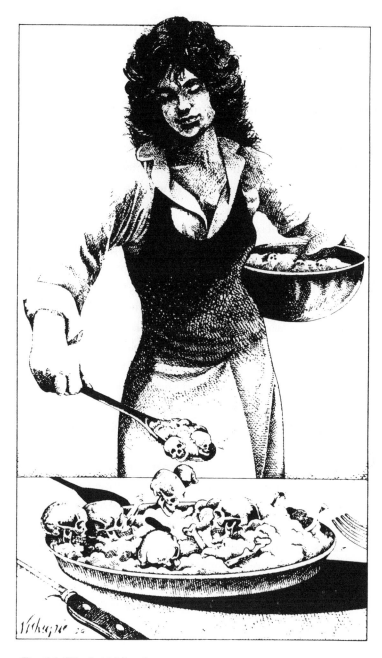

Fig. 7.6. *"Typhoid Mary" serving up skulls and bones, drawing, 1979.*

thorities to release Mary." Since Mallon's Irish heritage was always an issue in how she was perceived, her possible connection to a nationalist political movement is very intriguing. But there is no record of such a petition campaign in the Irish press, and sources at the *Irish Advocate* and the American Irish Historical Society as well as the National Historian of the Ancient Order of Hibernians in America have found no evidence of Mallon's political connections to an Irish national movement. It is probable that McLaughlin's informant remembered a different Mary Mallon.[15]

These popular accounts reveal only a small amount of sympathy for Mary Mallon in the decades following her death. With hints that Mallon herself might be innocent or an unwitting perpetrator, authors presented, albeit sometimes reluctantly, a negative picture of Typhoid Mary and her blameworthiness. Mallon's story sometimes was told to illuminate the progress of science and modern accomplishments of public health, but authors and illustrators did not endow her personally with many redeeming features. Instead, they underscored and reinforced the same kind of negative interpretations of her story and of the meaning of Typhoid Mary that had emerged in the media following her recapture in 1915.

From 1980 to the present, a stream of productions drawing on Typhoid Mary's story exemplify that its compelling narrative continues to have meaning in our end-of-the-century world. The newer renditions of Mallon's story differ from their immediate predecessors in some important ways. First, writers have increasingly shown sensitivity to the personal sadness in Mallon's story, a response that hearkens back to the sympathy for Mary Mallon expressed in the 1909 newspaper stories. Second, they explicitly connect her story with current worries about new viruses and old diseases reappearing in drug-resistant forms. And finally, they make efforts to understand Mallon's own position and to find some agency in her actions.

It was predictable that our experiences at the end of the twentieth century with a new epidemic of HIV infection and AIDS and an upsurge in drug-resistant tuberculosis, in addition to other emerging viruses like Hanta, Ebola, and Sabia, and Lyme disease, Legionnaire's disease, and toxic shock syndrome, would have inspired writers to use Mary Mallon's story to develop the human meaning in our new health worries. The first modern dramatic rendition of her story appeared on January 15, 1979, when BBC Radio 4 aired a new play by the award-winning play-wright Shirley Gee, called simply *Typhoid Mary*.[16] This play was the BBC entry for the Italia Prize and won the jury's Special Commendation. It won the Society of Authors/Pye Award for the Best Original Play of 1979, and it has been rebroadcast numerous times, including most recently in 1993.

Gee invents an Irish childhood for Mary Mallon, as Molly Malone, the poor daughter of a fishmonger immortalized by the song "Cockles and Mussels," whose days are spent working at the fish stall and bearing up under the taunts of the other children who do not like the lingering smell.[17] Molly's beloved brother dies of the fever (unspecified) while Molly nurses and cuddles him, presumably picking up the typhoid infection. At the age of sixteen, she escapes to America, where immigration officers change her name and provide her with the identity of a cook. She develops this skill to a fine art while working for elite New York families, but all the while she is bothered by a recurrent dream of children's whispers and scorn. One of their cruel taunts in partic-ular, "misbegotten Mary, misbegotten Mary," brings back the torments of her youth, sufferings she eventually associates with the treatment she gets at the hands of George Soper. When the sanitary engineer finds her and tries to explain her carrier state, Mary replies, "You're a quack or a crank or something, be accus-ing me of witchcraft next." Soper, who does not realize the dis-tance she places between them, urges, "Trust me. Come with me." To which Mary replies, "Trust you? Go with you? A man who says I'm dirty? I kill people?" The distance between them is an impassible moat.

When the health department isolates Mary, the playwright puts her in irons, and while she is in this helpless position Soper visits again, always asking questions. When he asks her where she is from, Mary explodes: "So that's it. I might have known. You think all immigrants are trash, don't you. Riffraff. You think we stink—that's why you call me dirty.... Stinking transients. We're supposed to pee on the stairs, aren't we, and drink, and kill." Misbegotten Mary. In America she cannot escape her Irish fishmonger heritage, her birth stigma.

Mary finds some redemption, but no true peace, in Shirley Gee's hands. At the end of the play and her life, she ponders the meaning of it all. She becomes resigned to her fate and her isolation. "My window has no bars," she muses. "The days go by." But more: "I've been a bit of a marvel. I've a place in the history books. I've had a destiny. That's more than you can say for some. Isn't it? It is. Isn't it?"

We learn much about the historical place of America's first identified healthy carrier of typhoid fever from playwrights like Gee, who have put Mallon's story to present-day use. Gee avoids the stigmatization of the Typhoid Mary label and presents instead a sympathetic portrayal of a woman trapped by circumstances. She is critical of Soper's lack of understanding of Mallon's point of view. She considers the problem, still relevant, of what to do with people like Mary Mallon who pose a risk to society, perhaps innocently, but who are still potentially deadly. Her play, by emphasizing sympathy for Mallon's plight, suggests that compassion should govern public health responses.

The social and public policy dilemma Mary Mallon's story posed was addressed repeatedly in the 1980s, as writers tried to help people come to terms with new health dangers and dilemmas. Vermont Royster, for example, in a piece for the *Wall Street Journal*, told Mallon's story to illuminate the controversy over compulsory drug tests for airline pilots who might endanger their passengers. He asked the "haunting" question: "Under what circumstances, if any, may society for the protection of all infringe on the rights of its individual members?" He remembered compulsory smallpox vaccination and thought that even though some religious beliefs might have been ignored in that case, "did not the end [the elimination of smallpox] justify the means?" But he acknowledged there were no simple answers to the difficult question of conflicting rights of individuals and society. "As we grapple with [the question]," he suggested, "we might give some thought to the sad story of Mary Mallon."[18]

J. F. Federspiel's widely read 1982 novel *The Ballad of Typhoid Mary* was an effort to come to terms with questions of individual responsibility.[19] Federspiel, a Swiss author, draws a psychological portrait of an alienated and lonely young woman, who cuts a sexual and culinary path across New York under the sympathetic eye of a physician, drawn as the present-day narrator's grandfather. Federspiel creates Mary Mallon as a Swiss émigré, Maria Caduff. While sailing to America Maria's family dies on board ship, and the ship's cook, Sean Mallon, befriends the twelve-year-old, initiating her sexually while imparting recipes.

By the time she arrives in New York, Maria has become Mary Mallon. Sean Mallon has died in the interim, and Mary is alone and free to develop her cooking and sexual skills in a series of escapades with unsavory characters, most of whom die after their encounter with this "avenging angel." Only two characters genuinely appreciate the young ambitious immigrant, and these two are immune to her form of "truly equalizing justice." One is a four-year-old retarded girl, for whom Mary cares lovingly for four years, despite her family's wish that Mary's curse would kill the child. The second is her chaste lover, anarchist intellectual Chris Cramer, who hunkers down in New York after throwing a bomb at the Haymarket riots in Chicago. Chris is loyal to a point: he always provides her refuge when she needs it, but he refuses to have a sexual relationship with her, possibly because he fears her disease.

The novel recounts Mary's isolation on North Brother Island and her release and return to her former life. When Chris dies, among his papers she finds a note, which speaks for both his bomb throwing and her cooking: "Either every human being is guilty of what he does; or, on the contrary: everyone is innocent, despite everything he has done. I can't decide. May I be forgiven."

Federspiel leaves his readers to decide for themselves if Mallon should be forgiven. Although he adopts a mode of verisimilitude—a present-day pediatrician writing the story from his grandfather's notes and his own research (one piece of which is one of Soper's articles)—the novelist changes Mary Mallon's roots and ethnicity, he makes people around her conscious of the danger she poses long before they could have been, and he portrays her as more lethal than any evidence suggests.[20] Perhaps the author altered Mallon's story in these ways to make a more universal statement about individual responsibility, the culpability of medicine, and the impotence of the state.

A 1984 story in *Current Health*, "The Tale of Typhoid Mary," takes a more positive approach. It begins with strong language: "Mary Mallon was a mass murderer—unknowingly."[21] The article touts modern medical advances to conclude that Mary Mallon's experiences will not be repeated. The unnamed author makes no direct reference to new infections and implies that typhoid fever itself is a problem only for developing nations. The illustration accompanying the story provides a strong example of how an AIDS-aware America might make use of the story of a healthy carrier from the past. Looking directly at the reader, a prim Mary Mallon carries a tea tray (see fig. 7.7). She is in uniform, her hair neatly pulled back. One might be prepared to sit down to her serving if it were not for the "wings" of pathogenic microbes that frame her, wings that propel the angel of death, bringing her within your home, ready to light on your food. Evil

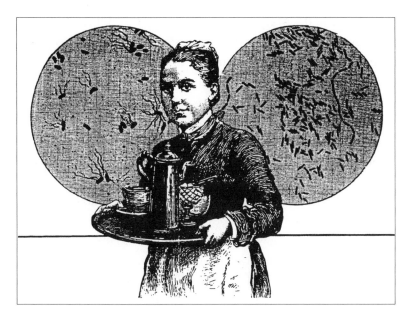

Fig. 7.7. *Mary Mallon, drawing, 1984.*

lurks all around, especially in unlikely places. The warning from the past is even more relevant today. A suspicious nation, untrusting and wary, is ready to see danger in every teapot, death in each pretty face.[22]

Boston-area playwright Tanya Contos in 1985 offered a stage presentation called *Typhoid Mary*, which directly confronts the problem of whether Mary Mallon knew about the danger she carried.[23] The question of the extent to which people who carry and spread disease are aware of the danger they pose has become an important one in our nation's response to people who test positive for HIV. Contos took on the challenge and found in Mary Mallon an excellent medium. In the first act of the two-act play, Mallon denies her guilt to three visitors, a priest, her physician, and a young kitchen maid. She is filled with her defenses, bitter and sad. The doctor says to her: "Every time there was an outbreak, you fled the house in the dead of night, only to surface somewhere else with a new alias. Is that the pattern of a victim, or of a criminal?" Mary replies, "I left because I didn't want to get sick myself." Refusing to take any responsibility, Mary lashes out at her captors: "Suddenly I'm the one to blame for everything that happens to me. Well, you can't wash your hands of me like that. I won't accept responsibility. . . . I'm a prisoner, not a patient, but I can be a patient prisoner."

The second act brings ghosts from Mary's past, ghosts of people who know her better than her earlier visitors: her former employer/lover, a teen-age girl who died in her care, and her own son. These characters urge her to remember and accept, which, by the end of the play, she does. With a roar, she says, "GUILTY. I had that power. I knew I had it, I knew how to use it, and I used it. Again and again and again. I cooked my way from house to house to hotel to hospital to hell." She is redeemed in her confession, and, surrounded by the ones she loved in the past, shouts (very much to a late-twentieth-century audience), "I'm FREE!" In this modern-day rendition of Mallon's story, the woman carrier accepts blame, and in the process is forgiven. Mary Mallon on stage emerges from the Typhoid Mary stigma.

Another experimental rendition of Mary Mallon's story is Joan Schenkar's 1986 play, *Fulfilling Koch's Postulate*, which the author calls a "comedy of menace."[24] The play is staged within the huge lips of an infected throat. The playwright has devised an inventive cross-Atlantic pairing. On one side of the stage, Mary Mallon holds forth in her kitchen; on the other, Robert Koch works in his laboratory. Koch was the German scientist whose postulates establishing proper bacteriology laboratory procedures helped lead to the realization of healthy carriers. In Schenkar's play he is also Mallon's employer and struggles to dictate her actions. More figuratively, he is her creator, but he is himself not immune to her influence. Mallon and Koch work in their separate laboratories on the two sides of the stage, dissecting culinary and scientific treats, both with a purpose. The play examines the power struggle between the laboratory and the kitchen:

MARY: Sooner or later, in every household I've ever worked in comes the same question: Who is to be cook in the kitchen? Is the master of the house to be cook in the kitchen? Or is the *cook* to be cook in the kitchen? That is always the question.

MAID: Is there an answer, Miss Mary?

MARY: To *that* question? There *is* an answer. (*Pause.*) *I am the cook.* That is the answer I always give.

Mary's power diminishes when no one will eat what she prepares, and Koch himself cannot control all that happens in his own house. He understands Mary's danger but cannot stop her from cooking. "You're Cooking Poison! You're Cooking Death!" Koch accuses. Mary responds, "The important thing is to keep cooking." Koch can only warn his laboratory assistant, "Nothing from the kitchen should ever go into your mouth." The assistant puts his finger in the pot anyway. "It's the cook's postulate," he laughs, as its potency overwhelms him.

One critic wrote that the play "mates the kitchen with a doctor's laboratory ... [and] contagion, sexuality, and scientific research [go] haywire." Schenkar's play, even though she denies it was about AIDS or about contemporary America at all, but rather says she was "waltzing the floor with history," has enormous significance today. "You can't blame a bug," she told her interviewer.[25] It seems, though, that Shenkar more emphatically does not want to blame the bug's carrier. As drama critic Vivian Patraka noted, "Schenkar undermines the traditional responses of revulsion for Mary as contaminated pariah" at the same time as she debunks an "idealization of Koch as hero of medicine."[26] The audience is left to conclude that menace can exist in both camps and that blame, either of the carrier or the science, is not the point. Schenkar subtly disposes of the question that hangs over the 1980s about what to do with people who carry the HIV virus by showing that neither side of her stage—carrier or scientist—can alone solve our problems.[27]

Barry J. Drogin, musical creator in 1988 of the theater dance production *Typhoid Mary*, and choreographer Peg Hill portray a complex Mary Mallon and, like Contos and Schenkar, move well beyond the common view of her as menace and demon. Drogin believed that Mallon's isolation and silence "forced [her] to become that which the public sees," as he put it in the production notes.[28] He felt haunted to get beyond the public representation and see inside Mallon, but he also worried whether his efforts were right, "primarily because of what I learned about Mary's fierce fight for privacy." He wrote, "As we delved further into our project, we found ourselves in a lose-lose position—by pointing out that Mary Mallon was not 'Typhoid Mary,' had we turned her into our vision of her instead? I continue to work in biographical forms . . . and to rub up against this problem of depicting people who do not want to be depicted."[29]

Drogin and Hill staged the production with the dancers dressed in "ghoulish" costumes, the brown streaks at the back of their union suits, a reviewer noted, "particularly graphic reminders that typhoid was spread through poor personal hygiene."[30] Here is *Dance Magazine*'s description of the play's opening scene: Mary Mallon is "supervising the preparation of a meal that is served to members of the audience by dancers whose faces are made up to resemble hollow-eyed death masks. We ate the pasta, salad, bread, and fruit somewhat warily as dancers were rapidly overcome by disease and dropped dead [in front of us]."[31] By having the audience actually eat a meal dramatically prepared, Drogin and Hill force people to confront their fears on the spot, in public.

The Drogin and Hill narrative dance-pantomime poses the dilemma of why Mary returned to cooking after her release from her original isolation. Either as a form of a "dangerous sense of denial or merely due to financial necessity," as the program notes put it, they feel the choice and the responsibility for that choice were hers. The misfortune, too, was Mary's. But it is also ours. Drogin's anguish becomes society's anguish. During the dance

Mallon is painted with a big red X. At the close of the evening, she stands alone, recaptured, "in a cloud of powder-puff dust." The problem she poses is solved only by separating her from society. The production stands as a challenge to the audience to find a better way, to move beyond stigma and isolation.

The premier performance of Drogin and Hill's *Typhoid Mary* was a benefit for People with AIDS Coalition. Drogin was "struck by the similarities between the way Mary was treated, her social position, and contemporary editorials and news articles about AIDS and prostitutes." He and Hill staged the production to speak to the similarities, a conscious contemporary use of history. Reviewers caught the significance for today's audiences: "The notion of a dance about Typhoid Mary is intriguing because it puts us in mind of threats of quarantine in connection with the AIDS crisis," wrote the *Village Voice* critic. *Dance Magazine*'s reviewer also saw the "bold but nonetheless valid comparisons between the public hysteria of the early twentieth century and contemporary reactions to the spread of AIDS."[32] Such a confrontation between history and the present forces audiences and readers to think about how the past might help us understand our current public health problems and also suggests how our present concerns shape our interpretation of the past.

The longest-running stage play of Mary Mallon's story to date is Mark St. Germain's 1989 *Forgiving Typhoid Mary.*[33] Produced multiple times, and once starring Estelle Parsons in the title role, the play has achieved recognition and critical praise. *Time Magazine* named it "one of the ten best plays of 1991."[34] Two scenes frame the action: one, Mary's memory of her loving relationship with a young girl in her care (who died from typhoid fever), and two, Mary's cottage on North Brother Island during her first isolation in 1909 and 1910. There is a short epilogue that takes place in the 1930s. Two physicians, one a sympathetic man and the other an angry and dismissive woman, and a priest, who is scared but caring, interact with Mary. The basic outline of Mallon's story unfolds during the play, and around it the playwright creates various responses to the problems posed by the healthy carrier, the most notable of which is, "What is to be done and who will be responsible?"

The characters demonstrate a range of attitudes toward Mallon from complete rejection and blame to fear to understanding. In turn, they try sympathy, isolation, radical medical treatments, release from quarantine, and again isolation to solve the problem Mallon poses. The priest loses confidence in the Church's ability to address such a thorny dilemma and ultimately leaves the priesthood. The male physician remains kindly but incapable of bringing about a lasting solution. The woman physician, whose job it is to obtain specimens and explain treatment procedures to Mary Mallon, is unable to let go of her rigid interpretation of what science demands until a touching scene toward the end of the play, which moves her toward understanding and warmth. Even so, she cannot bring herself to sit down and drink tea with Mary Mallon. Mallon herself evolves in the play from a dish-breaking, angry, resistant woman who only wants to get out of her confinement to one who gains insight, makes some concessions to the science she does not understand, and reveals a caring concern for the people who work with her. She slowly comes to terms with her complicity in the young girl's death: "I killed her. I killed my little girl." She understands why the doctor cannot sit down to tea. But despite her new insight, when they release her, she returns to her deadly cooking and demonstrates that she, too, cannot alone solve the problem her situation poses.

St. Germain sets up the dilemma of what to do about Mary Mallon very much in the context of the 1980s and 1990s. As the program notes for the 1995 Minneapolis production advised, "The life of the infamous cook who contaminated New York in the early part of this century has vital importance today." A post-show forum focused on "Rights and Responsibilities: The Dynamic Interface Between Individual and Public 'Health.'"[35] The play purposely leaves ambiguous how to reconcile Mallon's right to freedom and her doctors' need to protect the public's health so that St. Germain can engage his audiences in using Mary Mallon's early-twentieth-century story to think about what is, to him, an end-of-the-century problem.

Carolyn Gage's 1990 one-woman, one-act play, *Cookin' with Typhoid Mary*, gives another present-day vivid meaning to Mary Mallon's predicament. Gage transforms the view of Mallon as a public menace into a story that reveals the health department as the "real public enemy." In the play, Mallon calls George Soper "that devil of a doctor" and a "nasty little pig-eyed bastard holdin' his hat over his privates like he's got somethin' to be ashamed of." A strong and belligerent Mary Mallon preparing potatoes in the Sloane Maternity Hospital kitchen has a clear analysis of her situation: "If you're a woman and you're Irish, they think they can say anything they like, and you've got to take it. Not this woman. Not Mary Mallon." Gage's cynical and knowing Mallon laughs, "Made me sign a paper that I'd never cook for a livin' again. Now that was charitable of them, don't you think? Maybe they was hopin' I'd hire on as president of a bank." In Gage's mind, Mallon knows the health department did not do right by her and puts the blame back on the public officials. Gage speaks to a 1990s audience of women by presenting a resistant, strong-minded, foul-language version of Mary Mallon, democratically cooking potato stew for the masses, against a health department that protects the rich over the starving immigrants. Even as Gage strains against the common negative portrayals of Typhoid Mary, though, her own Mallon retains a nasty edge.[36]

Gage has given us a powerful, victimized, and innocent Mary Mallon. The contrast to Gage's characterization in John Steele Gordon's 1994 article on Mallon in *American Heritage* shows the range of interpretations still available in the 1990s. While sympathetic, Gordon implies that Mary Mallon deserved considerable blame for her situation. He likens her case, that of a cook not allowed to invite anyone to dinner, to that of a poet or a painter whose artistic compositions will remain forever unseen. He admits that "she probably had no knowledge of the latest theories about typhoid." But he cannot help wondering "if she did not, at some level at least, suspect something. Certainly the disease followed her about like an incubus."[37] In a radio interview, Gordon explained that Mary Mallon must have known she was a carrier of typhoid because she changed jobs so frequently, usually after typhoid fever broke out in the families for whom she had cooked. "It's hard for me to imagine that she didn't at least at some level understand that it must have been connected with her," Gordon concluded.[38]

Most recent renderings of Mary Mallon, especially the theatrical productions, try to cast her story in a positive or sympathetic frame. But the negative meaning of the phrase *Typhoid Mary* has continued to influence the tellings of her story. Indeed, the term has a life of its own and is increasingly called upon as an abstract referent. Sometimes the phrase is used in the popular press in directly analogous ways. For example, Jane E. Brody used it in her "Personal Health" column in the *New York Times* in an article on toxic shock syndrome. Brody noticed that it was very difficult to avoid the organism responsible because so many people carried the staphylococcal bacteria that produce the deadly toxin: "Most of these 'Typhoid Marys,' among them health care providers," Brody wrote, "are immune to the toxin but can spread the organism to others who are susceptible."[39]

The transference of the phrase outside of medicine is more telling of how deeply into our culture it reaches. *Typhoid Mary* has a dictionary definition as a noun, "A person from whom something undesirable or deadly spreads to those nearby." Or, "one that is by force of circumstances a center or focus from which something undesirable spreads."[40] The examples of how our language has adopted the symbol as part of the common lexicon are numerous. In the legal profession the term is applied to lawyers who move from one firm to another and in the process move to the opposite side of an active case. Such a lawyer becomes a "Typhoid Mary" because he or she can, because of previous knowledge, infect the new firm, which in turn might be disqualified from representation of their clients.[41]

A *New York Times* columnist wrote that a Senate Committee asking Richard Nixon if he thought presidents might for national security reasons undertake illegal activities was "a little like asking Typhoid Mary for advice on communicable diseases."[42] A *Wall Street Journal* editor praising the Republican party in 1988 for making specific and detailed proposals in its election-year platform wrote that conversely, "The Democrats in Atlanta last month issued a 4,500-word manifesto that treated specifics like Typhoid Mary."[43] A *Newsweek* story about how American urban violence affected Japanese-American trade talks, quoted one Japanese student saying, "You're like Typhoid Mary trying to cure the plague."[44] "Saturday Night Live" comedians joke, "I'm going to a banquet. It's being catered by Typhoid Mary."[45] Arthur M. Schlesinger, Jr., advised President Clinton not to appease the money markets: "You don't call on Typhoid Mary to stop a typhoid epidemic."[46]

Mystery readers encounter a character complaining about a police visit to another character who was in the hospital, "[They] wear surgical masks and stand back ten feet from his bed like he's Typhoid Mary" while they interview him.[47] A character in a Marge Piercy novel, noting the misfortunes surrounding his friend, laughs, "A sick cleaning lady in your bed, a sick kitten and a sick sister? What are you, Typhoid Mary?"[48] The term has relevance even on the newspaper sports page. When Dennis Rodman, the flamboyant and controversial National Basketball Association player, was in the news, a sports writer commented, "Madonna wanted to marry him, he says. Visualizing Rodman with Madonna is ... like trying to picture the Elephant Man dating Typhoid Mary."[49] In a sign of our technological times, an advertisement in a computer magazine depicts "Typhoid Carol," who, while processing the payroll and the mail, infected the communications network in her office with a computer virus.[50] And, perhaps the best measure of how far into our culture the term has reached, the epithet is featured in a children's jump-rope rhyme, part of which chants, "Typhoid Mary, What do you carry?"[51]

Russell Baker's *New York Times* Op Ed article on smoking and nonsmoking sections of restaurants encapsulated the term's enduring cultural meaning. He commiserated with the people who, when they go out to dinner, had to answer "smoking" to the question of which section they prefer. "Of all the nasty punishments for smoking nowadays," he wrote, "the worst must be the smoker's sense of being a Typhoid Mary. Imagine a whole society hating you, isolating you from the good, strong, healthy people whose lives you imperil, you smoke-drenched swine!" Baker well understood the negative judgment carried in the phrase, and he took its meaning an additional step by adding an article in front of the term. *Typhoid Mary* at the end of the century is generic.[52]

Mary Mallon was one among tens of thousands of Americans over the twentieth century who carried typhoid bacilli chronically within their bodies. She was one among thousands who refused to cooperate with authorities to follow set restrictions. She was one among many (possibly in the hundreds) who outright defied authorities by continuing to cook after being informed of their carrier status. Yet, as a culture, we still see Mary Mallon as unique. The retellings of her particular story indicate that she holds a special place in American life, worthy of recounting again and again. We do not, as a society, remember Alphonse Cotils or Tony Labella, who continued to cook food for others after being warned to stop. We do not remember Frederick Moersch, even though following his return to ice cream handling, he, like Mary Mallon, was isolated for years as a registered carrier. We do not remember other defiant carriers whose names are no longer recoverable. It is Mary Mallon's story alone that carries meaning today. It is the image of "Typhoid Mary" that our culture retains; to this day, one woman carries the burden of all that healthy carriers represent.[53]

Reflected in the media and the popular imagination, an initially benign descriptive term for a woman whose name was not known has become a widespread negative epithet. Typhoid Mary has a life of its own, no longer necessarily making a reference back to Mary Mallon and the specifics of her story.[54] The phrase has become a general metaphor for contagion and the inadvertent or purposeful spread of disease or infection and, more broadly, evil.

Marc L. Sherman, a California lawyer, has written a short story that demonstrates the use of the Typhoid Mary metaphor and dramatically illustrates the organizational theme of this book, that where you stand determines your perceptions and your understanding of what Mallon's story means. Receiving a recent Pushcart Award nomination, a "Diptych" of parallel stories entitled, "Until the Pill Kicks In" and "Till Morning Comes" ran in parallel columns down the pages and simultaneously tracked two people's perceptions of the same event. On the left side of the page, Sherman presented the woman's story and on the right, the teenage boy's.[55] The woman, lying on one side of a bed, reviews her upwardly mobile life and marriage, which she has just left for a country house, slower pace, and, last night, a sexual encounter with the teenage boy who helped her move in. The boy lies on the other side of the bed, thinking of this, his first sexual experience. It worries him and causes him some disgust. He remembers the high school health class where he has just learned about AIDS and sexually transmitted diseases. His mind buzzes, "And didn't this lady come from the city. She could be like that Typhoid Mary. Who knows with whom she has slept? Slut! Germs! . . . He's really anxious now. Maybe she does it on purpose—to get back at men. . . . He could get sick." He pictures his penis: "white, withered and flaccid, falling off while he climbs a rope in gym." The two wait for morning.

The Sherman story crystallizes the connections between Mary Mallon and the lasting legends of her created by our culture. Mary's is not a simple story of evil or of conscious intent to harm, although it sometimes may be that, but it is a complex story of meanings imposed and multiple possible responses. It is a story of real people and experiences, of grief and hurt, of life and destruction of life. It never occurs to the young suburban woman in Marc Sherman's story that she could be viewed as Typhoid Mary, yet that identity seems fearfully clear to the teenager on the other side of the bed. Danger lurks in the most unsuspecting places, and we are now a society on guard against it. Is there any way out? What should we do next?

A "Square Deal" for Public Health

*T*hroughout this book, I have reconstructed Mary Mallon's story and shown how she appeared from different standpoints. While the various perspectives overlap, they also sometimes diverge in significant ways. There can be no one way to understand Mary Mallon and her place in the history of medicine and our culture. There is no single truth about her. Instead there are various stories about her and multiple productions of her different meanings. Together the various perspectives challenge us to recognize the compelling dilemmas faced by those who tried to protect the public's health from the kind of dangers she posed. Just as point of view influences our comprehension and shapes our sympathy in fictional plots, history is also more richly understood through analysis that proceeds from different perspectives.[1] Examining the contrasting perspectives on Mary Mallon and looking back at the debate about the control of healthy carriers of typhoid fever will not reveal ready-made solutions to our current public health problems, but the exercise does, I think, remind us of important approaches to consider and pitfalls to avoid as we seek answers to similar health dilemmas today.

The story of how Mary Mallon became "Typhoid Mary" underscores the necessity of looking at public health problems from different stances. In her stories, a powerful negative image replaced the human being very early on—a negative image constructed by public health officials, medical writers, and the media, all of whom helped it become entrenched in American culture. In turn, the cultural meaning of the popular but stigmatizing phrase "Typhoid Mary" influenced the actual treatment of Mary Mallon, as well as her own responses to her situation. Scientists at the time accepted the medical perspective on healthy carriers in the new world of bacteriology and hoped for a world in which infectious diseases would no longer threaten human life. Health officials worried about how they were to carry out their job to protect the public's health against preventable diseases in a world in which many doubted their words and their methods. The law tried to balance medical and social concerns, struggling with the dilemma in which it seemed necessary to sacrifice an individual's civil liberty to a larger good. The media helped to construct a stylized Typhoid Mary who embodied the conflicts and the worries of a fearful public. Meanwhile, public actions were constantly influenced by the social and cultural values of a society that believed in limited roles for women, held stereotyped views of immigrants, and stigmatized the poor. Mary Mallon was caught in the middle of a web woven partly of her own actions but more strongly by science and society.

Mary Mallon's story has been used in medical textbooks primarily to illustrate the triumph of the new science of bacteriology in informing methods for public health protection. This is the story from the "winners'" point of view, and it has had a long historical appeal. But that telling differs from others; most significantly, it diverges from Mary Mallon's own perceptions, the narrative of the "loser." These contrasting perspectives, and the others explored in this book, are what James C. Scott called a "community of discourse," competing renditions of the same historical events, all of which are essential for understanding the past. Paul Farmer called such distinct points of view "positioned rhetoric" and demonstrated in his anthropological studies how multiple points of view are logically situated in particular historical contexts and necessary to construct a full remembrance of past events.[2]

It should be obvious, here at the conclusion of this book, that our lines of sight on Mary Mallon are intertwined. Without considering our cultural biases, we cannot fully understand how the medical and public health communities saw this defiant immigrant Irish cook, nor begin to comprehend their actions toward her. Without considering turn-of-the-century enthusiasm for bringing scientific advances into a public arena, we cannot understand why the particular symbol of "Typhoid Mary" has embedded itself in our history as deeply as it has.

Now that we have looked at several of the distinct but overlapping stories about Mary Mallon, I would like to join the various perspectives together again in a way that allows us to see how her example raises general issues that continue to concern public health today. The biggest questions raised by Mary Mallon's case remain: Would it have been possible to protect the health of New Yorkers without taking away Mary Mallon's liberty for twenty-six years? Is it possible, today, to protect the public from diseases such as drug-resistant tuberculosis and AIDS (and new ones that will yet emerge) without infringing on individuals' rights and liberties? There are at least three issues basic to Mary Mallon's story that present-day concerns echo and may help guide us in understanding the past as well as charting future paths. The three are: the identification and labeling of new categories of people who challenge the public's health; the question of isolation and its potential threat to personal liberty; and the attribution of blame and responsibility for the spread of disease. All of these issues emphasize the interdependence of medicine and society; all, too, revolve around a basic conflict between individual rights and the public's health.

Identification and Labels

The medical tests that led to the possibility of identifying healthy carriers of typhoid fever at the turn of the twentieth century developed in advance of public health policy about how to handle healthy people who could transmit disease. The bacteriological assays that detected *salmonella typhi* in the blood, urine, and feces of people recovered from their sickness led quickly to discovering the bacteria in people who thought they had never suffered from the disease at all, and to an understanding of the role such people played in perpetuating the disease. The healthy carrier concept initially contradicted the public's understanding of pathophysiology. The new category of healthy people who could be tested and labeled as dangerous to their families and friends was as exciting to physicians and scientists as it was perplexing to an incredulous lay population.

George Soper understood the concept, accepted it, and was determined to carry it into public actions. His initial interactions with Mary Mallon indicated how far his perceptions were from those of the public at large. "I was as diplomatic as possible," Soper explained, "but I had to say I suspected her of making people sick and that I wanted specimens of her urine, feces and blood."[3] He expected Mallon to cooperate with a close inspection of her body's fluids and discharges because she would understand the dangers she posed: "It must have looked as though it [typhoid fever] was pursuing her," Soper concluded. "Possibly she had even thought that she had produced the epidemics."[4] But this was not how Mary Mallon or those around her saw it. The disease did not pursue her; instead it looked as if a misguided and obsessive George Soper was himself irrationally in pursuit. This was new, a healthy person identified as a dangerous person; it was baffling and frightening to be so labeled and pursued, especially given the imbalance of power between Mallon and the health officials. Soper's desire to identify and test a healthy woman, which seemed to him a benign request, did not appear so innocent to the woman he approached.

Ethicist and philosopher Timothy Murphy explains the same phenomenon of denial and incredulity in those gay men first identified as transmitters of AIDS (then called GRID, Gay-Related Infectious Disease) in the early 1980s. Identification itself, with a new category and new conception of disease, seemed threatening. In looking at Randy Shilts's book, *And the Band Played On*, an early account of the epidemic, Murphy criticizes Shilts for not being sufficiently sensitive to the full meaning of identification. He sees Shilts as stacking the "narrative cards" against Gaetan Dugas, the Canadian "patient zero," by portraying him as a "one-dimensional scoundrel in a gothic novel, an occasion for lamentation about the evils of (gay) men." Instead, Murphy suggests, "Dugas's incredulity about the communicability of his condition—who had ever known cancer could be contagious?"—should have been sympathetically understood in terms of how hard it was at the time "to believe that medicine could produce new categories of disease."[5] To have expected Dugas, or any other early sufferer of AIDS, to understand immediately the ramifications of the disease that wracked his body or how his sexual behavior might be implicated and need to be changed was to ask too much. Judgment about initial responses must take into account, Murphy believes, the full social context in which they occur. What seem to be dissenting voices may merely be uncomprehending ones. How one tells the story affects how it is understood.

The big unknown, for Mary Mallon, Gaetan Dugas, and other first targets of new medical and public health conceptualizations, is what follows from the identification. The power to identify is intimately linked to the power to control. Mary Mallon, a single Irish immigrant woman at the turn of the century, already knew herself to be vulnerable and to rank low in the American social hierarchy. In her perception, the system was not on her side, but instead protected the native-born upper classes. Whether or not she was aware of people like Alphonse Cotils, male breadwinner healthy carriers who were not isolated following their identification, she clearly understood her social marginality and how her status contributed to her being scapegoated and blamed. Gaetan Dugas, too, as a gay man, understood his precarious position in the predominant heterosexual mainstream.

Obviously, identification as "dangerous to the public health," especially when added to existent social vulnerability, is a label to avoid. Mary Mallon's identification as a dangerous carrier brought with it police action, forcible hospitalization, and isolation. As in the example of AIDS, where the immediate identification of the disease with homosexual men narrowed official thinking about how to address the epidemic, the identification of Mallon came before health officials had time to think through the wider implications of such an identification.

Identification is not simply a benign act to promote medical understanding. It carries powerful social meaning and radically alters the world of the individuals, especially the first ones, to be so labeled. Before naming individuals as menaces to the public health, we must understand the full ramifications of such designations.[6]

When a medical identification is accompanied by a social label or equated with a specific social group, the results are especially complex and problematic. Labels too often become caricatures, and, like cartoons, are simplistic and one-dimensional. Mary Mallon's experience provides a stark example of how the stigmatization of people who suffer from or carry diseases can adversely affect ensuing events and actually make disease control more difficult. Mallon perceived herself as the brunt of cruel and unusual punishment when she was identified and carted off to her isolation. A working-class single immigrant woman, she felt defenseless against the powerful forces massed against her. Her position of having been "banished like a leper," in her words, was further compounded with the dehumanizing stigma of Typhoid Mary. She knew that city bacteriologist William Park would not appreciate the label "Typhoid William Park"; she understood the shame that society attached to the epithet and to her. In an effort to protect herself from the attacks aimed personally at her, she closed her mind against the health officials who put her on North Brother Island and refused to listen to them. She fought them, and the ideas they represented, vigorously.

"Typhoid Mary" originally was simple description. Rosenau used the phrase, no doubt, merely as a way to refer to a woman whose real name had not been released. But the convenience and vivid imagery of Typhoid Mary captured public imagination and allowed for easy public reference to a complex health concept. Once the phrase was in the public sphere, it was arguably in the interest of the health department and in the public's interest to allow, and even to encourage, the spread of the image of Typhoid Mary in the hope that its negativity might discourage other carriers from cooking and spreading disease. But the cost to Mary Mallon herself was incalculable. It took away her individuality, her personhood, her self: it replaced her person with a symbol. In the public's mind, Mary Mallon ceased to exist, even when her body continued to inhabit the world.

If protection of the public health is our aim, we must move in the direction of diminishing the use of labels that stigmatize and separate. "Stigma and discrimination are the enemies of public health," reminds Jonathan Mann, Director of the International AIDS Center. We can learn from Mary Mallon how such identification, especially if carried out within a public health program that is not perceived to be fair and equitable, will only escalate the problems of disease control and make matters worse. We have already experienced the singling out and stigmatizing of HIV-infected gay men, minorities, and immigrants; many Americans today hold these groups responsible for the spread of AIDS and label them promiscuous and immoral. We must instead try to avoid the creation of an "AIDS Mary," or an "Ebola Mary," demonizing labels, and learn from the Mallon example that stigma can actually work against protecting the public's health.[7]

Mallon's words bear repeating: "I lived a decent, upright life under the name of Mary Mallon until I was seized ... locked up in a pest-house and rechristened 'Typhoid Mary.'" The transformation imposed on her made her believe there were "two kinds of justice in America," and it embittered her. Her initial treatment at the hands of the health officials itself fueled her resistance.[8] Mallon's story reminds us that when people who are infected are treated as if they are polluted and deviant because a virus or bacterium is attached to them, they are forced to defend themselves and resist public health restraints. On the other hand, if people who are infected are treated with respect and empathy for their personal stories, it should be possible to foster cooperation with public health measures and help stem dangerous epidemic crises.

Isolation

In thinking about how far the government might take disease control actions today, isolation emerges as one of the most comprehensive, and to many, most frightening, possibilities. Some states have considered quarantining people with AIDS, and others have actually placed in isolation individuals who violate orders to refrain from unprotected sexual encounters. As Ramon Perez, an attorney with the California Department of Health Services, commented when his department began developing explicit policy to allow for such isolation, "For anyone with any civil libertarian inklings, the kind of power that health authorities could exercise is horrifying. . . . We have to balance the right to privacy against the right of the public to be protected." Isolation of people with AIDS, Perez realized, "could continue [for an indefinite period] until a person died."[9]

The seriousness of the dilemma today is well illustrated in an exchange between Stephen C. Joseph, New York City's health commissioner from 1986 through 1989, and Sandor Katz, a New York–based writer and AIDS activist. In a *New York Times* Op Ed article, Joseph articulated two general objectives of public health work: "the care of the sick and the protection of the uninfected." He understood that these sometimes come into conflict—"especially ... in the city of Typhoid Mary"—and when they do, he thought that "concern for the individual liberties of those currently infected must take second place to the protection of the uninfected and the larger community." He understood public health authority to allow forcible isolation for those people whose actions make them "a clear and present danger to the health of others," and he concluded: "The issue, then, is not whether quarantine is a legitimate tool for protecting the public health. The issue is: Under what circumstances should it be employed, and with what safeguards against its abuse?" Joseph thought the best groups to decide such policy terms would be "a combination of professional expertise, mayoral leadership and court oversight."[10]

Sandor Katz responded in a lengthy article in *The Nation* worrying that unless civil liberties could be guaranteed, the sick would be driven underground and problems would escalate. Katz believed testing, identification, labeling, and possible isolation were all efforts at "social control in the name of public health." He continued, "Given the stigma of AIDS and the vulnerability of the groups hardest hit by it so far—gay men, drug addicts and their partners and children—there is an ever-present danger that public health officials will trample on civil liberties in their zeal to do something." He said that "virtually every AIDS service-providing agency in the city" condemned Joseph's plans to compile lists of people who test positive for HIV because testing "raised the specter of discrimination in employment, housing, health insurance and other areas." Katz found quarantine a "chilling" prospect, and he evoked by analogy Hitler's control of syphilis as outlined in *Mein Kampf*: "there must be no half-measures; the gravest and most ruthless decisions will have to be made. It is a half-measure to let incurably sick people steadily contaminate the remaining healthy ones." In an example closer to home, Katz quoted North Carolina Senator Jesse Helms: "I think somewhere along the line we are going to have to quarantine, if we are really going to contain [AIDS]."[11]

Both Joseph and Katz wanted to protect the health of New Yorkers, and both understood that civil liberties and public health, which they agreed are valuable, can come into conflict. The two disagreed about what process should decide policy when that conflict occurs—Joseph's plan, for example, did not include any shared decision making with people infected with HIV. Most significant, they did not share ideas about when in the process isolation should be invoked, and Katz particularly worried that too early a use of quarantine might produce resistance. The differences between Joseph and Katz seem minor when Hitler is held up as the extreme position, but the general priority Joseph was willing to articulate in favor of the uninfected over the currently infected significantly distinguishes the two.

The delicate balance between personal liberty and public health as it applies to our current health crises in the United States can be explored further through a look at Cuba's policies for people infected with HIV. In 1986 Cuba initiated a national program to contain AIDS, including systematic screening, isolating all HIV-positive people in sanatoriums, and requiring all HIV-positive pregnant women to abort. The plan was comprehensive and not voluntary for Cuban citizens. In the sanatorium, people who tested positive for HIV and those suffering from AIDS received aggressive medical treatment and care, more than might be available to them outside. This "odd blend of care and coercion," as anthropologist Nancy Scheper-Hughes calls it, has resulted in an extremely low incidence rate of the disease in Cuba.[12]

There are other factors that help explain the apparent Cuban success in containing AIDS. Since Castro's revolution, intravenous drug use, a significant contributor to HIV transmission, has been severely curtailed. Cuba also maintains a strict sexual code, which discourages another common route of AIDS transmission. Because of its economic isolation in the hemisphere, Cuba also is relatively underexposed to the disease. Nonetheless, those who studied the situation agree that isolation of HIV-positive people can be credited with helping Cuba to keep the disease at bay.

But at what political and personal cost? The Cuban government forced a group of citizens to leave their work and communities abruptly and move into settlements of the infected, behind barbed wire. Is this what we in the United States envision as necessary to protect the health of the uninfected? If containing a disease that, for now, can be limited only through prevention is a high priority for the United States, we must examine the Cuban experience. Indeed, Scheper-Hughes, who made multiple visits to Cuba to study their AIDS-control activity, concludes that Western democracies should take note and reevaluate their own thinking: "Individual liberty, privacy, free speech, and free choice are cherished values in any democratic society but they are sometimes invoked to obstruct social policies that favour universal health care, social welfare, and equal opportunity."[13]

Writer Karen Wald interviewed Cubans inside and outside the walls of the sanatorium to examine whether the barriers represented a "golden cage" or a prison. She insists that those inside receive good care in a "super luxurious setting that includes everything from high protein diet to air conditioners and color televisions in resort-like cottages and modern apartments." But, she acknowledges, "for those who value personal liberty over all else—even life—the Cuban requirement that HIV carriers relocate to a health care facility ... is on a par with placing them in a concentration camp."[14] Wald is convinced that most Cuban people believe the risks to the general population are great enough to justify the forced incarceration. According to Wald, those who have themselves undergone the isolation feel a "sense of security" within the walls and understand that AIDS itself is their worst problem, not where they live or work. Cubans who do not test positive for HIV feel a lot safer because the infected ones are inside: "Well, I'm safe as long as they're in there."[15]

Whether or not Wald's and Scheper-Hughes's assessments are overly positive, more recent economic hardships in Cuba preclude optimism about the maintenance of the quality of physical care within the institutions. The economic constraints coupled with the rise in the numbers of HIV-infected people isolated in the special sanatoriums have led to some deteriorating conditions and greater dissatisfaction of the inmates. While there are continuing reports that some people infect themselves in order to escape the escalating deprivations outside the barbed-wire confines, many of those inside find significant reason to be dissatisfied. One told *New York Times* reporter Tim Golden, "It is very difficult to be just sitting here waiting to die." Isolated and depressed, another inmate realized, "We have lost our freedom; that is the most important thing there is."[16]

Recent Cuban experience illustrates another very significant outcome of the forcible isolation policy: It has not been effective in stopping the epidemic. The confidence and safety that people have felt outside the walls of the sanatoriums have been demonstrated to be false. The numbers of people infected with HIV in Cuba continue to grow despite the policy, especially as the country opens to more foreign tourism and investment. As one observer put it, "The isolation of people in the sanitariums [*sic*] has given everyone else a mistaken idea. They think that AIDS is in the sanatoriums, not out on the street." Because of their sense of security, Cubans generally do not adopt practices, like the use of condoms, that would stem the spread of infection. Although arguably slowing the spread of the epidemic, forcible isolation has not been able to stop it.[17]

Considering Cuba's experience alongside New York's history with Mary Mallon may help us begin to resolve United States' priorities. Officials in New York immediately isolated Mallon in 1907, but they did not repeat the policy with most other carriers, even other noncooperative carriers. By comparison, Cuba's example of AIDS control, however much we might condemn its totalitarianism, is at least in appearance consistent and even-handed, applying equally to all who test positive. The question remains, though: Are lower disease rates and equity sufficient measures of the value of a public health program?

It is fair to say, I think, that what is most jarring to some Americans about both the Cuban example and Mary Mallon's experience is that individual liberty seems to be irrevocably and maybe too quickly overridden by the perceived larger good of protecting the public's health. Health officials went immediately to what even their own policies said should be their last resort when they isolated Mary Mallon without trying possible alternatives, and they were supported in their arbitrary actions two years after the fact by the court of law and even later by the court of public opinion. The actions of the officials—establishing indefinite and involuntary permanency to her isolation—were condoned even though they had not initially included due process procedures and rehabilitative measures. By devaluing Mallon with the label of "Typhoid Mary," society helped to cast her aside to an island where her risk to social order and health could be contained. A health policy that emphasizes a custodial as much as a health-keeping function makes it easier to dismiss individuals from the social polity, but these custodial aspects are also the ones we find so perplexing and problematic as we develop public health policies at the end of the twentieth century.[18]

If health officials at the time could have more convincingly argued that Mallon was such a unique menace to those around her that there was no choice but to apply the harshest penalty, historical judgment might be kinder. But the hundreds or thousands of other carriers remaining on the streets of New York, both unidentified and registered, belied such a conclusion, especially in light of other carriers who had caused more typhoid fever than Mary Mallon and had shown equal resistance to restraint. There were other ways to keep Mary Mallon from transmitting typhoid fever short of leaving her on an island for twenty-six years. If health officials could have initially approached her without force, if they could have initially—in 1907—retrained her for a job of equal or higher status and pay that did not involve food preparation, she might not have continued to be a risk to others. If she had been provided with a subsidy to help her survive until such time as she could have become economically independent, she might have been of a mind to try to learn prescribed sanitary routines. Clearly, these and other alternatives are easier for us to see now than for New York health officials early in the century. But the fact that some of these alternatives were strongly supported by public health experts such as Charles V. Chapin of Rhode Island and Health Commissioner Ernst Lederle in New York suggests that other possibilities were within reach at the time and could have been applied to Mallon.

This is not to suggest that Mallon herself should remain blameless in historical judgment. While it seems that health officials acted too precipitously and without sufficient tact or understanding of her situation, it also seems that Mallon herself overreacted to their advances. Mallon felt that public health officials discriminated against her, and her perception made her resistance to public health authority all the stronger. Her ire, once raised, could not be contained again, and it contributed to escalating the chain of events and in part to her long-term incarceration. But she was the one who was the most vulnerable, and, in the face of a powerful health authority, she paid the highest price.

If we can use history to explore the various aspects of identification and isolation, even though the analogy with the past is imperfect, perhaps we can avoid some of the mistakes health officials made in Mallon's case and act more judiciously today. We can learn to pay careful attention to the injury that is caused by stigmatizing labels. If public health law were to be applied more equitably, then people might begin to trust it not to discriminate in their particular cases. A more highly trusted public health system could more effectively educate people who carry disease to refrain from activities that put others at risk, making isolation truly a last resort. There might remain a few individuals who would need to be forcibly separated from society in order to stop them from willfully transmitting disease, but with an equitably applied public health policy, we might expect the number to be small.

People who have the potential for putting others at risk need, probably more than anything else, to be made aware of their infectivity and taught how to minimize or prevent it. This argument is made, for example, by Johan Giesecke, an infectious disease specialist in Stockholm who studied and participated in Sweden's efforts to control AIDS. Giesecke believes that "strong public confidence in a benevolent and non-discriminatory state and health care system" is more valuable than "repressive legislation."[19] This is also the conclusion that emerges from our study of Mary Mallon's experiences. If she had had confidence in a benevolent system, she would have been more inclined to cooperate with authorities. Instead, she had reason to believe the system would work against her, that who she was—a poor, immigrant, single, middle-aged woman—made her vulnerable to harm by the system rather than protection by it.

Unfortunately, there are numerous examples in twentieth-century U.S. public health history that lead people to conclude, with Mary Mallon, that policies have been discriminatory and have not been fairly applied. In 1900, San Francisco health authorities literally strung a quarantine rope around Chinatown in their efforts to stem an outbreak of the plague, blatantly relying on prejudices and stereotypes to identify the group blamed for putting the population at risk.[20] In the 1930s, the U.S. Public Health Service began an experiment in Macon County, Alabama, to trace the natural development of syphilis in African-American males, and in the process denied the participants the benefits of effective therapy.[21] The Tuskegee experiment, now notorious, lasted forty years. It is no accident, according to historian Alan Kraut, that immigrants and racial minorities have historically felt the strongest pressure from the discriminatory application of health policies. Nativist beliefs lead society to attach the stigma of disease to such already marginalized individuals, isolating them even further from the mainstream. Immigrants have been consistently despised and feared—and then labeled— as harbingers of disease and death to the native-born.[22]

Fairness in health policy is not just a matter of uniform and consistent application of the laws. If so, the Cuban example of incarcerating all people who test positive for HIV would be our model for creating a system that could be trusted. Process and method are also crucial to our thinking about equity in health policy. How we as a society decide which of the myriad health issues facing us will receive our priority attention, and how we talk about, identify, and treat those individuals we consider to put others at risk reflect our cultural values and our strength as a nation. What Mary Mallon's story contributes to our efforts to create a more just health system is exemplary pitfalls to avoid and signposts for flagging important individual issues.

Early experience with HIV infection indicates that American public health has not yet moved very far away from some of the social insensitivities evident in Mallon's day. In the early 1980s, the infection's initial association with gay men and Haitian refugees allowed the marginalization of homosexuality and race to shape an emerging disease-associated stigma and exacerbate what seemed to many an unfair distribution of blame. The response from gay men was rapid. Believing the governmental response flawed and inadequate, gay activists, predominantly white, middle-class men accustomed to working within the system despite the homophobia they felt daily, organized to combat the disease within their own communities. The combination of local organization and public efforts proved beneficial, and in cities like San Francisco, where AIDS initially hit hardest, incidence rates began to fall.[23] But other groups affected by HIV— "gay/bisexual black and Hispanic men ... many black and Hispanic i.v. drug users; black and Hispanic women and black and Hispanic babies born to these women"—could not offer effective, organized responses, and they continued to suffer greater social stigma and higher rates of disease.[24] The initial thinking and early actions to combat AIDS provide a powerful example of how public health policy still falls short of equitable judgment and treatment for all.

The United States can legally decide, as the Cuban government did, that protection of the public health is a higher national priority than are individual rights and the liberty of the stricken. Or it can instead choose to continue to consider civil liberty an equally dominant national priority and work to establish a policy of fair nondiscriminatory health reform that will earn the confidence of all American citizens and provide them genuine, cooperative, long-term protection. Such changes would move the country in a direction that will foster the public's health and at the same time show maximum respect for individual rights. As I write, millions of uninsured Americans continue to feel that they are outsiders to the health system. Perhaps Mary Mallon's story of the confusion, anger, and final bitter denial of an outsider should be in the minds of those who will determine our future public health strategies.

Blame and Responsibility

Public support plummeted and opinion turned against Mary Mallon in 1915 because of her conscious return to cooking when people believed she should have learned her lesson. "The chance was given to her five years ago to live in freedom," editorialized the *New York Tribune*, and "she deliberately elected to throw it away."[25] Historians have since that time been no more lenient in their assessment of Mallon's informed return to cooking. In 1994, Robert J. T. Joy put it directly: "Consider that Mallon disappeared for five years, and used several aliases and went straight back to cooking! . . . Now, as far as I am concerned, this verges on assault with the possibility of second degree murder. Mallon knows she carries typhoid, knows she should not cook—and does so."[26]

To be sure, Mary Mallon was not entirely blameless when she knowingly returned to cooking in 1915, but the blame must be more broadly shared. Much of what Mallon did can be explained by events greater than herself and beyond her control. It is only in the full context of her life and the actions of the health officials and the media that we can understand the personal position of Mary Mallon and people like her—people whom society accuses of endangering the health of others—and can hope to formulate policies that will address their individual needs while still permitting governments to do what they are obligated to do, act to protect the public's health.

Mallon was not a free agent in 1914, when she returned to cooking. Consider her circumstances. She had been abruptly, even violently, wrenched from her life, a life in which she found various satisfactions and from which she earned a decent living. She was physically separated from all that was familiar to her and isolated on an island. She was labeled a monster and a freak. She was not permitted to work at a job that had sustained her, but she was not retrained for any comparable work. If Lederle helped her find a job in a laundry, it did not provide the wages or job satisfaction to which she had previously become accustomed. Nor did it provide the social amenities, as limited as they were, of domestic work in the homes of New York's upper class. The health department, for all of Lederle's words of obligation to help her in 1910, did not provide her with long-term gainful employment. Neither did health officials, who precipitously locked Mallon up, succeed in convincing Mallon that her danger to the health of people for whom she cooked was real and lifelong. The medical arguments that carried weight among the elite at the time and have become more broadly convincing since did not resonate with her. There was no welfare system to support her. There was no viable "safety net," practical or intellectual, for an unemployed middle-aged Irish immigrant single woman.

So she did what many other healthy carriers since have done: returned to work to support herself. And the health department responded by doing what it felt it had to do when faced with a now very public uncooperative typhoid carrier: returned her to isolation. As we have seen, New York health officials did not isolate all the recalcitrant carriers it identified; many who had disobeyed health department guidelines were out in the streets during the years Mallon remained on the island. But officials had reason to act as they did. And so did Mary Mallon.

In other words, there were choices for both the health officials and Mary Mallon, and judgment, when we make it, should take this full context into account. Events could have evolved in a different pattern. If tempers had not been raised to fever pitch in 1907, and positions not solidified, various compromises and possibilities would have been available for education, training, employment, all of which might have led to decreasing the potential of Mallon's typhoid transmission. Health officials, who certainly held the reins of power most tightly, chose not to deal with their first identified healthy carrier in a flexible way. They chose to make an object lesson of her case. But it was a choice. If they had shown some personal respect for how difficult it was for Mary Mallon to cope with what happened to her, it is conceivable that she would have responded in kind, and come to respect their position. As it happened, neither side considered the other, and communication was stopped short.

Warren Boroson, who studied Mary Mallon's case, and Barry Blackwell, a psychiatric authority on noncompliant patients, have also concluded that her story could have been different, and happier, if "health authorities had been [immediately] more understanding and had given her [in Blackwell's words] 'a well paying job that would have fulfilled her need to care for others, that would have made her feel competent and appreciated, clean and healthy[.]'" These observers believe that health authorities held the power to create an atmosphere in which Mary Mallon could have become compliant, regardless of whether she accepted the theory of healthy carriers.[27]

But factors determining patient compliance have only recently been studied seriously, and health officials in the first decades of this century understandably focused their concerns elsewhere. Lederle, seemingly alone among New York health officials (although he had company elsewhere in the country), did see a public obligation to help Mary Mallon find satisfying work once they took away her regular employment, but his observation came too late in her history and came with too little force to solve the dilemma. From the vantage point of today, it seems clear that the blame heaped on Mary Mallon in 1915 when she returned to cooking, and by observers since, is more fairly a shared blame.

Not every case of carrier or patient noncompliance can be avoided. The evidence points to potential alternative endings for Mary Mallon's story which were not realized, but there are instances in which the maximum penalty of law, long-term or even lifetime denial of liberty, have been and will continue to be necessary. Mary Mallon's resistance came in part because she did not understand how she, a healthy woman, could be a threat to health. But some people who resist public health policy do so with full understanding of the medical theory of disease transmission and choose consciously to transmit disease anyway. It may not always be possible to prevent the involuntary restraint and isolation of individuals who want to use their illnesses to harm others. But our public policy should aim toward protecting individuals as well as society. It is important that we educate ourselves in alternatives, that we stress the human side of public health dilemmas, in order to prevent as much as possible the denial of personal liberty even as we work diligently to protect the health of the people.

In 1922, A. J. Chesley, who was then the executive officer of the Minnesota State Board of Health, clearly expressed the conflicting nature of the dilemma then confronting public health authorities in the control of typhoid fever. His insights can help us today. Chesley saw two parts to the effort to reduce the health threat of typhoid. First, the public had to be convinced that it was "good business" to support the use of public funds for health work. Second, hearkening to the language of President Theodore Roosevelt's progressive reforms, he urged his colleagues, "the typhoid carrier must be given a square deal." Chesley explained, "This means compensation for his losses incurred as the inevitable result of strict and logical enforcement of the measures necessary to prevent the swallowing by other people of his infectious bowel and bladder discharges."[28]

Chesley heeded the personal stories of typhoid carriers that bespoke the hardships and personal loss of the carrier condition. There was "Mrs. M. S.," a fifty-year-old widow, who supported her eight-year-old foster child and herself by doing housework and cooking until she was identified as a typhoid carrier and "forbidden to engage in the only kind of employment which have [*sic*] enabled her to keep soul and body together." Chesley concluded, "No safe employment has been provided for her. Is this a square deal for the carrier?"[29] There was "A. D. W." and his family, who rented a farm and produced milk for their livelihood, "compelled to sell his cows at a sacrifice and to give up the dairying business permanently. This is a very serious financial loss to him and his family." There was "Mr. A. S.," a fifty-two-year-old cook for a railway construction crew, who was barred from cooking when identified as a carrier. "However, he was unable to make a living at other work, so in June, 1920, against the orders of the State Board of Health, he opened a restaurant." When the health department found him again and "caused him to close his restaurant," he promised once again not to engage in the occupation that put others at risk. But "after trying to get work he became discouraged and purchased a resort on a small lake and was about to act as guide and cook for fishermen at this resort" when health officials again banned him from the work. Chesley realized, "Mr. A. S. has become discouraged. His age and physical condition make it impossible for him to find work other than of the type which he is forbidden to do. This man is broken in spirit."[30]

How, Chesley asked, is the carrier to be treated more fairly, to get a "square deal"? "Unquestionably, the public must demand protection against the typhoid carrier menace," he realized. But he also understood, "When an individual suffers for the benefit of the community as a whole as in war service no one questions the justice of his claim against the community." Thus, "social conscience" demanded that the state similarly compensate "persons whose means of earning are interfered with for the public good." Only by fulfilling both sides of the equation, both encouraging public officials to do their job by identifying carriers and at the same time understanding the carriers' difficulties and providing them realistic alternatives to cooking, could typhoid be eliminated.[31]

How *can* we address the problem that is now, still, again, before us? Shall we insist on locking up the people who are sick or who are at risk of becoming sick because they threaten the health of those around them? The representations of Mary Mallon and of Typhoid Mary reviewed in this book and the range of meanings that continue to resonate from the beginning of the century to its close indicate that our own situation in large part determines how we think about these questions and informs our various responses to this public health dilemma. We can view people who carry disease as if they consciously bring sickness and death to others—like the demon breaking skulls into the skillet. We can view such people as inadvertent carriers of disease, as innocent victims of something uncontrollable in their own bodies. We can see disease carriers as instruments of others' evil, as victims of society's or science's perversity.

Wherever we position ourselves, as individuals and as a society, we must come to terms with the fundamental issue that whether we think of them as guilty or innocent, people who seem healthy can indeed carry disease and under some conditions may menace the health of those around them. We can blame, fear, reject, sympathize, and understand: withal, we must decide what to do. Optimally, we search for responses that are humane to the sufferers and at the same time protect those who are still healthy.

Mary Mallon's captivity and the stories of other individual sufferers and carriers demonstrate the need for policies that, when health needs and personal rights conflict, put the least restriction on individual lives compatible with protecting the public's health. Programs that seek to stem preventable diseases at the price of stigmatizing or impoverishing people, or that employ Cuban-style coercive mass isolation, are unjust, undemocratic, and ultimately not effective. The conflict between competing priorities of civil liberties and public health will not disappear, but we can work toward developing public health guidelines that recognize and respect the situation and point of view of individual sufferers. People who can endanger the health of others would be more likely to cooperate with officials trying to stem the spread of disease if their economic security were maintained and if they could be convinced that health policies would treat them fairly. Equitable policies applied with the knowledge of history should produce very few captives to the public's health.

Events in Mary Mallon's Life

September 23, 1869	Born in Cookstown, County Tyrone, Ireland
1883	Immigrated to America
March 19, 1907	Apprehended by health department; isolated at Willard Parker Hospital; thereafter sent to North Brother Island
June–July, 1909	Habeas corpus hearing, New York Supreme Court
July 16, 1909	Remanded back to North Brother Island
February 19, 1910	Signed affidavit and released from North Brother Island
December, 1911	Tried to sue city for damages
October, 1914	Hired as cook at Sloane Maternity Hospital
March 26, 1915	Apprehended for second time by health department and sent back to North Brother Island
March 1, 1918	Employed by city as Riverside Hospital helper
June 11, 1918	Granted off-island privileges
1925–1932	Worked in Riverside Hospital laboratory
December 4, 1932	Suffered a stroke, becoming bedridden
November 11, 1938	Died at Riverside Hospital
November 13, 1938	Buried from St. Luke's Church; interred in St. Raymond's Cemetery, Bronx, N.Y.

Notes

INTRODUCTION

1. The term "Typhoid Mary" should always appear in quotation marks because it is a phrase applied to Mary Mallon and not her real name and in acknowledgment of its negative connotation. However, because the consistent use of quotation marks becomes too cumbersome and because the phrase appears without them so frequently in common parlance, I will use the term alone throughout the book. I urge readers to remember that the term is a creation of circumstances and not a given name.

2. The most recent, although brief, historical look at her is Alan M. Kraut, *Silent Travelers: Germs, Genes, and the "Immigrant Menace"* (New York: Basic Books, 1994), pp. 98–103.

3. *Milwaukee Journal*, January 25, 1994, p. 1.

4. *Wisconsin State Journal*, December 22, 1993. I use these local examples knowing that similar stories are published throughout the country.

5. The phrase is Wade Oliver's, from his biography of William H. Park. See Wade W. Oliver, *The Man Who Lived for Tomorrow: A Biography of William Hallock Park, M.D.* (New York: E. P. Dutton & Co., 1941), p. 266. See pp. 262–66 for his full section on Mary Mallon.

6. In the Matter of the Application for a Writ of Habeas Corpus for the Production of Mary Mallon, New York Supreme Court (June 28–July 22, 1909), Return to Writ. Available at the New York County Courthouse.

7. *New Yorker*, January 26, 1935, p. 21.

8. *New York American*, April 2, 1907, p. 2.

9. *New York American*, June 30, 1909, p. 18.

10. The phrase "microbes into infinity" is from Nicholas Wade, "Ebola's Vengeance: Microbes into Infinity," *New York Times*, May 15, 1995.

CHAPTER ONE: "Rigorous Spirit of Science"

1. Parts of this and the next chapter are derived from Judith Walzer Leavitt, " 'Typhoid Mary' Strikes Back: Bacteriological Theory and Practice in

Early Twentieth-Century Public Health," *Isis* 83 (1992): 608–29, and are reprinted here with permission.

My conclusion that Mary Mallon was the first healthy carrier to be identified and followed in North America rests on Soper's work (see n. 3) and on the subsequent renditions of her story. See, for example, Milton J. Rosenau, *Preventive Medicine and Hygiene*, 6th ed. (New York: D. Appleton-Century Co., 1935), p. 141. I looked for identification or charting of specific healthy carriers in the United States before Mary Mallon because the knowledge of such people had existed and been in use for about ten years previous, but I could not find other individuals so identified. See, for example, Walter Reed, Victor C. Vaughn, and Edward O. Shakespeare, *Abstract of Report on the Origin and Spread of Typhoid Fever in U.S. Military Camps During the Spanish War of 1898* (Washington, D.C.: Government Printing Office, 1900), pp. 178–79. My thanks to Robert J. T. Joy for reminding me of this source. Gordon Jones posited that a carrier was responsible for a seventeenth-century outbreak in Virginia, but even the identification of illness as typhoid fever is problematic in that period, retrospectively without bacteriological confirmation. See Gordon W. Jones, "The Scourge of Typhoid," *American History Illustrated* 1 (1967): 222–28.

2. The social connection between the Thompsons and the Sopers was suggested to me by Tom Wenzell, the Thompsons' grandson, in a telephone interview from his home in New York City, October 27, 1994. I am grateful to Gerard Fergerson for putting me in touch with Mr. Wenzell, and to Mr. Wenzell for his help.

3. See George Soper, "[The Epidemic at Butler, Pa.]" *Engineering News* 50 (1903): 542; "Filtration and Typhoid," *Engineering Magazine* 26 (1904): 754–55; "The Epidemic of Typhoid Fever at Ithaca, N.Y.," *Journal of the New England Water Works Association* 18 (1905): 431–61; and "The Management of the Typhoid Fever Epidemic at Watertown, N.Y., in 1904," ibid. 21 (1908): 87–163. The last was published after Soper's initial work on Mary Mallon, but the work reported in it was carried out and known earlier. On the Ithaca investigation see Heather Munro Prescott, " 'How Long Must We Send Our Sons Into Such Danger?' Cornell University and the Ithaca Typhoid Epidemic of 1903," Paper presented at the Conference on New York State History, June 11, 1988. I am grateful to Professor Prescott for sending me a typescript of this paper. Soper's biography in brief is available in *Who's Who in America* 24 (1946–47): 2215. Soper later went on to work on sewerage problems, on air and ventilation in subways, and on street cleaning methods.

Soper's investigations of Mary Mallon were published in three main articles. The first, "The Work of a Chronic Typhoid Germ Distributor," *Journal of the American Medical Association* (hereafter *JAMA*) 48 (1907): 2019–22, was the first published account tracing Mary Mallon. See also his "Typhoid Mary," *The Military Surgeon* 45 (July, 1919): 1–15; and "The Curious Career of Typhoid Mary," *Bulletin of the New York Academy of Medicine* 15 (October, 1939): 698–712. In his 1939 article, Soper identified the renters as the family of General William Henry Warren, instead of Charles Henry Warren as he had done elsewhere (p. 699). He identified the investigators that the Thompsons first hired as "experts." His only specific naming of them occurred in the 1907 article, when he wrote the water samples were analyzed by E. E. Smith and D. D. Jackson (p. 2020). In one case Soper identified the person who hired him as Mrs. Thompson ("Curious Career," p. 699). Mrs. Thompson's role was confirmed by Tom Wenzell (see n. 2).

It is not entirely clear when Soper began his investigation of the Oyster Bay outbreak. In a few accounts, he wrote it was during the "winter" and also claims it was four months after the August outbreak, which would place his start sometime in December, 1906. When he wrote he worked on the investigation "for some months" before locating Mary Mallon in March, 1907, it suggests that he began his investigations in November, 1906. In yet another rendition, he claims he was "not called for more than six months after the outbreak," which would date the beginning of his investigation in February, 1907, only one month before her apprehension. ("Winter" is stated in "Chronic Typhoid Germ Distributor," p. 2019 and in "Typhoid Mary," p. 2; the four-month interval is given in "Curious Career," p. 704; the more than six months claim is in a letter to the *British Medical Journal*, January 7, 1939, p. 38.) See chap. 4 for more on Soper's involvement.

4. Soper had not sought healthy carriers in his earlier typhoid fever work in Ithaca, Butler, or Watertown, but in his first published article on Mary Mallon he did refer to the German word for chronic carriers, "typhusbazillentragerin," indicating his familiarity with the literature. See "Chronic Typhoid Germ Distributor," p. 2022. When he first presented his work on the Mallon case to the Biological Society of Washington, D.C., on April 6, 1907, he called attention to the work of pioneer bacteriologist Robert Koch. See the discussion of the meeting in "Chronic Typhoid Fever Producer," *Science* n.s. 25 (1907): 863. I am grateful to John Q. Barrett for helping me locate the minutes of this meeting in the Smithsonian Archives, Record Unit 7815. In his 1919 recounting of Mary Mallon's discovery, Soper wrote: "Somewhat similar investigations had been made in Germany, and I make no claim of originality or for any other credit in her discovery. My interest and experience in the epidemiology of typhoid had been of long standing. I had read the address which Koch had delivered before the Kaiser Wilhelm's Akademic, November 28, 1902, and his investigation into the prevalence of typhoid at Trier, and thought it was one of the most illuminating of documents. In fact it had been the basis of

much of the epidemic work with which I had been connected." See Soper, "Typhoid Mary," p. 14. The peaches are mentioned in "Curious Career," p. 702.

5. An excellent study tracing epidemiology to its prebacteriology roots is William Coleman, *Yellow Fever in the North* (Madison: University of Wisconsin Press, 1987).

6. The seven outbreaks that Soper attributed to Mary Mallon are listed at the end of the laboratory reports submitted by the New York City Health Department to the New York Supreme Court at Mallon's habeas corpus hearing in July, 1909. See In the Matter of the Application for a Writ of Habeas Corpus for the Production of Mary Mallon, New York Supreme Court (June 28–July 22, 1909). Available at the New York County Courthouse. Soper details the cases in "Chronic Typhoid Germ Distributor," p. 2020; "Typhoid Mary," pp. 5–7; and "Curious Career," pp. 702–4. The following discussion is garnered from all of the above. The employment agency from which Soper received most of his information was called Mrs. Strickers', although it was run by a man (unnamed in the extant records).

7. "Typhoid Mary," p. 6. Soper introduces an error, no doubt typographical, in this account of the Mamaroneck outbreak, giving the date here as 1904, when he means 1900. He also misspells Hermann M. Biggs's name (as "Herman M. Briggs," p. 9). See also "Curious Career," p. 702.

8. The court records give nine as the number infected in the Drayton group, but cite the source as Soper, who indicates seven sufferers in the family and the addition (which he does not always note) of a day nurse and household worker.

9. In one account of this outbreak, Soper added two other individuals, a nurse and a "woman who came to work by the day," as also afflicted with typhoid fever; in another account he added just one. "Curious Career," p. 703, adds the two; "Typhoid Mary," p. 6, adds one.

10. R. J. Wilson later was one of the physicians who helped supervise Mallon's stay on North Brother Island. Soper refers to him as R. L. Wilson in "Curious Career,"p. 703, and in "Chronic Typhoid Germ Distributor," p. 2021, but gets his name right in "Typhoid Mary," p. 9.

11. Quoted in Soper, "Chronic Typhoid Germ Distributor," p. 2019–20.

12. The list of cases that Soper traced to Mary Mallon is presented in " 'Carriers' of Infectious Disease," *School Health News* 4 (February, 1918), p. 1, but it wrongly attributes seven cases to the Oyster Bay outbreak. It goes on to list the other outbreaks that Soper thought could be traced to Mallon in 1913–1915.

13. Soper, "Chronic Typhoid Germ Distributor," p. 2022.

14. Soper presents the seven outbreaks and the numbers as provided above, and concludes: "In all there have been twenty-six cases and one death," in "Chronic Typhoid Germ Distributor," p. 2021; he repeats the information in "Typhoid Mary," p. 9. William Park repeats it in his 1908 article, "Typhoid Bacilli Carriers," *JAMA* 51 (1908): 981, and in the 1914 textbook he wrote with Anna Williams, *Pathogenic Microorganisms: A Practical Manual for Students, Physicians, and Health Officers* (New York: Lea & Febiger, 1914), pp. 360–61. The New York City Health Department gives the same count in its 1907 *Annual Report* (p. 321); and I am guilty of repeating the same mistake in "'Typhoid Mary' Strikes Back." There is a hint that two more people might have been infected at the Drayton home (see nn. 8 and 9), but I will use twenty-two as the number of cases, since that is the figure for which Soper actually provides evidence.

Typhoid inoculations, which were developed based on Almroth Wright's work in 1896 and work by R. Pfeiffer and Wilhelm Kolle in the same year, were first recommended for use in the United States army in 1909 and made compulsory for troops in 1911. Immunity achieved through inoculation is not lifelong. Such vaccinations became common during a threat of an epidemic, but during the years before Mary Mallon was incarcerated in 1907, we can safely assume that none of the members of the families for whom she worked had been inoculated. Many might have achieved permanent immunity from having recovered from a case of typhoid fever.

15. Minutes of the Biological Society were printed in *Science* n.s. 25 (1907): 863–65. See also the Minutes of the 429th meeting of the Biological Society of Washington, April 6, 1907, Record Unit 7185, Smithsonian Archives. I am grateful to John Q. Barrett for helping me locate the archival minutes.

16. See, for example, Alan M. Kraut, *Silent Travelers: Germs, Genes, and the "Immigrant Menace"* (New York: Basic Books, 1994), p. 98; and Mary C. McLaughlin, "Mary Mallon: Alias Typhoid Mary," *The Recorder* (American Irish Historical Society) 40 (1979): 44–57. On pages 47–48, Dr. McLaughlin writes: "Most of the cases of typhoid were in the servants. It is postulated that the food prepared by Mary for members of the various families was mostly cooked and thus the typhoid bacillus killed. The uncooked desserts were probably prepared and served by the butlers or maids. The chances of Mary handling desserts of the servants was greater."

17. For example, the Daniels and Starr investigation of the Dark Harbor, Maine, outbreak concluded that either the footman alone or the first three (of seven) cases simultaneously had been infected outside the home and brought the infection into the house. Soper, when reviewing the evidence, concluded, "On checking over [Daniel's] report I could not agree with him. I found that

the three had not eaten the same food or drunk the same water." See "Curious Career," p. 703.

18. Soper relates this story in "Typhoid Mary," pp. 7–8; and in "Curious Career," pp. 704–5. I analyze it more closely in later chapters.

19. The early years of Mallon's incarceration can be found in the Soper articles listed in n. 3 and in Park, "Typhoid Bacilli Carriers," p. 981. The published health department reports for the year 1907 note merely that "special studies were made during the year on the so-called typhoid carriers. . . . A woman who had served as cook in various families during the past five years is known to have infected at least twenty-six people and has caused at least two deaths. This patient was examined from week to week." *Annual Report of the Board of Health of the Department of Health of the City of New York for the Year Ending December 31, 1907* (New York: Martin E. Brown Co., 1908), p. 321. (Hereafter Board of Health *Annual Reports* are cited NYCDH, *AR*, followed by the year. The actual titles of reports varied from year to year.) Any unpublished health department material for this period, with the exception of some Minutes which are here used, is either destroyed or not available at the present time.

20. The legal aspects of the story are described in detail in chap. 3.

21. The classic epidemic during which the city officials fled is the yellow fever epidemic that struck Philadelphia in 1793. See John Powell, *Bring Out Your Dead: The Great Plague of Yellow Fever in Philadelphia in 1793* (Philadelphia: University of Pennsylvania Press, 1949); and Martin S. Pernick, "Politics, Parties, and Pestilence: Epidemic Yellow Fever in Philadelphia and the Rise of the First Party System," *William and Mary Quarterly* 29 (1972): 559–86.

22. Nineteenth-century public health work can be followed best through local studies. See, for example, John Duffy, *A History of Public Health in New York City, 1625–1866* (New York: Russell Sage Foundation, 1968); John Duffy, *A History of Public Health in New York City, 1866–1966* (New York: Russell Sage Foundation, 1974); Judith Walzer Leavitt, *The Healthiest City: Milwaukee and the Politics of Health Reform* (Princeton: Princeton University Press, 1982); Stuart Galishoff, *Newark, the Nation's Unhealthiest City, 1832–1895* (New Brunswick, N.J.: Rutgers University Press, 1988), and his *Safeguarding the Public Health: Newark, 1895–1918* (Westport, Conn.: Greenwood Press, 1975).

23. Louis P. Cain, "Raising and Watering a City: Ellis Sylvester Chesbrough and Chicago's First Sanitation System," *Technology and Culture* 13 (1972): 353–72. See also, Heman Spalding and Herman N. Bundesen, "Control of Typhoid Fever in Chicago," *American Journal of Public Health* 8 (1918): 358.

24. Although some historians have seen bacteriology as a complete break with the filth theory of disease, and have treated this discovery as a paradigmatic revolution in medicine, a number of recent studies have described the "new" public health more as an integration of old and new. For example, see Allan M. Brandt, *No Magic Bullet: A Social History of Venereal Disease in the United States since 1800* (New York: Oxford University Press, 1985); John Ettling, *The Germ of Laziness: Rockefeller Philanthropy and Public Health in the New South* (Cambridge: Harvard University Press, 1981); Nancy Tomes, "The Private Side of Public Health: Sanitary Science, Domestic Hygiene, and the Germ Theory, 1870–1900," *Bulletin of the History of Medicine* 64 (1990): 509–39; Naomi Rogers, *Dirt and Disease: Polio in America before FDR* (New Brunswick, N.J.: Rutgers University Press, 1992); and Barbara Bates, *Bargaining for Life: A Social History of Tuberculosis, 1876–1938* (Philadelphia: University of Pennsylvania Press, 1992). For earlier studies along these lines, consult, for example, Lloyd Stevenson, "Science Down the Drain: On the Hostility of Certain Sanitarians to Animal Experimentation, Bacteriology and Immunology," *Bulletin of the History of Medicine* 29 (1955): 1–26; William Rothstein, "Bacteriology and the Medical Profession," in his *American Physicians in the Nineteenth Century* (Baltimore: Johns Hopkins University Press, 1972), pp. 261–81; Phyllis Allen Richmond, "American Attitudes Toward the Germ Theory of Disease (1860–1880)," *Journal of the History of Medicine* 9 (1954): 428–54; Howard D. Kramer, "The Germ Theory and the Early Public Health Program in the United States," *Bulletin of the History of Medicine* 22 (1948): 233–47; Barbara Rosenkrantz, "Cart Before Horse: Theory, Practice, and Professional Image in American Public Health 1810–1920," *Journal of the History of Medicine and Allied Sciences* 29 (1974): 55–73. See also Leavitt, " 'Typhoid Mary' Strikes Back," pp. 608–29.

25. James H. Cassedy, *Charles V. Chapin and the Public Health Movement* (Cambridge: Harvard University Press, 1962). Chapin served as superintendent of health for the city of Providence from 1884 through 1931. I focus on him in this section to illustrate a public health officer who represented an extreme of support for bacteriology; most health officials of the period more likely adopted some of the newer ideas alongside the older ones and saw that germ theory and filth theory had some things in common.

26. Charles V. Chapin, "Dirt, Disease and the Health Officer," in *Papers of Charles V. Chapin, M.D.: A Review of Public Health Realities*, ed. Clarence L. Scamman (New York: The Commonwealth Fund, 1934), pp. 20–26; quotations from pp. 21, 22. Chapin maintained this position throughout his long career. He wrote after his retirement from public life about the changes he had witnessed during his career in public health: "When I was first drawn into public health I had to accept the teachings of our English friends as to the

close dependence of disease upon dirt. I soon found that these ideas were for the most part erroneous and were so strongly entrenched in this country that they have proved to be one of the greatest hindrances to the development of public health. A large part of my own time has been occupied in getting English rubbish out of American heads. So far as I can see there is very little 'dirt' that is really dangerous to health." Charles V. Chapin to George Soper, June 10, 1932, John Hay Library, Brown University, Providence, Rhode Island. Chapin continued, echoing directly words he had used before: "The removal of garbage, street cleaning and even the control of dumps are most important from an esthetic standpoint but in my opinion have practically no influence upon public health. I have never seen any evidence that they have." Chapin died in 1941.

27. Chapin, "The Fetich of Disinfection," *Papers*, pp. 65–75. Chapin first presented this paper as an address to the American Medical Association in Boston, June, 1906. It was first published in *JAMA* 47 (August 25, 1906): 574–77.

28. See, for example, Charles V. Chapin, *The Sources and Modes of Infection* (New York: John Wiley & Sons, 1910), pp. 93–94.

29. Charles V. Chapin, *How to Avoid Infection*, Harvard Health Talks (Cambridge: Harvard University Press, 1918), p. 21.

30. Ibid., pp. 60–61.

31. Chapin created a "score card" delineating the relative value of various public health activities to give his fellow workers a practical guide. On a scale with a total of city activities at 100, he rated communicable disease work 36 and sanitation 9. Charles V. Chapin, "Effective Health Work," in *Papers*, pp. 37–45; the scale appears on pp. 41–42.

32. Chapin, "Dirt, Disease" p. 25.

33. Leavitt, *The Healthiest City.*

34. C.-E. A. Winslow, *The Evolution and Significance of the Modern Public Health Campaign* (New Haven: Yale University Press, 1923), p. 36. Quotation from third printing, July, 1984.

35. There are fewer than 500 sporadic cases of typhoid fever per year in the United States today. Richard C. Harruff, *Pathology Facts* (Philadelphia: J. B. Lippincott Co., 1994), p. 118.

36. See, for example, Michael P. McCarthy, *Typhoid and the Politics of Public Health in Nineteenth-Century Philadelphia* (Philadelphia: American Philosophical Society, 1987). See also Ronald K. Huch, " 'Typhoid' Truelsen, Water, and Politics in Duluth, 1896–1900," *Minnesota History* 47 (1981): 189–99; Reimert T. Ravenholt and Sanford P. Lehman, "History, Epidemiol-

ogy, and Control of Typhoid Fever in Seattle," *Medical Times* 92 (1964): 342–52; and Terra Ziporyn, "Typhoid Fever: A Disease of the Indifferent," in *Disease in the Popular American Press* (Westport, Conn.: Greenwood Press, 1988), pp. 71–111. On the medical understanding of the disease, see Leonard G. Wilson, "Fevers and Science in Early Nineteenth Century Medicine," *Journal of the History of Medicine and Allied Sciences* 33 (1978): 386–407; Lloyd G. Stevenson, "Exemplary Disease: The Typhoid Pattern," ibid. 37 (1982): 159–81; and Dale C. Smith, "Gerhard's Distinction between Typhoid and Typhus and Its Reception in America, 1833–1860," *Bulletin of the History of Medicine* 54 (1980): 368–85.

37. Abram S. Benenson, ed., *Control of Communicable Diseases in Man* 14th ed. (Washington, D.C.: American Public Health Association, 1985), pp. 420–24.

38. The available evidence suggests to me that typhoid fever was, in fact, one of the diseases most responsive to public health sanitation projects at the end of the nineteenth century. Of twenty-one cities analyzed by George A. Johnson in 1916, twenty showed significant reduction (between 28 and 85 percent) in typhoid mortality after the introduction of water filtration systems. See his "The Typhoid Toll," *Journal of the American Water Works Association* 3 (1916): 249–326, especially pp. 304–10. See also Edward Meeker, "The Improving Health of the United States 1850–1915," *Explorations in Economic History* 9 (1972): 353–73; and Eric Ashby, "Reflections on the Costs and Benefits of Environmental Pollution," *Perspectives in Biology and Medicine* 23 (1979): 7–24. For a slightly less optimistic reading of these data, see Gerald N. Grob, "Disease and Environment in American History," in *Handbook of Health, Health Care, and the Health Professions*, ed. David Mechanic (New York: Free Press, 1983), p. 18.

39. Leavitt, *The Healthiest City*, p. 61. In coastal cities, contaminated shellfish continued to constitute a risk even after city water works had been adequately protected.

40. Duffy, *A History of Public Health in New York City, 1866–1966*, passim.

41. Johnson, "The Typhoid Toll," pp. 249–326, graph is on p. 308. See also John Duffy, *The Sanitarians: A History of American Public Health* (Urbana: University of Illinois Press, 1990), chap. 13, "Bacteriology Revolutionizes Public Health"; and Christopher Hamlin, *A Science of Impurity: Water Analysis in Nineteenth-Century Britain* (Bristol: Adam Hilger, 1990).

42. C. L. Overlander, "The Transmission of Typhoid Fever," *Interstate Medical Journal* 21 (1914): 133–144.

43. The first to document the carrier state, with regard to bacteria in his

own saliva, was George M. Sternberg in 1881. See his "A Fatal Form of Septicaemia in the Rabbit Produced by the Subcutaneous Injection of Human Saliva," Special Report to the National Board of Health (Baltimore: John Murphy & Co., 1881), first published in the *National Board of Health Bulletin* 2 (1881): 781–83. I am grateful to Robert J. T. Joy for alerting me to this reference. In 1884 Fredrich Loeffler, the German bacteriologist, posited the concept of a healthy carrier of disease for diphtheria, and in 1893 Robert Koch did the same for cholera. In New York City, Hermann M. Biggs, William H. Park, and A. L. Beebe convincingly established the carrier principle in cases of diphtheria in 1893, finding virulent diphtheria bacilli in about 1 percent of the healthy throats in New York. Hermann M. Biggs, William H. Park, and Alfred L. Beebe, *Report on Bacteriological Investigations and Diagnosis of Diphtheria From May 4, 1893 to May 4, 1894*, Scientific Bulletin No. 1, Health Department, City of New York, From the Bacteriological Laboratory (New York: Martin B. Brown, 1895); available in Arno Press Reprint, *The Carrier State* (New York, 1977). Some 1890s studies uncovered typhoid bacilli in convalescent typhoid patients, sometimes years after initial infection, and by 1900 studies revealed that typhoid fever, too, could be transmitted by healthy recovered persons. See Reed, Vaughn, and Shakespeare, *Abstract of Report*, pp. 178–79. In 1902, Robert Koch published a paper on the subject, and during subsequent years a few typhoid carriers were discovered and described in Europe. See, for example, D. S. Davies and I. Walker Hall, "Typhoid Carriers, with an account of Two Institution Outbreaks traced to the same 'Carrier,'" *Proceedings of the Royal Society of Medicine*, 1907–8, pp. 175–91; and Alex Ledingham and J. C. G. Ledingham, "Typhoid Carriers," *British Medical Journal* 1 (January 4, 1908): 15–17. The most succinct account of the work on healthy carriers is C.-E. A. Winslow, *The Conquest of Epidemic Disease* (Madison: University of Wisconsin Press, 1980), pp. 337–46. The book was first published in 1943 by Princeton University Press. For specific carriers, see for example, Charles Bolduan and W. Carey Noble, "A Typhoid Bacillus-Carrier of Forty-Six Years' Standing, and a Large Outbreak of Milk-Borne Typhoid Fever Traced to This Source," *JAMA* 58 (1912): 7–9; C. W. Gould and G. L. Qualls, "A Study of the Convalescent Carriers of Typhoid," *JAMA* 58 (1912): 542–46; Frederick G. Novy, "Disease Carriers," *Science* n.s. 36 (July 5, 1912): 1–10; and C. L. Overlander, "The Typhoid Carrier Problem," *Boston Medical and Surgical Journal* 169 (1913): 37–40. See also Mazyck Ravenel, "History of a Typhoid Carrier," *JAMA* 62 (1914): 2029–30; O. McDaniel and E. M. Wade, "The Significance of Typhoid Carriers in Community Life, with a Practical Method of Detecting Them," *American Journal of Public Health* 5 (1915): 764–65; F. M. Meader, "The Detection and Control of Typhoid Carriers of Disease," *Medical Times*, September, 1916, p. 278; and A. J. Chesley *et al.*, "Three Years' Experience in the Search for Typhoid Carriers in Minnesota," *JAMA* 68 (1917): 1882–85. For a lengthy exploration of the early work on healthy carriers, see John Andrew Mendelsohn, "Typhoid Mary: Medical Science, the State, and the 'Germ Carrier,'" undergraduate thesis, Harvard University, 1988. I thank Mr. Mendelsohn for his permission (granted through his advisor, Barbara Gutmann Rosenkrantz) for me to read this paper.

New diagnostic techniques aided in the discovery of people who had typhoid and ultimately of those who, although symptomless, could transmit the disease. In 1896, with the help of the newly developed Widal agglutination reaction test, a bacteriological assay for typhoid bacilli in the blood, New York City began offering free diagnoses for New Yorkers in health centers around the city. See Duffy, *A History of Public Health in New York City, 1866–1966*, pp. 105, 247. See also, for example, Thomas G. Hull, "The Widal Test as Carried Out in Public Health Laboratories," *American Journal of Public Health* 16 (1926): 901–4.

44. This history is pieced together from the sources cited in n. 43. See also, "Typhoid Bacillus Carriers: Their Importance and Management," *JAMA* 52 (May 8, 1909): 1501; and "Typhoid Carriers," *JAMA* 50 (June 13, 1908): 1986–87. Other factors that led to a better understanding of typhoid emerged by the 1940s. For example, while early investigators noted the predominance of women carriers, health officers usually attributed this to the fact that more women than men handled food (Chesley *et al.*, "Three Years' Experience," p. 1884). In the 1940s studies began to document more women carriers in the population at large, not just among those found in food-handling jobs, as transmitting the disease. In a New York state study published in 1943, the investigators concluded, "The rate of development of the carrier state at all ages is almost twice as high for females as for males." The most striking sex difference found in that study occurred in the group aged forty to forty-nine, in which 16 percent of female cases and only 3.5 percent of male cases resulted in the chronic carrier state. Wendell R. Ames and Morton Robins, "Age and Sex as Factors in the Development of the Typhoid Carrier State, and a Method for Estimating Carrier Prevalence," *American Journal of Public Health* 33 (1943): 223. Medical science in 1990 acknowledges similar sex and age differentials. I want to thank Dennis Maki, Head of the Section of Infectious Diseases, Department of Medicine, University of Wisconsin Medical School, and Herbert Dupont, Chief of Infectious Diseases at the University of Texas, Houston, for consulting with me on this issue.

45. On Hermann Biggs and the New York City laboratory, see C.-E. A. Winslow, *The Life of Hermann M. Biggs, M.D., D.Sc., LL.D.: Physician and Statesman of the Public Health* (Philadelphia: Lea & Febiger, 1929); David A. Blancher, "Workshops of the Bacteriological Revolution: A History of the Lab-

oratories of the New York City Department of Health," unpublished Ph.D. thesis, City University of New York, 1979; and Evelynn Maxine Hammonds, "The Search for Perfect Control: A Social History of Diphtheria, 1880–1930," unpublished Ph.D. thesis, Harvard University, 1993.

46. Chapin, quoted in Winslow, *Conquest*, p. 340.

47. On William Park, see W. W. Oliver, *The Man Who Lived for Tomorrow: A Biography of William Hallock Park, M.D.* (New York: E. P. Dutton & Co., 1941); Winslow, *Conquest*; Winslow, *The Life of Hermann M. Biggs* (Philadelphia: Lea & Febiger, 1929); and Hans Zinsser, "William Hallock Park, 1863–1939," *Journal of Bacteriology* 38 (1939): 1–3. For more on the significance of the laboratory, see Jon M. Harkness, "The Reception of Pasteur's Rabies Vaccine in America: An Episode in the Application of the Germ Theory of Disease," unpublished M.A. paper, History of Science Department, University of Wisconsin, 1987; and John Harley Warner, "The Fall and Rise of Professional Mystery: Epistemology, Authority, and the Emergence of Laboratory Medicine in Nineteenth-Century America," in *The Laboratory Revolution in Medicine*, ed. Andrew Cunningham and Perry Williams (Cambridge: Cambridge University Press, 1992). On Park's laboratory-based contributions to typhoid fever investigations, see, for example: "The Bacteriology of Typhoid Fever," *Medical News* 75 (December 16, 1899): 792–96; "Typhoid Bacilli Carriers," *JAMA* 51 (1908): 981–82; and "The Importance of Ice in the Production of Typhoid Fever," *JAMA* 49 (1907): 731–32.

48. Charles F. Bolduan is quoted in the William Hallock Park Papers, "Miscellaneous Information" file at the Public Health Research Institute, New York City. I am grateful to Shirley Chapin, the Institute Librarian, for her help in locating this material. Of course, New York City followed other carriers, and used the data they provided as well. See, for example, Bolduan and Noble, "A Typhoid Bacillus-Carrier of Forty-Six Years' Standing."

49. All the laboratory reports are filed with In the Matter of . . . Mary Mallon (1909).

50. Mary Mallon's letter, no date, in her own hand, is filed with ibid.

51. Soper, "Curious Career," p. 706.

52. Mr. Briehof (once spelled Nriehof) was the man Soper visited in his efforts to learn more about Mary Mallon. See chaps. 2 and 4.

53. George Ferguson to Mary Mallon, April 30, 1909, In the Matter of . . . Mary Mallon (1909), laboratory reports.

54. On laboratories and typhoid diagnoses, see Thomas G. Hull, "The Widal Test as Carried Out in Public Health Laboratories," *American Journal of Public Health* 16 (1926): 901–4; Fred Berry and R. E. Daniels, "Comparative

Studies in Typhoid Stool Examinations," ibid. 18 (1928): 883–92; Marion B. Coleman, "Serological and Bacteriological Procedures in the Diagnosis of Enteric Fevers," ibid. 25 supplement (1935): 147–51; and T. F. Sellers, "Practical Procedures in the Laboratory Diagnosis of Typhoid and Clinically Related Fevers," ibid. 27 (1937): 659–66. On transporting fecal specimens to the laboratory, see Th. M. Vogelsang, *Typhoid and Paratyphoid B Carriers and Their Treatment: Experiences from Western Norway* (Arbok: Universitetet I. Bergen, 1950), pp. 81–82. The legal issues in the case are discussed in greater detail in chap. 3.

55. In the Matter of . . . Mary Mallon (1909), Return to Writ.

56. In the Matter of . . . Mary Mallon (1909), Proposed Order and Notice of Settlement. It is probable that the judge did not understand the difficulty of quantifying bacterial counts in this era, nor their unreliability, and he might also have been baffled by the different reports of the two laboratories. The important point, no doubt, is that health department officials who testified to Mallon's dangers convinced the judge and he merely accepted the laboratory results at face value. I am grateful to bacteriologist Thomas Brock at the University of Wisconsin for his discussion of the quality of the procedures to measure bacilli in stools in this period.

57. In the Matter of . . . Mary Mallon (1909), Return to Writ.

58. Mary Mallon's undated letter is filed with ibid. Westmoreland and Mary Mallon refer to the same drug: hexamethylenamin is methenamine, a condensation product of ammonia and formaldehyde, $(CH_2)_6N_4$, a urinary antiseptic. Urotropin is a proprietary brand of methenamine.

59. Mary Mallon's letter describing the times physicians offered her surgery is discussed further in chap. 6. The letter can be found in In the Matter of . . . Mary Mallon (1909). On the surgical cure for typhoid fever, see Thomas J. Leary, "Surgical Method of Clearing Up Chronic Typhoid Carriers," *JAMA* 60 (1913): 1293–94; H. J. Nichols *et al.*, "The Surgical Treatment of Typhoid Carriers," *JAMA* 73 (1919): 680–84; Edwin Henes, "Surgical Treatment of Typhoid Carriers," *JAMA* 75 (1920): 1771–74; Walter H. Vosburgy and Anna E. Perkins, "The Surgical Treatment of Typhoid Carriers in the Gowanda State Hospital," *Surgery, Gynecology & Obstetrics* 40 (1925): 404–6; George H. Bigelow and Gaylord W. Anderson, "Cure of Typhoid Carriers," *JAMA* 101 (1933): 348–52; and Herman F. Senftner and Frank E. Coughlin, "Typhoid Carriers in New York State with Special Reference to Gall Bladder Operations," *American Journal of Hygiene* 17 (1933): 711–23.

60. William Hallock Park and Anna Williams, *Pathogenic Microorganisms: A Practical Manual for Students, Physicians, and Health Officers* (New York: Lea & Febiger, 1914), p. 361. The health officials could not force Mary

Mallon to undergo the surgical procedure. See, for example, Charles E. Simon, *Human Infection Carriers: Their Significance, Recognition and Management* (Philadelphia: Lea & Febiger, 1919), p. 101.

61. See the NYCDH, *AR*, 1921, p. 53. See also, for example, Eilif C. Hanssen, "The Present Status of the Typhoid Carrier Problem," *New York State Journal of Medicine* 39 (July 15, 1939): 1347–52.

62. In the Matter of . . . Mary Mallon (1909), Writ.

63. Note recorded on Mary Mallon Carrier Card #36, one of several different carrier cards, copies of which are in the Hoffman/Marr Collection. I am grateful to Ida Peters Hoffman and John S. Marr for their permission for me to visit their homes and to use the information collected in their own research.

64. The 1907–1909 numbers are computed from the laboratory reports filed with In the Matter of . . . Mary Mallon (1909), and the figures for 1915 through 1936 are computed from the various carrier cards in the Hoffman/Marr Collection.

65. See Cassedy, *Charles V. Chapin*, pp. 54–56, and Frederic P. Gorham, "The History of Bacteriology and Its Contribution to Public Health Work," in *A Half Century of Public Health*, ed. Mazyck Porcher Ravenel (New York: Arno Press Reprint ed., 1970), pp. 66–93. Originally published in 1921 by the American Public Health Association. Chapin's use of the new methods to trace typhoid fever carriers is illustrated in the case of Margaret Hurley, a Brown University fraternity house cook who infected at least four students with typhoid fever, one of whom died. See the Charles Value Chapin Scrapbooks, Collections of the Rhode Island Historical Society, February-March, 1929. My thanks to Sarah A. Leavitt for calling my attention to this case.

66. Winslow, *Evolution and Significance*, p. 36. Winslow identified the two decades from 1890 to 1910 as the "period of scientific control of communicable disease by the applications of bacteriology," a period he and others referred to as ushering in the "new public health" (p. 49). See also, for example, Philip D. Jordan, *The People's Health: A History of Public Health in Minnesota to 1948* (St. Paul: Minnesota Historical Society, 1953).

CHAPTER TWO: "Extraordinary and Even Arbitrary Powers"

1. For a general overview of public health departments and their work in this period consult John Duffy, *The Sanitarians: A History of American Public Health* (Urbana: University of Illinois Press, 1990).

2. For a full history of the New York City Health Department, see John Duffy, *A History of Public Health in New York City, 1625–1866* (New York:

Russell Sage Foundation, 1968) and John Duffy, *A History of Public Health in New York City, 1866–1966* (New York: Russell Sage Foundation, 1974). To understand how New York events influenced the hinterland, see, for example, Judith Walzer Leavitt, *The Healthiest City: Milwaukee and the Politics of Health Reform* (Princeton: Princeton University Press, 1982).

3. On this latter point, see Daniel M. Fox, "Social Policy and City Politics: Tuberculosis Reporting in New York, 1889–1900," *Bulletin of the History of Medicine* 49 (1975): 169–95.

4. On Hermann Biggs, see C.-E. A. Winslow, *The Life of Hermann M. Biggs, M.D., D.Sc., LL.D.: Physician and Statesman of the Public Health* (Philadelphia: Lea & Febiger, 1929).

5. Hermann Biggs's editorial from the *Monthly Bulletin*, March, 1911, quoted in Winslow, *Life of Hermann M. Biggs*, pp. 230–31.

6. A. W. Freeman, "Typhoid Fever and Municipal Administration," *U.S. Public Health Reports* 32 (1917): 642–55, quotation from p. 642.

7. Hermann M. Biggs, "The Preventive and Administrative Measures for the Control of Tuberculosis in New York City," *The Lancet* 2 (August 6, 1910): 371. See also John S. Billings, "Principles of Adminstrative (*sic*) Control of Communicable Diseases in Large Cities," *American Journal of Public Health* 5 (1915): 1204–8.

8. William H. Welch, "Foreword" to Winslow, *Life of Hermann Biggs*, pp. xi–xii.

9. George Soper, "Curious Career of Typhoid Mary," *Bulletin of the New York Academy of Medicine* 15 (October, 1939): 704.

10. Hoobler later became head of Children's Hospital, Detroit.

11. George Soper, "Typhoid Mary," *The Military Surgeon* 45 (July, 1919): 8.

12. Soper, "Curious Career," p. 705.

13. In Baker's account, she was not requesting fecal specimens at this time.

14. On the history of women in medicine, see Regina Morantz-Sanchez, *Sympathy and Science: Women Physicians in American Medicine* (New York: Oxford University Press, 1985).

15. S. Josephine Baker's autobiography *Fighting for Life* (New York: Macmillan Co., 1939) remains the best source for Baker's life story. See also the short biography written by Leona Baumgartner in *Notable American Women* vol. 1, ed. Edward T. James (Cambridge: Belknap Press of Harvard University Press, 1971), pp. 85–86. In her efforts to differentiate herself from the jazz

singer with the same name, Baker adopted the use of the initial of her first name, Sara.

16. Isabelle Keating, "Dr. Baker Tells How She Got Her Woman," *Brooklyn Daily Eagle*, May 8, 1932, p. A17. I am grateful to Ida Hoffman for leading me to this reference.

17. Baker, *Fighting for Life*, p. 74.

18. Ibid., p. 74.

19. Ibid., p. 75.

20. Mary Mallon to George Francis O'Neill (editor of the *American* crossed out and O'Neill's name added), In the Matter of the Application for a Writ of Habeas Corpus for the Production of Mary Mallon, New York Supreme Court (June 28–July 22, 1909). Available at the New York County Courthouse. This letter is fully discussed in chap. 6.

21. William H. Park, "Typhoid Bacilli Carriers," *JAMA* 51 (September 19, 1908): 982.

22. See, for example, ibid., pp. 981–82, and William Hallock Park and Anna Williams, *Pathogenic Microorganisms: A Practical Manual for Students, Physicians, and Health Officers* (New York: Lea & Febiger, 1914), pp. 355–73.

23. Charles V. Chapin, *The Sources and Modes of Infection* (New York: John Wiley & Sons, 1910), p. 110.

24. Milton J. Rosenau, *Preventive Medicine and Hygiene* (New York: D. Appleton-Century Co., 1935), pp. 137–38. See also William Saphir, Walter H. Baer, and Frederic Plotke, "The Typhoid Carrier Problem," *JAMA* 118 (1942): 964–67. According to one observer, there were over 35,000 deaths each year from typhoid fever in the United States. C. L. Overlander, "The Transmission of Typhoid Fever," *Interstate Medical Journal* 21 (1914): 133–44.

25. Cecil K. Blanchard, "Typhoid Carriers: Their Detection and Control," *Public Health News* (New Jersey State Department of Health) 9 (1924): 250–58.

26. M. Dorthy Beck and Arthur C. Hollister, *Typhoid Fever Cases and Carriers: An Analysis of Records of the California State Department of Public Health from 1910 through 1959* (Berkeley: State of California Department of Public Health, 1962), pp. 14, 18.

27. James G. Cumming, "Should the Barriers Against Typhoid be Continued?" *JAMA* 98 (1932): 94; and Saphir, Baer, and Plotke, "Typhoid Carrier Problem," p. 964. By 1930, Washington officials estimated only 671 carriers per 100,000 population.

28. Editorial, "A Pressing Problem," *American Journal of Public Health* (1915): 313.

29. Numbers of cases as reported in the New York City Health Department *Annual Reports*. See, for example, the table in the 1939 *Report* summarizing department data for the years 1898–1939.

30. A. L. Garbat, "Typhoid Carriers and Typhoid Immunity," Monograph 16, Rockefeller Institute for Medical Research, New York, 1922. See also, Eilif C. Hanssen, "The Present Status of the Typhoid Carrier Problem," *New York State Journal of Medicine* 39 (July 15, 1939): 1347–52.

31. Hanssen, "Present Status of the Typhoid Carrier Problem," p. 1347. Likewise, in Connecticut, new typhoid cases could not be traced to water or milk supplies but were blamed on healthy carriers. M. Knowlton, "The Typhoid Carrier Problem in Connecticut" (1936), as cited in Saphir, Baer, and Plotke, "Typhoid Carrier Problem," p. 964.

32. James G. Cumming, "Should the Barriers Against Typhoid be Continued?" *JAMA* 98 (January, 1932): 94.

33. Beck and Hollister, *Typhoid Fever: California*, pp. 12–16; Herman F. Senftner and Frank E. Coughlin, "Typhoid Carriers in New York State with Special Reference to Gall Bladder Operations," *American Journal of Public Hygiene* 17 (1933): 711. According to William Best, deputy health commissioner of New York City, city officials showed 727 carriers by 1937, of which 270 "were listed as the result of persistence of positive stools after recovery from typhoid." I cannot verify these numbers from other sources. See William H. Best, "Is Routine Examination and Certification of Food Handlers Worth While?" *American Journal of Public Health* 27 (1937): 1005. See also Stephen M. Friedman, "Chronic Fecal Typhoid Fever Carriers in New York City," unpublished M.P.H. thesis, Columbia University School of Public Health, 1978. I am grateful to Dr. Friedman for permission to use his paper in my research.

34. California located 94 percent of its registered carriers between 1910 and 1919 this way. See Beck and Hollister, *Typhoid Fever: California*, and Senftner and Coughlin, "Typhoid Carriers in New York State." See also, "Typhoid in the Large Cities of the United States in 1922," *JAMA* 80 (1923): 691–94. The latter article was part of an ongoing series in *JAMA* on typhoid in large cities. The editors concluded that tracing group outbreaks was virtually the only way to detect carriers, otherwise finding "an almost impossible epidemiologic tangle" (p. 692).

35. Charles Bolduan and W. Carey Noble, "A Typhoid Bacillus-Carrier of Forty-Six Years' Standing, and a Large Outbreak of Milk-Borne Typhoid Fever Traced to This Source," *JAMA* 58 (1912): 7–9. Carriers in dairies were particularly dangerous, leading one public health official to write that Mary Mallon "constituted a decided menace to the community, but it is safe to say that the morbidity produced by her was numerically insignificant compared

with what it would undoubtedly have been had she been employed as a milker on a farm, or in handling milk at a large municipal dairy." J. W. Trask to Charles V. Chapin, December 15, 1908, in response to Chapin questionnaire. See also same to same, January 5, 1909, and E. C. Levy to Charles V. Chapin, December 7, 1908, "I would certainly take extreme measures if a carrier were found on any of our milk producing farms." Letters found in the Chapin Papers, Rhode Island Historical Society, Box 1, Folder "Management of Milk Outbreak of Typhoid Fever, 1908–1909."

36. Friedman, "Chronic Fecal Typhoid Fever Carriers," p. 24. See also John C. Welton, John S. Marr, and Stephen M. Friedman, "Association Between Hepatobiliary Cancer and Typhoid Carrier State," *The Lancet* 1, no. 8120 (1979): 791–94.

37. Best, "Routine Examination," pp. 1003–6. See also Louis I. Harris and Louis I. Dublin, "The Health of Food Handlers: Results of 1,980 Physical Examinations in the New York City Department of Health," Department of Health Monograph no. 17, a Cooperative Study by the Department of Health, Metropolitan Life Insurance Company, and the American Museum of Safety, (New York, 1917).

38. See Beck and Hollister, *Typhoid Fever: California*, p. 41; and Senftner and Coughlin, "Typhoid Carriers in New York State," p. 712.

39. Best, "Routine Examination," p. 1004. For a more optimistic view of the examination of food handlers and a brief discussion of other detection methods, see Charles F. Bolduan and Samuel Frant's review, "The Typhoid Carrier Situation in New York City," *Medical Officer*, February 13, 1937, pp. 66–67.

40. Best, "Routine Examination," p. 1006. A fourth way of identifying healthy carriers involved discovery of the carrier state during surgery or medical treatment undergone for other reasons. This was haphazard and could not be relied upon for locating substantial numbers of carriers. See, for example, Beck and Hollister, *Typhoid Fever: California*, pp. 37, 40.

41. New York State Department of Health, *Annual Report*, 1920, p. 66. Two excellent articles addressing this question are: L. L. Lumsden, "What the Local Health Officer Can Do in the Prevention of Typhoid Fever," *Public Health Reports* 25 (1910): 111–20; and C. L. Overlander, "The Typhoid Carrier Problem," *Boston Medical and Surgical Journal* 169 (1913): 37–40.

42. NYCDH, *AR*, 1913, p. 84. Family members of such people were provided with free immunizations. In 1913, 1,710 such immunizations were provided.

43. NYCDH, *AR*, 1915, p. 51.

44. NYCDH, *AR*, 1916, p. 56. See also, reports for 1918–1922. The New York rules followed national guidelines closely. Milton J. Rosenau advised in his textbook: "The proper place to care for typhoid fever is in a suitable hospital. A private home is a poor makeshift for a hospital, and it is unreasonable to turn a household into a hospital for four to eight weeks or longer." He further advised that convalescents should be kept until "the danger of bacillus carrying has passed." Rosenau, *Preventive Medicine and Hygiene*, pp. 156–57, 158. See also, for example, *Transactions of the Tenth Annual Conference of State and Territorial Health Officers with the United States Public Health and Marine-Hospital Service*, Washington, D.C., June 1, 1912, Public Health Bulletin no. 59 (Washington, D.C.: Government Printing Office, 1912), p. 65. Chicago used regulations similar to New York's, also requiring, "The family must be sufficiently intelligent and willing to carry out the rules." See Heman Spalding and Herman N. Bundesen, "Control of Typhoid Fever in Chicago," *American Journal of Public Health* 8 (1918): 358–62, quotation from p. 361. The New York rules appear in "Typhoid Carriers and Their Control in New York City," *Weekly Bulletin of the Department of Health, City of New York* 11 (1922): 289–90, which also lists (without names) the 107 chronic carriers then under department observation. The Minutes of the Board of Health provide the names and addresses of 106 healthy carriers of typhoid fever then on department rolls. *Minutes*, Board of Health of the City of New York, New York Municipal Archives, Box 3948, vol. 43, May 24, 1923, pp. 19–22. Names are added to the list, passim, through the 1920s and 1930s. See also May 3, 1922, *Minutes*, Box 3947, vol. 40, for the 1922 alterations to the Sanitary Code; and June 30, 1915, *Minutes*, Box 3939, vol. 2 in the box for the initial alteration to address the carrier state (as it applied to various diseases, including cholera, dysentery, polio, diphtheria, and typhoid fever).

45. These carrier cards can be found at the National Archives, Washington, D.C. Unfortunately, it seems that the city did not continue to send its carrier records to the national office. I am grateful to John Parascondola and Aloha Smith for their help in locating these records, and to Lian Partlow who, during a research trip of her own to Washington, brought me copies.

46. NYCDH, *AR*, 1918, p. 56. One of the three was Mary Mallon; the other two cannot be named by current available sources but it is clear from the subsequent records that these individuals were not hospitalized on an indefinite basis.

47. See, for example, NYCDH, *AR*, 1918, p. 53. In 1919, officials declared, "Unfortunately with the facilities at our disposal, we have not been able to do more than merely scrape the surface in the examination of approximately three-quarter million of food handlers in this city" (NYCDH, *AR*, 1919, p. 82).

48. F. M. Meader, "The Detection and Control of Typhoid Carriers of Disease," *Medical Times*, September, 1916, p. 278. For New York state rules about typhoid carriers, see Charles E. Simon, *Human Infection Carriers: Their Significance, Recognition and Management* (Philadelphia: Lea & Febiger, 1919), pp. 230–32. See also John W. Brannan, "Hospitals and Typhoid Carriers," *American Journal of Medical Sciences* 144 (1912): 347–50.

49. Friedman, "Chronic Fecal Typhoid Fever Carriers," p. 30. Bolduan and Frant concluded similarly: "In an overwhelming proportion, the carriers having once been told of their carrier state are very eager to co-operate and are willing to do everything within their power to prevent the spread of the disease to anybody else. With the exception of the well-known Typhoid Mary and two others, we have had but 24 cases of the disease that could be traced to typhoid carriers already known to be such." Bolduan and Frant, "Typhoid Carrier Situation," p. 67.

50. Freidman, "Chronic Fecal Typhoid Fever Carriers," p. 28. The high number of females among carriers was noted by health officials nationwide. See, for example, sources in n. 44 in chap. 1 and Th. M. Vogelsang, *Typhoid and Paratyphoid B Carriers and Their Treatment: Experiences from Western Norway* (Arbok: Universitetet I Bergen, 1950), pp. 119–20. In New York City, three-quarters of the 675 chronic carriers identified between 1907 and 1936 were female. See Bolduan and Frant, "Typhoid Carrier Situation," p. 66.

51. Charles E. Simon, *Human Infection Carriers: Their Significance, Recognition and Management* (Philadelphia: Lea & Febiger, 1919), p. 101.

52. NYCDH, *AR*, 1919, p. 81. Similar optimism about carrier policy can be seen in, for example, Stanley H. Osborn and Edith A. Beckler, "Once a Typhoid Carrier, Always a Typhoid Carrier," *Journal of Infectious Diseases* 27 (1920): 145–50. See also Mark W. Richardson, "Dirty Hands and Typhoid Fever," *American Journal of Public Health* 4 (1914): 140–44, which suggests that carriers be kept under "competent supervision" and not be allowed to handle food, "but a period of quarantine which might necessitate individual restraint for a period covering forty or fifty years, is, of course, not to be thought of" (p. 143). Some of the problems in getting carrier cooperation are discussed in Overlander, "Typhoid Carrier Problem," pp. 37–40.

53. NYCDH, *AR*, 1922, p. 92. The department list of chronic carriers included 112 people. See also, *New York Times*, October 13, 1922, and January 21, 1923.

54. NYCDH, *AR*, 1922, p. 92.

55. The *Minutes* of the Board of Health of the City of New York occasionally noted the detention of a typhoid carrier (once, a month late, when sanctioning his release), but we can assume these were temporary isolations be-

cause when counts of carriers at the city hospitals were made, these carriers were not included. I located nine carriers detained in the decade of the 1920s. See, for example, *Minutes*, November 21, 1923, when Thomas Flood was detained at Riverside Hospital, Box 3949, vol. 45; February 11, 1924, when Walman Cardoza was isolated at Kingston Avenue Hospital, designated "temporary," Box 3949, vol. 46; April 29, 1924, when May Josephs was taken to Riverside Hospital as a "suspected chronic typhoid carrier," Box 3950, vol. 47; and passim through the 1920s. Philip Ebel of Brooklyn was sent to Kingston Avenue Hospital on September 24, 1929, and released on October 8, 1929, when a health department investigation revealed "that the conditions at proposed residence of the Carrier are satisfactory" Box 3956, vol. 67.

56. *New York Times*, March 14, 1924, p. 19; March 15, 1924, p. 13. Quotations from the March 15 article. Cotils was added officially to the city carrier list on February 11, 1924. See *Minutes*, Board of Health of the City of New York, Box 3949, vol. 46, February 11, 1924.

57. Beck and Hollister, *Typhoid Fever: California*, p. 68.

58. Ibid., p. 87.

59. See ibid. for a discussion of noncooperation.

60. "Hunting the Typhoid-Carrier," *The Literary Digest* 65 (May 1, 1920): 115. See also New York State Department of Health, *Annual Report*, 1920, p. 68.

61. Senftner and Coughlin, "Typhoid Carriers in New York State," p. 718. See also New York State Department of Health, *Annual Report*, 1931, p. 150.

62. J. W. Kerr and A. A. Moll, "Communicable Diseases: An Analysis of the Laws and Regulations for the Control Thereof in Force in the United Sates," *Public Health Bulletin* no. 62 (July, 1913) (Washington, D.C.: Government Printing Office, 1914), pp. 66–67.

63. No family was mentioned in the news stories about Tony Labella, and in general the health department did not record personal details about the registered carriers.

64. Rosenau, *Preventive Medicine and Hygiene*, p. 638.

65. See reports in the *New York Times*, March 14, 15, 1924, and further discussion in chap. 4.

66. Chapin, *Sources and Modes* (1910), p. 110; 2d ed., 1912, p. 152.

67. Ibid. (1910), p. 93.

68. Freidman, "Chronic Fecal Typhoid Fever Carriers," p. 31.

69. Overlander, "Typhoid Carrier Problem," p. 39.

70. Chapin concluded (even with regard to the sick) that "isolation in our

prevailing contagious diseases is carried farther than is necessary; that less rigorous measures would accomplish practically as much good, and that there would be less temptation to conceal cases and to interpret doubtful symptoms in line with the patient's desires." See his *Sources and Modes* (1910), p. 110.

71. "Chronic Typhoid Fever Producer," *Science* n.s. 25 (1907): 864.

72. Chapin, *Sources and Modes* (1910), p. 37. For more criticism of the New York City health department's treatment of Mary Mallon, see W. H. Hamer, "Typhoid Carriers and Contact Infection. Some Difficulties Suggested by Study of Recent Investigations Carried out on 'Living Lines.'" *Proceedings of the Royal Society of Medicine* 4 (1911): 105–46.

73. The work of epidemiology itself precluded narrow approaches to disease control. A science that emerged in the pre-bacteriological 1840s, it searched all aspects of communicable diseases in its efforts to determine the reasons for the occurrence of epidemics. Epidemiologists, such as George Soper, added germ theory to their list of factors to be considered at the turn of the twentieth century. Although historian William Coleman concluded that bacteriology "greatly reduced" the scope of epidemiological investigations, the Mary Mallon case indicates the reduction was not so great. See William Coleman, *Yellow Fever in the North: The Methods of Early Epidemiology* (Madison: University of Wisconsin Press, 1987). Quotation from p. 173.

74. Lederle is quoted in the *New York Times*, February 21, 1910, p. 18.

75. *New York American*, February 21, 1910, p. 6.

76. Ernst J. Lederle, Ph.D., Commissioner of Health, to Mayor Gaynor, February 26, 1910. In the William L. Gaynor subject files, "welfare" box, GWJ-95, New York Municipal Archives.

77. Lederle is quoted in " 'Typhoid Mary' is Free; Wants Work," *New York American*, February 21, 1910, p. 6. Mallon's release agreement is also noted in the Hoffman/Marr Collection, which contains a copy of a memo from the Clerk of the Division of Epidemiology to the Director of the Health Department, which itself cited the *Minutes*, Board of Health of the City of New York, February 9, 1910.

78. Baker is quoted in Isabelle Keating, "Dr. Baker Tells How She Got Her Woman," *The Brooklyn Eagle*, May 8, 1932.

79. Soper, "Curious Career," p. 710.

80. "Hospital Epidemic From Typhoid Mary," *New York Times*, March 28, 1915, sec. 2, p. 11. Media descriptions of Mallon's recapture are examined in chap. 5.

81. An account of the hospital outbreak, without naming Mary Mallon, is M. L. Ogan, "Immunization in a Typhoid Outbreak in the Sloane Hospital for

Women," *New York Medical Journal* 101 (March 27, 1915): 610–12. See the stories in the *New York Times*, March 28, 1915, sec. 2, p. 1; and March 31, 1915, p. 8; the *New York American*, March 28, 1915, p. 1; and the *New York Tribune*, March 28, 1915, p. 7. The official remanding of Mary Mallon, "who had broken her parole and violated her agreement," back to North Brother Island can be found in *Minutes*, Board of Health of the City of New York, Box 3939, vol. 1 in the box, March 30, 1915.

82. Soper, "Typhoid Mary," p. 13. The *New York Tribune* editorialized similarly, "The sympathy which would naturally be granted Mary Mallon is largely modified for this reason: The chance was given to her five years ago to live in freedom, and ... she deliberately elected to throw it away.... It is impossible to feel much commiseration for her" (March 29, 1915, p. 8).

83. Baker, *Fighting for Life*, pp. 76, 75.

84. In the Matter of ... Mary Mallon (1909), Return to Writ.

CHAPTER THREE: "Menace to the Community"

1. NYCDH, *AR*, 1907, p. 299.

2. William H. Park, "Typhoid Bacilli Carriers," *JAMA* 51 (1908): 981.

3. "Woman Cook a Walking Typhoid Fever Factory," *The World*, April 1, 1907, p. 1.

4. *New York American*, April 2, 1907, p. 2.

5. In the Matter of the Application for a Writ of Habeas Corpus for the Production of Mary Mallon, New York Supreme Court (June 28–July 22, 1909), Memorandum. Available in the New York County Courthouse.

6. *New York American*, April 2, 1907, p. 2.

7. A *New York American* reporter claimed she was moved to the island after one month (June 30, 1909). This cannot be verified in extant health department records.

8. George A. Soper, "The Work of a Chronic Typhoid Germ Distributor," *JAMA* 48 (1907): 2019–22. He read the paper before the Biological Society of Washington, D.C., on April 6, 1907. The discussion following it was printed in *Science*, n.s. 25 (1907): 863–65 and is also available in the Smithsonian Archives, Record Unit 7185. Approximately fifty people attended the meeting. Park, "Typhoid Bacilli Carriers," pp. 981–82. Park first presented his paper at the Joint Meeting of the Section on Practice of Medicine and the Section on Pathology and Physiology of the American Medical Association, 59th Annual Session, Chicago, June, 1908. It was during the discussion of Park's paper that M. J. Rosenau used the term *typhoid Mary*, the first published instance.

9. NYCDH, *AR*, 1907, p. 321.

10. George Edington to author, January 18, 1994, quoting his mother who worked in the Riverside Hospital doctors' dining room, in response to Author's Query, *New York Times*, Book Review sec., January 16, 1994; Emma Rose Sherman, telephone interview with author, from her home in New York City, June 14, 1993: the cottage on the outside was "darling" but on the inside was like a "pig sty and had a bad stench;" and (New York) *Sun*, March 28, 1915.

11. The term is from the Latin, *habeas*, from *habere*, which means to have and *corpus*, or body, and literally requires the restrainer to bring the body of the restrained person to court. As legal expert James Tobey explains, "When a person has been arrested or deprived of his liberty by quarantine, isolation, or commitment to a hospital, jail, or institution, he is entitled to have the legality of his detention passed upon by a court of record. This he may do by means of a writ of habeas corpus, a command by the court to produce or 'have the body' of the person in court at a specified time." James A. Tobey, *Public Health Law* (New York: The Commonwealth Fund, 1947), p. 355.

12. "'Typoid [*sic*] Mary' Never Ill, Begs Freedom," *New York American*, June 30, 1909, p. 3.

13. Hearst's biographers do not provide any information that would verify his possible participation in the Mallon case. See, for example, John K. Winkler, *William Randolph Hearst: A New Appraisal* (New York: Hastings House, 1955), and W. A. Swanberg, *Citizen Hearst* (New York: Scribner's Sons, 1961). Swanberg notes other occasions when Hearst got financially involved with the people whose cases his newspaper covered. In 1897, the *New York Morning Journal* (previous name of the *New York American*) editorially defended Elizabeth Sommers, who had been jailed for accosting a police officer while drunk. Hearst hired an attorney who secured a writ of habeas corpus for Sommers, and she was ultimately released (p. 120).

14. George Ferguson to Mary Mallon, April 30, 1909, In the Matter of . . . Mary Mallon (1909), laboratory reports.

15. All the Ferguson laboratory reports are included in In the Matter of . . . Mary Mallon (1909) at the New York County Courthouse. It is also possible that Mallon had already planned the court appearance when the *New York American* learned of her plans and advertised them. There is no evidence that O'Neill took this as a pro bono case.

16. "'Typhoid Mary' The Extraordinary Predicament of Mary Mallon, a Prisoner on New York's Quarantine Hospital Island, Not Because She is Sick, But Because She Breeds Typhoid Fever Germs and Scatters Them Wherever She Goes," *New York American*, June 20, 1909, American Magazine sec., pp. 6–7. The depiction of the victims was slightly out of line with information

provided by Soper. (See discussion of the count in chap. 1.) I am grateful to Dawn Corley for locating this issue for me.

17. *N. W. Ayer & Son's American Newspaper Annual* (Philadelphia: N. W. Ayer & Son, 1907), p. 605, gives the circulation figure as 778,205, and here I estimate 1909 figures. The daily *New York American* garnered only 300,000 in 1907.

18. *New York American*, June 20, 1909. There are some errors in Park's statement which leads one to think he was not directly quoted. First, he twice refers to Mallon as a "typhus" carrier—a different disease, even though once thought to be the same: Park certainly knew the difference and would not have made this mistake. Second, he claimed that Mallon was "of course, segregated with the typhoid patients," when he knew she was the only person with typhoid isolated on North Brother Island, where almost every inmate was a tuberculosis sufferer. Third, he wrote that "examination is made each day," when it was made at the most three times a week and often not more than once a week. Fourth, he intimated that Mallon was unique among the small numbers of carriers, when the literature already posited that 3 percent of recovered cases became life-long carriers. See chap. 1 for the state of medical knowledge.

19. George Francis O'Neill's biography was pieced together from various newspaper notes about him and from the city directories; his admission to the bar was verified in a letter from Joe Murphy, Senior Assistant Appellate Court Clerk, to Sarah Pfatteicher, my research assistant, December 29, 1993. See his obituary in the *New York Times*, December 24, 1914. On his expertise, see, for example, the *New York Times*, December 3, 1911: "The lawyer who will prosecute Mary's case against the city is the same one who appeared for her before the Supreme Court in 1909, when her freedom was denied. He is George Francis O'Neill of 5 Beekman Street, and he is a specialist in medico-legal questions." The address given for Mallon's lawyer, 5 Beekman Street, corresponded to the office address of the specific O'Neill who died in 1914 and whose home address was 502 E. 89th Street. When he defended Albert Patrick, O'Neill's office moved to 291 Broadway, but his home address remained the same. On the Patrick case, see, for example, the *New York Times*, December 18, 1910; May 4, 1911; November 28, 1912. No papers of O'Neill's have been located. I have not been able to verify his standing for state senate. I would like to thank the New York Bar Association for their help in my efforts to learn more about this attorney.

20. Fred S. Westmoreland, the resident physician at Riverside Hospital, admitted that the health department received from Soper a report "similar" to his printed one, "with the exception that in the [printed] report the names are eliminated." O'Neill probably would not have seen this until after filing his pe-

tition. See In the Matter of . . . Mary Mallon (1909), Return to the Writ. I cannot absolutely verify that the notes quoted were written by O'Neill, but the context strongly suggests it.

21. The notes were written on the back of one of the pages of Mary Mallon's undated letter and are part of In the Matter of . . . Mary Mallon (1909).

22. In the Matter of . . . Mary Mallon (1909), Petition for Habeas Corpus.

23. On habeas corpus proceedings in public health matters, see Tobey, *Public Health Law*, pp. 354–56.

24. In the Matter of . . . Mary Mallon (1909), Memorandum.

25. See any of the newspapers cited above during June and July, 1909. For example, the *New York Times* reporter wrote on July 17, 1909: "Mary Mallon, known to fame as 'Typhoid Mary,' and once the cook in the family of J. Coleman Drayton of 56 East Seventy-ninth Street." Or the (New York) *Sun* of June 30, 1909: "She is Mary Mallon and in her day cooked in the homes of J. Coleman Drayton, Henry Gilsey, and others in New York."

26. Larry Gostin, "Traditional Public Health Strategies," in *AIDS and the Law: A Guide for the Public*, ed. Harlon L. Dalton, Scott Burris, and the Yale AIDS Law Project (New Haven: Yale University Press, 1987), pp. 47–65, quotations from p. 50.

27. Jacobson v. Massachusetts (1905), 197 U.S. 11. The decision is reproduced in its entirety in Tobey, *Public Health Law*, pp. 238–40, and the quotations here are from that printing.

28. Tobey, *Public Health Law*, p. 240.

29. Gibbons v. Ogden (1824), 9 Wheat. 1, 6 L. Ed. 23, quoted in Tobey, *Public Health Law*, p. 42.

30. In the Matter of . . . Mary Mallon (1909), Memorandum.

31. NYCDH, *AR*, 1919, p. 81. The department of health traced sixty-seven typhoid carriers in 1919, of which Copeland described four as "refractory, requir[ing] special care in order to make them comply with our requirements," two sentences after he states the laws on the books did not apply to healthy carriers.

32. NYCDH, *AR*, 1921, p. 52.

33. There is some confusion in the record about when New York law actually allowed health officials to consider carriers as sick in terms of health policy. According to one report of New York's regulations, on March 30, 1915, section 86 of the health code was revised to allow for carriers to be "subject to the regulations governing clinical cases" of typhoid fever and other infectious diseases. Similarly, a revision of regulation 3 was recognized by the Board of

Health *Minutes* on June 30, 1915, to the effect that "any person who is a 'carrier' of disease germs of Asiatic cholera, bacillary dysentery, epidemic cerebrospinal meningitis, poliomyelitis, diphtheria or typhoid fever, shall be subject to the regulations governing clinical cases of these respective diseases." *Minutes*, Board of Health of the City of New York, New York Municipal Archives, Box 3939, vol. 2 in the box. But Commissioner Copeland and other New York officials before 1921 did not see this as helpful in their own attempts to control carrier behavior (since they were not attempting to hospitalize or isolate every carrier they found), and their response is most critical for understanding events. See Charles E. Simon, *Human Infection Carriers: Their Significance, Recognition and Management* (Philadelphia: Lea & Febiger, 1919), pp. 238–39.

34. In the Matter of . . . Mary Mallon (1909), Traverse to the Return to the Writ.

35. George Soper, "Typhoid Mary," *Military Surgeon* 45 (1919): 10.

36. Despite the sound of the name of the court, this is a first-level city court that heard the case. See Randolph E. Bergstrom, *Courting Danger: Injury and Law in New York City 1870–1910* (Ithaca: Cornell University Press, 1992), p. 13: "In New York City the Supreme Court was the primary court of initial jurisdiction, while the highest State Court was the Court of Appeals."

37. *New York Evening Post*, July 16, 1909, p. 1.

38. *New York American*, June 30, 1909, p. 3.

39. Quoted in the *New York Times*, December 3, 1911, p. 9.

40. Quoted in the *New York American*, December 3, 1911, sec. 5, p. 6.

41. Letter to the editor, July 2, 1909.

42. On Progressive urban politics see David P. Thelen, *The New Citizenship: Origins of Progressivism in Wisconsin, 1885–1900* (Columbia: University of Missouri Press, 1972); Robert H. Wiebe, *The Search for Order, 1877–1920* (New York: Hill & Wang, 1967); John D. Buenker, *Urban Liberalism and Progressive Reform* (New York: W. W. Norton & Co., 1973); and a host of single-city studies including Zane L. Miller, *Boss Cox's Cincinnati: Urban Politics in the Progressive Era* (New York: Oxford University Press, 1968) and Melvin G. Holli, *Reform in Detroit: Hazen S. Pingree and Urban Politics* (New York: Oxford University Press, 1969). For the effects of reform on public health, see Judith Walzer Leavitt, *The Healthiest City: Milwaukee and the Politics of Health Reform* (Princeton: Princeton University Press, 1982).

43. Quoted in the *New York Evening Post*, July 16, 1909, p. 1.

44. Ibid.

45. *New York World*, July 20, 1909, p. 18.

46. Quoted in the *Brooklyn Daily Eagle*, June 29, 1909, p. 1. The identification of specific strains of typhoid bacilli that could have connected Mallon specifically to her victims—phage testing—did not exist in 1909. While the new science of bacteriology had uncovered ways to identify pathogenic bacteria within Mallon's body, it could not definitively state that her germs were the same type that had infected or killed her twenty-two alleged victims. Indeed, the victims' bacteria had not received the same laboratory scrutiny that Mallon's had undergone. My thanks to Thomas Brock for his discussion of serotypes, phage types, and bacteria strains.

On phage typing and its use in connecting case to carrier, see for example, M. Dorthy Beck and Arthur C. Hollister, *Typhoid Fever Cases and Carriers: An Analysis of Records of the California State Department of Public Health from 1910 through 1959* (Berkeley: State of California Department of Public Health, 1962), pp. 60–66. For an example of the debate on these issues, see W. H. Hamer, "Typhoid Carriers and Contact Infection: Some Difficulties Suggested by Study of Recent Investigations Carried out on 'Living Lines.'" *Proceedings of the Royal Society of Medicine* 4 (1910–11): 105–46. Mary Mallon specifically is discussed on p. 109.

47. For a general argument against detaining healthy carriers, see C. L. Overlander, "The Typhoid Carrier Problem," *Boston Medical and Surgical Journal* 169 (1913): 37–40.

48. The words isolation and quarantine were often used synonymously, as I tend to do here, but it should be noted that they have technically different meanings. Isolation refers to the separation of infected people during their period of infectivity to prevent them from spreading their disease; quarantine refers to the detention or separation of people who might be at risk for becoming sick, by virtue of, for example, being exposed to disease, to keep them from in turn exposing others. Because of Mary Mallon's ambiguous legal and new medical definition, it could be argued that she falls into both camps. See Tobey, *Public Health Law*, p. 138.

49. In the Matter of . . . Mary Mallon (1909), Memorandum.

50. Ibid.

51. In the Matter of . . . Mary Mallon (1909), Return to Writ.

52. In the Matter of . . . Mary Mallon (1909), Proposed Order and Notice of Settlement.

53. S. Josephine Baker, *Fighting for Life* (New York: Macmillan Co., 1939), p. 77.

54. This position was in line with national thinking at the time. Charles Simon, for example, wrote, "while operative treatment may be urged upon every fecal carrier . . . the vast majority of the cases will not come to operation

of their own free will, nor can they be compelled to subject themselves to the dangers incidental to such treatment." *Human Infection Carriers*, pp. 100–1.

55. Another example of the law abridging individual rights in the name of science can be found in Susan E. Lederer, *Subjected to Science: Human Experimentation in America before the Second World War* (Baltimore: The Johns Hopkins University Press, 1995). I explore the lure of science in this period as it became evident with regard to childbirth in *Brought to Bed: Childbearing in America 1750–1950* (New York: Oxford University Press, 1986).

56. "Guide to a Walking Typhoid Factory," *New York Times*, December 2, 1910.

57. *New York American*, March 15, 1924, p. 8. See also, the *New York Tribune*, which quotes Judge Cobb, "Any punishment I would impose would be in the hope that it would be a deterrent." March 15, 1924, p. 20.

58. The healthy carrier case that did become the weathervane of how health departments might act in similar circumstances was Illinois *ex rel.* Barmore v. Robertson, 302 Ill. 422 (1922), a ruling by the Illinois Supreme Court, in which Clarence Darrow defended healthy typhoid carrier Jennie Barmore (unsuccessfully) in her plea for release from house quarantine. The result was the same as Mallon's case in that it furthered health department authority to isolate carriers without systematic consideration of due process and personal liberty. I have written about this case in "Gendered Expectations: Women and Public Health in the Early Twentieth Century," in *U.S. History as Women's History: New Feminist Essays*, ed. Linda K. Kerber, Alice Kessler-Harris, and Kathryn Kish Sklar (Durham: University of North Carolina Press, 1995). I am grateful to Sarah Pfatteicher and Bob Conlin for helping me understand the legal traditions in publishing cases.

59. The Cuban response to HIV infection is examined in the Conclusion. See Karen Wald, "AIDS in Cuba: A Dream or a Nightmare?" *Z Magazine*, December, 1990, pp. 104–9; Nancy Scheper-Hughes, "AIDS, Public Health, and Human Rights in Cuba," *The Lancet* 342 (1993): 965–68; and Scheper-Hughes, "AIDS, Public Health and Human Rights in Cuba," *Anthropology Newsletter* 34 (October, 1993): 46, 48.

60. Charles V. Chapin, *The Sources and Modes of Infection* (New York: John Wiley & Sons, 1910), p. 110; Milton J. Rosenau, *Preventive Medicine and Hygiene* (New York: D. Appleton-Century Co., 1935), p. 144.

CHAPTER FOUR: "More Like a Man than a Woman"

1. Charles V. Chapin, "The Clinic," newspaper clipping (probably from the *Boston Transcript*) in Charles V. Chapin Papers, 1909 Scrapbook, Rhode Island Historical Society, Providence, Rhode Island.

2. Parts of this chapter are derived from my essay, "Gendered Expectations: Women and Early Twentieth-Century Public Health," in *U.S. History as Women's History: New Feminist Essays*, ed. Linda K. Kerber, Alice Kessler-Harris, and Kathryn Kish Sklar (Durham: University of North Carolina Press, 1995), pp. 147–69, and are used here with permission.

3. A 1916 Minnesota study found twenty-five of thirty identified carriers were women. The investigators noted that because women cook for their families and friends, as well as take many low-paying jobs in food handling occupations, it was natural to find more women than men among healthy carriers. Men were less likely to be discovered, and were also less likely to become public health hazards, because their daily tasks and their occupations did not center upon food preparation. Chesley *et al.*, "Three Years' Experience in the Search for Typhoid Carriers in Minnesota," *JAMA* 68 (1917): 1884. A Boston study similarly concluded that "we have a preponderance of women on our carrier list, this is largely because they handle food more frequently and are therefore more frequently discovered in connection with outbreaks." George H. Bigelow and Gaylord W. Anderson, "Cures of Typhoid Carriers," *JAMA* 101 (1933): 348–52. It was not until the 1940s that studies began to document more women carriers in the population at large, and not just among those found in food handling jobs, transmitting the disease. See sources given in chap. 1, nn. 43 and 44.

4. This is the only year, other than 1916, when the city submitted its carrier cards to the federal government, for which records allow us to definitely identify the carriers by sex. See the list in *Minutes*, Board of Health of the City of New York, New York Municipal Archives, Box 3948, vol. 43, May 24, 1923.

5. Soper is quoted in the *New York Times*, April 4, 1915, sec. 5, p. 3. Soper was not alone in focusing on domestic laborers as potentially dangerous in this regard. See, for example, William Royal Stokes, "Typhoid Fever Spread by Chronic Carriers," *U.S. Public Health Reports* 32 (1917): 1926–29. Stokes concludes, "We believe that whenever possible domestics in private service ... should not be admitted to such positions until a careful inquiry has been made into their previous medical history as to a possible former attack of typhoid fever" (p. 1929).

6. Charles F. Bolduan and Samuel Frant, "The Typhoid Carrier Situation in New York City," *The Medical Officer*, February 13, 1937, p. 66.

7. The only other historian I know of who has studied Mary Mallon and considered the role gender might play is Andrew Mendelsohn, whose Harvard undergraduate thesis was on the subject. Mendelsohn wrote (in a footnote): "Mary was not directly discriminated against for her class, religion, ethnicity, or gender." John Andrew Mendelsohn, "Typhoid Mary: Medical Science, the State, and the 'Germ Carrier,'" B.A. thesis, History of Science, Harvard Uni-

versity, December, 1988, p. 115. Alan Kraut discussed the ethnic component of the story effectively in *Silent Travelers: Germs, Genes, and the "Immigrant Menace"* (New York: Basic Books, 1994), pp. 97–103.

8. Apparently Mary Mallon used two employment agencies, one called Mrs. Strickers', the one Soper relied upon, and one called Mrs. Seeleys'.

9. On single working domestics, consult Susan Strasser, *Never Done: A History of American Housework* (New York: Pantheon Books, 1982), chap. 9; Barbara Mayer Wertheimer, *We Were There: The Story of Working Women in America* (New York: Pantheon Books, 1977); *America's Working Women*, comp. and ed. Rosalyn Baxandall, Linda Gordon, and Susan Reverby (New York: Vintage Books, 1976); David M. Katzman, *Seven Days a Week: Women and Domestic Service in Industrializing America* (New York: Oxford University Press, 1978); Faye E. Dudden, *Serving Women: Household Service in Nineteenth Century America* (Middletown, Conn.: Wesleyan University Press, 1983); Daniel E. Sutherland, *Americans and Their Servants: Domestic Service in the United States 1800 to 1920* (Baton Rouge: Louisiana State University Press, 1981); and Phyllis Palmer, *Domesticity and Dirt: Housewives and Domestic Servants in the United States, 1920–1945* (Philadelphia: Temple University Press, 1989).

10. Soper's account of his first encounter with Mary Mallon is in Soper, "The Work of a Chronic Typhoid Germ Distributor," *JAMA* 48 (1907): 2019–22. See also his "The Curious Career of Typhoid Mary," *Bulletin of the New York Academy of Medicine* 15 (October, 1939): 698–712, and his "Typhoid Mary," *The Military Surgeon* 45 (July, 1919): 1–15. S. Josephine Baker's account is in her autobiography, *Fighting for Life* (New York: Macmillan Co., 1939), pp. 73–75. See also Isabelle Keating, "Dr. Baker Tells How She Got Her Woman," *Brooklyn Eagle*, May 8, 1932.

11. See, as an example, *Science Citation Index*, 1961 to the present.

12. Susan Soper, Soper's great-granddaughter, told me that she checked with other family members and that none knew of any unpublished records. Telephone conversation from Atlanta, November 9, 1993.

13. Gilbert Wersan, pseud. for Warren Boroson, "The Truth (For a Change) About Typhoid Mary," *MD*, September, 1985, pp. 91–92, 97, 101, 109, quotation from p. 92. I am grateful to Mr. Boroson for sending me this article, and for his informative telephone conversations with me exploring these issues. See also his "Learning from Typhoid Mary," *Science Digest* 92 (March, 1984): 91.

14. One letter, in typescript, is available in the health department records, dated November 12, 1938, immediately following Mary Mallon's death and in

anticipation of articles about her; the second is the letter to the editor cited in n. 15 below.

15. Letter to the Editor, *British Medical Journal*, January 7, 1939, pp. 37–38.

16. George Soper, Great Neck, New York, letter without salutation, November 12, 1938, in the files of the New York City Health Department, copy in the Hoffman/Marr Collection. It may be that a member of the AAAS recommended Soper, but it is unlikely that the association did so formally.

In his later career, Soper continued to have strong opinions about how to solve health problems. In 1923 he began a six-year job as the managing director of the Cancer Society, in which he was described as "a vigorously unconventional thinker" and "disputatious" because he believed in using "heroic methods" to gain public attention. See Richard Carter, *The Gentle Legions* (New York: Doubleday & Co., 1961), pp. 146–50. I am grateful to Barron Lerner for pointing out this description.

17. I use "progressive" with a small *p* to mean that Soper fit the characteristics consistent with the reform movement in this period. I do not know if Soper actually affiliated with the Progressive Party, the third party whose candidate for the presidency in 1912 was Theodore Roosevelt.

18. See, for example, George Soper, *The Air and Ventilation of Subways* (1908); *Modern Methods of Street Cleaning* (1909).

19. Rosalyn Baxandall and Linda Gordon, with Susan Reverby, eds., *America's Working Women: A Documentary History 1600 to the Present*, rev. and updated ed. (New York: W. W. Norton & Co., 1995), pp. xxii–xxiii. For a general history of women and work patterns, see Sara M. Evans, *Born for Liberty: A History of Women in America* (New York: Free Press, 1989).

20. Soper was born in 1870, Mallon in 1869. Biographical information on George Soper is available in *Who's Who in America* 24 (1946–47): 2215. His obituaries can be found in the *New York Times*, June 18, 1948, p. 23, and the *New York Herald Tribune*, June 18, 1948, p. 30.

21. Soper's articles on the subject were published in 1907, 1919, and 1938; in all of them he referred, he said, to notes taken at the time of the actual events.

22. These simple descriptors can be found in all of Soper's publications, including the 1907 initial article.

23. Soper, "Curious Career," p. 698.

24. Ibid.

25. Soper never described Mallon in completely negative terms. He some-

times even seemed to acknowledge a grudging admiration for her strength, and he openly admitted to her cooking talents. But he saw Mallon foremost as a public health problem, and her characteristics as an uncooperative carrier outweighed any positive personal traits he noticed.

26. Soper, "Curious Career," p. 698.

27. This photograph, which appeared in the newspapers of the period, has been reproduced in various health department publications and in some recent historical studies. The earliest use of it, as far as I have been able to determine, was in the *New York American*, June 20, 1909. The most recent is in Kraut, *Silent Travelers*, p. 102. Emma Rose Sherman was surprised when she saw this photograph, as it did not seem to resemble the Mary Mallon she had known in the 1930s. Of course, aging can change physical appearance considerably, and the Mary Mallon that Sherman knew was in her sixties whereas the photograph depicts Mallon at thirty-seven. Emma Rose Sherman, Interview with author, New York City, July 16, 1993. There is always the possibility that the photograph was of another woman in the Willard Parker Hospital, but its authenticity was not questioned at the time by the people who had seen both the photograph and Mary Mallon herself.

28. Soper, "Curious Career," pp. 704–5.

29. I have concluded that the man whose apartment Soper visited was A. Briehof, or Breshof, although Soper does not use his name, because that is the man who brought Mary Mallon's stool samples to the Ferguson Laboratory and the one who died during the time between her incarcerations. Mallon sometimes used the name Marie Breshof. Their relationship is further explored in chap. 6.

30. Soper, "Typhoid Mary," p. 11.

31. On the status of single working domestics, including cooks, see the sources given in n. 9 above.

32. Soper, "Typhoid Mary," p. 13.

33. See, for example, "She was not particularly clean" ("Curious Career," p. 701) or "No housekeeper ever gave me to understand that Mary was a particularly clean cook" ("Typhoid Mary," p. 10). Soper, of course, was not alone in his thinking about cleanliness being class related. See, for example, A. W. Freeman, "Typhoid Fever and Municipal Administration," *U.S. Public Health Reports* 32 (1917): 642, who writes that the standards for cleanliness necessary for typhoid carriers are reasonable and "in line also with our inherited ideas of decency and cleanliness."

34. "A Typhoid Fever Carrier," *Medical Record* (June 1, 1907): 924. See also *Medical Record* (May 18, 1907): 818.

35. Soper, "Curious Career," p. 705.

36. Ibid., p. 705.

37. Ibid., p. 708.

38. Ibid. See also, "Typhoid Mary," p. 9.

39. Soper, "Curious Career," p. 711. Emma Rose Sherman agreed that Mary Mallon's temper was known and feared on North Brother Island. People rarely saw it, but stories abounded, and those who knew her tried not to arouse her. Sherman viewed Mallon as "tightly bottled up" and said she "pussyfooted around her." Telephone conversation from her home in New York, with author, June 26, 1994. In chap. 6 I take a closer look at Mallon's temperament and her responses to her incarceration. I am grateful to Tom Archdeacon for his confirmation that temper was considered stereotypical of the Irish in this period (February, 1995).

40. Soper, "Typhoid Mary," p. 8.

41. Ibid., pp. 7, 4.

42. Soper is quoted in the *New York Times*, April 4, 1915. This sentiment is echoed by some recent observers of Mary Mallon's situation, most recently by John Steele Gordon, "The Passion of Typhoid Mary," *American Heritage* 45 (May/June, 1994): 118–21.

43. Soper, "Typhoid Mary," p. 12.

44. Soper, *New York Times*, April 4, 1915.

45. L. L. Lumsden, "What the Local Health Officer Can Do in the Prevention of Typhoid Fever," *Public Health Reports* 25 (1910): 111–20, quotations on p. 118.

46. Soper, "Typhoid Mary." Soper did continue in his interest in Mary Mallon. In 1919, for example, he wrote to the health department asking for information about her. See copy of a memo in the Hoffman/Marr Collection (in private hands), from Clerk, Division of Epidemiology, to the Director, May 9, 1919, providing "information for reply to Dr. Soper's inquiry re: Mary Mallon." Soper continued to write about her until 1939.

47. Soper, "Typhoid Mary," p. 12.

48. Baker, *Fighting for Life*. Baker gave a press interview about her role in bringing Mallon into the hospital in the *Brooklyn Eagle*, May 8, 1932. There is no full-length biography of Baker (and we need one), but a good account of her life by someone who knew and worked with her is the entry by Leona Baumgartner in *Notable American Women*, ed. Edward T. James, vol. 1 (Cambridge: Belknap Press of Harvard University Press, 1971), pp. 85–86.

49. Baker, *Fighting for Life*, p. 13.

50. For an excellent discussion of the simultaneous democratic and elitist parts of the reform movements in this period, especially with regard to women, see Linda Gordon, *Pitied but Not Entitled: Single Mothers and the History of Welfare 1890–1935* (New York: Free Press, 1994).

51. Baker, *Fighting for Life*, p. 48.

52. Ibid., pp. 57–58; see also p. 70.

53. Ibid., pp. 73–74.

54. Ibid., p. 74.

55. Ibid., p. 75.

56. Kraut, *Silent Travelers*, p. 97. Of all New York City typhoid carriers who died and were registered in or before 1940, 62.3 percent were foreign-born. See John C. Welton, John S. Marr, and Stephen M. Friedman, "Association Between Hepatobiliary Cancer and Typhoid Carrier State," *The Lancet* 1, no. 8120 (1979): 791–94.

57. Kraut, *Silent Travelers*, p. 103. Kraut distinguishes Mary Mallon's treatment from that of the Chinese in San Francisco during the 1900 outbreak of plague, in which the Chinese were singled out as a group. See also, Charles McClain, "Of Medicine, Race, and American Law: The Bubonic Plague Outbreak of 1900," *Law and Social Inquiry* 13 (1988): 447–513. During the years of Mallon's incarceration, the United States considered adding the category of healthy typhoid fever carrier to the list of reasons to exclude immigrants to this country. But in May, 1916, Surgeon General Rupert Blue wrote to John Shaw Billings, then deputy commissioner of the New York City Health Department, that the abilities of the immigration service were already taxed to capacity and that examination for typhoid carriers could be deferred. See Billings to Blue, May 26, 1916, and Blue to Billings, May 29, 1916, in the National Archives, RG 90 Records of the Public Health Service, Central File, 1897–1923, Box 459, Folder labeled 4141 1916.

58. In March, 1907, the same month Mary Mallon was apprehended, reporters from the *New York Tribune* uncovered in Katonah, in the Croton watershed, "two fine, big, rich cesspools overflowing . . . and emptying in a direct line for the city's water supply" (March 31, 1907, p. 2). Investigators connected the cesspools to a camp of Italian laborers, who were constructing a new dam in the waterworks, a few of whom became infected with typhoid fever. "The greatest source of contamination for any community," wrote one reporter, "is a colony of foreigners, who, with their unregulated and primitive ideas of hygiene, are breeders of every one of the most dangerous diseases that affect communities" (March 30, 1907, p. 1).

Today, our immigration policy explicitly excludes people who carry the HIV virus or who suffer from other infectious diseases, such as tuberculosis, from immigrating to the United States. Haitians, most publicly, have been quarantined and excluded under this policy.

59. Cotils, then forty-two years old, and his wife, Felicia, age forty-eight, also a Belgian immigrant, lived at 242 Sixteenth Street with their son, Robert, then twelve and born in New York. U.S. Census, 1920 Soundex Index. See also the city directories, 1920, 1922–23, which list him as a baker at the above address. Alphonse Cotils is still listed as a baker at the Sixteenth Street address in the 1925 City Directory. He (and his wife) are still listed at that address in the 1933–34 City Directory, although that is a residential directory and does not specify businesses.

60. NYCDH, *AR*, 1922, p. 92. See also the *New York Times*, October 13, 1922, and January 21, 1923. Tony Labella's name does not appear in the Minutes of the Board of Health in which the carriers for 1923 are listed. We do not know if this is because he absconded again. I could not find him in the city directory listings for these years. See also the Newark *Evening News*, October 13 and 14, 1922, p. 1.

61. At times, breadwinners received greater latitude in public health regulations. See, for example, a national study of laws and regulations controlling infectious diseases, in which researchers noted that "exceptions in favor of breadwinners ... may be made by local health authorities." J. W. Kerr and A. A. Moll, "Communicable Diseases: An Analysis of the Laws and Regulations for the Control Thereof in the United States," *Public Health Bulletin*, no. 62 (July, 1913) (Washington, D.C.: Government Printing Office, 1914), pp. 66–67. There was precedent for finding other means of support for healthy carriers instead of isolating them. At the Pasteur Institute in Paris, bacteriologist Ilya Metchnikoff had found employment in a library for a healthy carrier whose case interested him. See the *New York Times*, March 30, 1913. In 1918 New York state began subsidizing the incomes of those carriers who were having difficulty finding adequate employment outside the food industry. See Herman F. Senftner and Frank E. Coughlin, "Typhoid Carriers in New York State with Special Reference to Gall Bladder Operations," *American Journal of Hygiene* 17 (1933): 711–23. The health department did ultimately retrain Mary Mallon, years after her second incarceration. She was employed in the hospital laboratory at Riverside Hospital, but not released from her isolation.

62. The story is reported in the *New York Times*, December 2, 1923, sec. 2, p. 2; the quotations are from this story.

63. Voigt is identified by his carrier card, which the New York City Department of Health submitted to the United States Public Health Service in 1916, along with twenty-three others, all twenty-four of which are now available at the National Archives. This submission was noted in NYCDH, *AR*, 1915, p. 52. A Richard Voigt, possibly the same man, although then seventy-

three years old, is listed in the 1933–34 City Directory as a waiter at Hunts Point Palace, living in Ozone Park (p. 3372). Richard Voidt (different spelling) is listed as a "temporary carrier" in a 1916 letter in the health department files. (Chief of Division of Epidemiology to Director of the Bureau of Infectious Diseases, February 14, 1916; copy in Hoffman/Marr Collection.

Of the twenty-four carriers identified by the health department in 1916, when Voigt sought his medical treatment, only Mallon and Voigt (who was there only for one month) were then in city institutions. There were ten men and fourteen women listed; nine of them worked directly with food, another four were domestic workers, and one was a laborer. Four were inmates in mental hospitals; the others were employed in retail or their occupations were not known. Of the 106 carriers listed in 1923, two were residents of the Manhattan State Hospital, two (Mary Mallon and May Newton) of Riverside Hospital, two at Long Island State Hospital, and one at Long Island College Hospital; all others provided home addresses. *Minutes*, Board of Health of the City of New York, New York Municipal Archives, Box 3948, vol. 43.

64. See Will F. Clarke, "City Watches 208 Typhoid Carriers," *New York World*, October 14, 1928, p. 6.

65. His first name was occasionally given as George; spelling of his last name varied, too, sometimes given as Morsch. The outbreak he was blamed for may have been in Park Slope in 1914, as the newspapers say, or it may have been an August, 1915, outbreak in Bay Ridge. It is listed as February, 1915, on the copy of the carrier card in the Hoffman/Marr Collection. See the *New York Times*, August 4 and 5, 1915. Fred Moersch is listed as a candy maker in the 1913 Brooklyn City Directory, at 577 Atlantic Avenue, Brooklyn. The health department card gives his address as 5606 Third Avenue, Brooklyn. I am grateful to Rebecca Walzer for her help in tracing Fred Moersch.

66. It is possible that over time (and by 1928 New York public health officials had had considerable time to think about and deal with healthy typhoid carriers) procedures were more matter-of-factly applied. Thus, health officials could lock up Moersch, even indefinitely, without stating any causes other than the bare fact of his causing an outbreak after being identified as a carrier. But this did not mean that they needed to lock up all carriers who continued to pursue their trade. Cotils, for example, appears to have continued in his bakery even after the court case. Officials had the freedom to determine by whatever subjective means they wanted to apply who they would trust and who they would not. Some flouting of the law by some carriers could be allowed, but there would be limits. In Mary Mallon's case these limits came into play sooner and lasted longer than they did for other carriers.

67. Memo from G. L. Nicholas to Director of the Bureau of Infectious Diseases, Department of Health, February 14, 1916. Copy in the files of Hoff-

man/Marr Collection. See also Moersch's carrier card in the National Archives.

68. The word "official" was originally typed. It was crossed out with a pen, and the word "special" written above it.

69. Memo, Nicholas to Director, February 14, 1916.

70. Acting Director of the Bureau of Infectious Diseases to the Health Commissioner, February 15, 1916. Copy in the files of Hoffman/Marr Collection.

71. The treatment involved subcutaneous injections of autogenous vaccine. The results, according to the Chief of the Division of Epidemiology, were "nil." (Chief, Division of Epidemiology to Director, Bureau of Infectious Diseases, February 14, 1916; copy in the Hoffman/Marr Collection.) Moersch may have been in Kingston Avenue Hospital in Brooklyn or at Riverside for a time. NYCDH, *ARs* from 1918 to 1922 indicate more than one carrier held on North Brother Island: in 1918, three carriers; in 1919, two; in 1920, several; in 1921, some taken but not held; in 1922, two. Moersch's carrier card seems to indicate that his stools were examined at Kingston Avenue Hospital. He was detained at Riverside Hospital by official action of the Board of Health on October 23, 1928. See *Minutes*, Board of Health of the City of New York, Box 3955, vol. 63, October 23, 1928. He was released to his home in 1944 and he died in Kingston Avenue Hospital on August 15, 1947.

72. Chief, Division of Epidemiology to Director, Bureau of Infectious Diseases, February 14, 1916; Hoffman/Marr Collection. See the 1923 listing of registered healthy carriers. "Fred Morsch [*sic*] 244 — 5th Avenue, Brooklyn." *Minutes*, Board of Health of the City of New York, Box 3948, vol. 43, May 24, 1923.

73. *New York Times*, October 7, 1928, indicated eighteen cases and on October 10 reported two more. The *Daily Mirror* reported fifty cases (October 8, 1928); the *New York World* claimed that sixty were ill in the neighborhood (October 7, 1928). The health department records do not allow a clear count. Moersch's health department carrier card attributes 144 cases and 6 deaths to him. His stool samples showed an intermittent pattern of positives and negatives, similar to Mallon's.

74. *New York Times*, October 7, 1928.

75. *Herald Tribune*, October 7, 1928, p. 10. See also *New York World*, October 7, 1928, p. 1, and Clarke, "City Watches," p. 6.

76. According to the *New York Times*, October 10, 1928, "George Moersch, the typhoid carrier, . . . is now in Riverside Hospital." See also *New York Times*, October 7, 1928, in which the reporter states that the carrier was

isolated in Riverside Hospital. His carrier card indicates specimens were examined at Kingston Avenue Hospital. Unfortunately, the information on the card was grouped, making it impossible to know the exact dates or places of the laboratory tests. For example, we learn that between October, 1916, and May, 1934, eighty-four specimens were shown to be positive; between February, 1918, and February, 1934, forty-four stool cultures were found to be negative. Dates during the 1940s are more specific and indicate infrequent examination, suggesting he was not then hospitalized. The city directories for 1931 and 1933 list Fred Moersch as a "helper" at Riverside Hospital (1931, p. 687; 1933–34, p. 2336).

77. Emma Rose Sherman, Interview with author, New York City, July 16, 1993, followed up with telephone query, July 13, 1994. Sherman is very sure she would have known if another carrier were on the island, since she was responsible for the laboratory analyses. Even if his specimens had been sent downtown, and Sherman indicated they would have been sent to Willard Parker Hospital where better equipment was available, she would have been the one to label and send the specimens.

78. Unfortunately, much remains ambiguous about Moersch's story. We do not know for sure if he stayed at Riverside after 1928 for treatment voluntarily or if he was kept against his will. This is a significant distinction, but the records do not allow us to answer it except by inference. Moersch's employment status as a "hospital helper" is also vague. Was the job part of the agreement to isolate him so that he could continue to support his family? For more on his story, see chap. 6.

79. Moersch's city employment record can be traced in the Civil Lists, available on microfilm at the New York Municipal Archives. He was first listed in the 1931–32 Civil List, with the date February 10, 1930, provided as his start of employment. He continues on the list until his death. His move to Kingston Avenue Hospital in 1944, with a home address in Brooklyn at 156 Butler Street, can be found in the 1944–45 Civil List.

80. Illinois *ex rel.* Barmore v. Robertson, 302 Ill. 422 (1922). Quotation from the Application for Rehearing, pp. 4, 9.

81. See, for example, the discussion in Baker, *Fighting for Life*, p. 75. A California study of healthy typhoid fever carriers revealed that in that state a full 25 percent of identified carriers did not cooperate with authorities. See the discussion in chap. 2 and M. Dorthy Beck and Arthur C. Hollister, *Typhoid Fever Cases and Carriers: An Analysis of Records of the California State Department of Public Health from 1910 through 1959* (Berkeley: State of California Department of Public Health, 1962).

CHAPTER FIVE: "This Human Culture Tube"

1. M. J. Rosenau is quoted in the discussion section following William H. Park, "Typhoid Bacilli Carriers," *JAMA* 51 (1908): 81–82, on p. 82. "Typhoid Mary" appears in print with the small "t" typhoid, although later it is more frequently capitalized. Warren Boroson also concluded that this was the first printed use of the term. See his "Learning from Typhoid Mary," *Science Digest* 92 (1984): 91.

2. George C. Whipple, *Typhoid Fever: Its Causation, Transmission and Prevention* (New York: John Wiley & Sons, 1908), p. 20. Park had reported twenty-six cases of typhoid traced to Mary Mallon, which was the number Soper used, even though Soper's evidence pointed to only twenty-two (see chap. 1). Whipple changed the figure to twenty-eight, and the 1907 *New York American* story raised it to thirty-eight.

3. *New York American*, March 13, 1907, p. 4.

4. Ibid., April 2, 1907, p. 2.

5. Ibid.

6. *New York World*, April 1, 1907, p. 1. The *New York Tribune* ran front-page stories on a typhoid fever outbreak in Katonah in the Croton watershed at the end of March and through the first half of April, 1907, but never mentioned the issue of healthy carriers or "Mary Ilverson." They did blame the outbreak on the Italian workers, described as "saturated with contagion.... the descendants of Caesar's legions ... have lost the hygienic instincts which the great master of the Roman empire inculcated" (April 12, 1907, p. 2).

7. Paul H. Weaver, "Selling the Story," *New York Times*, Op-Ed, July 29, 1994, p. A13. See also his *News and the Culture of Lying* (New York: Free Press, 1994).

8. W. A. Swanberg, *Citizen Hearst: A Biography of William Randolph Hearst* (New York: Bantam Books, 1967), pp. 68, 192–93.

9. *New York American*, Sunday Magazine sec., June 20, 1909, pp. 6–7.

10. John Andrew Mendelsohn characterizes the news accounts as raising curiosity more than fear. I agree with him with regard to the July, 1909, stories of Mallon, but, as the following discussion indicates, I read the ensuing reports as raising a host of emotions. See his "Typhoid Mary: Medical Science, the State, and the 'Germ Carrier,'" B.A. thesis, Harvard University, 1988.

11. "'Typoid [*sic*] Mary' Never Ill, Begs Freedom," *New York American*, June 30, 1909, p. 1. The Sunday edition boasted almost 800,000 readers. For newspaper circulation, see *N. W. Ayer & Son's American Newspaper Annual* (Philadelphia: N. W. Ayer & Son, 1907), p. 605.

12. Terra Ziporyn, *Disease in the Popular American Press* (Westport, Conn.: Greenwood Press, 1988). See, especially, chap. 3, "Typhoid Fever: A Disease of the Indifferent," pp. 71–111. For Adams's contributions, see, for example, Samuel Hopkins Adams, "Typhoid: An Unnecessary Evil," *McClure's Magazine* 25 (1905): 145–56. Paul De Kruif's most famous book was *The Microbe Hunters* (New York: Harcourt, Brace, 1926).

13. *New York World*, July 20, 1909, p. 18.

14. *New York American*, July 21, 1909, p. 2; and July 23, 1909, p. 5.

15. *New York Tribune*, July 17, 1909, p. 4.

16. *New York Times*, July 1, 1909, p. 8. See also July 17, 1909, p. 3.

17. (New York) *Evening Sun*, July 16, 1909, p. 10. See also June 29 and 30, 1909.

18. "'Typhoid Mary' in Cry for Liberty," *New York Herald*, June 30, 1909.

19. *New York Call*, June 30, 1909, p. 2. See also July 17, 1909, p. 1. For other newspaper accounts, see *New York Evening Post*, July 16, 1909, p. 1; and the *Brooklyn Eagle*, June 29 and July 16, 1909.

20. *Ayer American Newspaper Annual*, p. 629, provides the circulation figures. The *World*, July 20, 1909, p. 18. On Pulitzer's influence on American newspapers, see W. A. Swanberg, *Pulitzer* (New York: Scribner's Sons, 1967) and George W. Juergens, *Joseph Pulitzer and the New York World* (Princeton: Princeton University Press, 1966).

21. *New York Call*, February 21, 1910, p. 1.

22. *New York Times*, February 21, 1910, p. 18. See also *New York Herald*, February 20, 1910, p. 1; *New York Daily Tribune*, February 21, 1910, p. 5; and *New York American*, February 21, 1910, p. 6.

23. "'Typhoid Mary' at Large," *Boston Medical and Surgical Journal* 162 (March 3, 1910): 294.

24. "The Average Individual as a Carrier of Typhoid," *Current Literature* 47 (1909): 569. See also C. L. Overlander, "The Transmission of Typhoid Fever," *Interstate Medical Journal* 21 (1914): 133–44.

25. *New York American*, February 21, 1910, p. 6.

26. Arthur B. Reeve, *The Silent Bullet* (New York: Harper & Bros., 1910). I am grateful to Gerard Fergerson for leading me to this novel.

27. The comparison with Sherlock Holmes must have occurred to contemporary readers, since Arthur Conan Doyle's stories were popular at the turn of the century.

28. "The Germ-Carrier," *Punch, or the London Charivari* 37 (July 7, 1909): 2.

29. (New York) *Sun*, March 28, 1915, p. 1.

30. "Caught at Last," ibid., March 31, 1915, p. 6. For the *Sun's* coverage, see also March 27, April 2 and 4, 1915.

31. " 'Typhoid Mary' Is Again a Captive," *New York World*, March 28, 1915, p. 1 of Classified section. See also March 29, 1915, p. 16. The character of Mary Mallon's walk was also commented upon in the *New York Times*, March 28, 1915, sec. 2, p. 11.

32. " 'Typhoid Mary' Reappears," *New York Tribune*, Editorial, March 29, 1915, p. 8. See also March 28, 1915, p. 7.

33. " 'Typhoid Mary' Has Reappeared: Human Culture Tube, Herself Immune, Spreads the Disease Wherever She Goes," *New York Times*, sec. 5, April 4, 1915, pp. 3–4, quotation from p. 3. See also the *New York Herald*, March 28, 31, 1915.

34. *New York Times*, April 4, 1915, p. 3.

35. "Typhoid Fever," *Scientific American* 112 (May 8, 1915): 428.

36. *New York Times*, October 13, 1922, p. 19. See also January 21, 1923, p. 22. A Newark newspaper did mention his "native Italy" when wondering if Labella could be deported, and described the situation: "He has been warned repeatedly to stay away from places where food is handled, and persistently returns." *Newark Evening News*, October 14, 1922, p. 1.

37. See, for example, *New York World*, January 21, 1923, p. 9. See also the *Annual Reports* of the Department of Health of the State of New Jersey, 1922, p. 40, and 1923, p. 21; and NYCDH, *AR*, 1922, p. 92; and *Newark Evening News*, October 13, 1922, p. 1 and October 14, p. 1. In January, 1923, Labella was released from surveillance in New Jersey, and New York health officials issued a warning that he might have returned to New York City. *New York Times*, January 21, 1923, p. 22.

38. *New York Times*, March 14, 1924, p. 19. See also ibid., March 15, 1924, p. 13. The possibility that Cotils returned to cooking comes from the fact that he is listed at his bakery in the 1925 City Directory.

39. *New York Tribune*, March 15, 1924, p. 20.

40. Ibid., March 14, 1924, p. 24.

41. *New York World*, March 14, 1924, p. 15, and March 15, 1924, p. 13.

42. Gene Fowler, "Health Board Bars Robust Baker, Typhoid Carrier," *New York American*, March 14, 1924, p. 13. See also March 15, 1924, p. 8.

43. *New York World*, March 15, 1924, p. 13.

44. *Daily Mirror*, October 8, 1928. This newspaper wrote, " 'Typhoid Freddie' Moersch, isolated on suspicion of causing nearly 50 typhoid cases in

Greenwich Village, probably will be committed for life to a city hospital.... His daughter, Mrs. Fredericka Kraus, a young widow, will begin a desperate fight to free him today believing he is the victim of a 'frame-up.'" For other articles on Frederick Moersch, see *Sunday News*, October 7, 1928, p. 6; *Daily News*, October 7, 1928, p. 8; and *New York American*, October 7, 1928, pp. 1, 36, and October 7, 1928.

45. *New York World*, October 7, 1928.

46. Will F. Clarke, "City Watches 208 Typhoid Carriers," ibid., October 14, 1928.

47. "I Wonder What's Become of—'Typhoid Mary,'" *Sunday Mirror*, Magazine sec., December 17, 1933, p. 19.

48. According to the 1931 and 1933 City Directories, Fred Moersch was employed as a "helper" at the hospital during those years.

49. Stanley Walker, "Profiles: Typhoid Carrier No. 36," *New Yorker* 10 (January 26, 1935): 21–25. Mary Mallon became number 36 in 1923, when the health department began a new registry of typhoid carriers and listed the ones then under observation alphabetically. Frederick Moersch was number 46.

50. Soper's real complaint was that he did not receive enough credit in the article. See Soper's letter to the editor, "The Discovery of Typhoid Mary," *British Medical Journal*, January 7, 1939, pp. 37–38, quotations from p. 37.

51. Walker, "Typhoid Carrier," p. 21.

52. Ibid., p. 25.

53. An example of a distortion in a medical article is the report by C. L. Overlander, of Harvard, that in 1914 Mallon had caused twenty-seven cases of typhoid fever "with three or four deaths" when Soper had reported twenty-six cases, with one death, and I reconstruct (see chap. 1) twenty-two cases and one death. Overlander, "Transmission of Typhoid Fever," p. 139.

54. *New York Times*, November 12, 1938, p. 17. See also, *New York Herald Tribune*, November 12, 1938, p. 12; *New York Journal and American*, November 12, 1938, p. 4; (New York) *Sun*, November 12, 1938, p. 4; and *Daily Mirror*, November 12, 1938, p. 5.

55. *New York World-Telegram*, November 12, 1938, p. 26 (story begins on p. 1).

56. The California longitudinal study of healthy typhoid carriers concluded that 25 percent of 753 carriers they studied were uncooperative. Among 175 food handlers the investigators traced, 89 were cooperative and 78 were not (8 could not be determined). M. Dorthy Beck and Arthur C. Hollister, *Typhoid Fever Cases and Carriers: An Analysis of Records of the Califor-*

nia State Department of Public Health From 1910 through 1959 (Berkeley: State of California Department of Public Health, 1962), pp. 85, 89.

57. The usual date given for Mary Mallon's major stroke is Christmas day, 1932, a date that seems to have originated in one of George Soper's articles. The *Daily Mirror*, December 17, 1933, dated the stroke to sometime in October, 1933. Emma Sherman, who found Mary Mallon in her cottage after the stroke, knows for certain that it did not occur on Christmas day, because she did not work on the holiday. On the day of Mallon's stroke, Sherman was at work and expecting Mary to come in. When she did not appear, Sherman went looking for her and found her disabled by the stroke. Emma Rose Sherman, Interview with author, New York City, July 16, 1993. December 4, 1932, is the date given on her death certificate, as the day she was admitted to the hospital for the final time. I have accepted this as the correct date for her last stroke.

58. The phrase is from the headline for the article in the *New York World-Telegram*, November 12, 1938, p. 1 ("Nine Mysterious Mourners Pay Last Tribute to Typhoid Mary").

59. *New York American*, November 12, 1938, p. 4. For an out-of-town obituary, see, for example, "Typhoid Mary Pardoned by Death," *Minneapolis Journal*, December 11, 1938. I am grateful to Nina Ackerberg and Peter Ackerberg for recovering this article for me.

CHAPTER SIX: "Banished Like a Leper"

1. Cotils was quoted in Gene Fowler, "Health Board Bars Robust Baker, Typhoid Carrier," *New York American*, March 14, 1924, p. 13.

2. *New York World*, July 20, 1909, p. 18.

3. The information is provided on her death certificate, Number 1137-1935, Bureau of Records, Department of Health of the City of New York, Register No. 9799. Copy in Hoffman/Marr Collection, in private hands. Mary Mallon sometimes claimed that she had been born in the United States, but her noted Irish brogue and the frequent reference to her Irish birth convinced me that the information on the death certificate is correct. A search of birth records in New York turned up no record. See Carlyle R. Bennett, Director of the Municipal Archives and Records Center, to John S. Marr, May 5, 1975, in Hoffman/Marr Collection.

The identification of her place of birth as Cookstown, County Tyrone, is provided by John Concannon, National Historian of the Ancient Order of Hibernians in America in an enclosure to his letter to author, November 22, 1993. I am grateful for his help, especially since the town and county of her place of birth does not appear on her death certificate and is not otherwise confirmable. See also, for example, Mary C. McLaughlin, "Mary Mallon: Alias Typhoid Mary," *The Recorder* 40 (1979): 44–57. The name Mallon can be found in many of the northern counties, including Tyrone, Antrim, and Armagh. See the "Mallon" entry in the *Garvin-Mallon Family History Newsletter*, no. 2, p. 19.

4. Adelaide Jane Offspring, "Petition to the Surrogate's Court of the County of Bronx," November 15, 1938. Filed with the Last Will and Testament of Mary Mallon, number P894-1938, Surrogate's Court, Bronx County, New York.

5. Death Certificate. Reproduction of the death certificate is prohibited by Section 3.21 of the New York City Health Code. The certificate carries the notice that the city "does not certify to the truth of the statements made thereon." Hoffman/Marr Collection.

6. Emma Rose Sherman, Interview with author, New York City, July 16, 1993.

7. The land ownership system in Ireland reduced and delayed marriage in the post-famine period, thus encouraging young women to emigrate. See Janet A. Nolan, *Ourselves Alone: Women's Emigration from Ireland 1885–1920* (Lexington: University Press of Kentucky, 1989).

8. Patrick J. Blessing, "Irish," *Harvard Encyclopedia of American Ethnic Groups*, ed. Steven Thernstrom (Cambridge: Harvard University Press, 1980), p. 531.

9. Nolan, *Ourselves Alone*, p. 68. See also Hasia Diner, *Erin's Daughters in America: Irish Immigrant Women in the Nineteenth Century* (Baltimore: Johns Hopkins University Press, 1983), especially chap. 4, and Kerby A. Miller, *Emigrants and Exiles: Ireland and the Irish Exodus to North America* (New York: Oxford University Press, 1985).

10. Blessing, "Irish," pp. 524–45.

11. Ibid., p. 532. See also Alan M. Kraut, *Silent Travelers: Germs, Genes, and the "Immigrant Menace"* (New York: Basic Books, 1994), passim.

12. See, for example, Inez Goodman, "A Nine-Hour Day for Domestic Servants," *The Independent* 54 (February 13, 1902), excerpted in *America's Working Women*, comp. and ed. Rosalyn Baxandall, Linda Gordon, and Susan Reverby (New York: Vintage Books, 1976), pp. 213–14. See also other documents in this collection.

13. Mary Heaton Vorse, "Making or Marring, The Experiences of a Hired Girl," 1901, excerpted in Baxandall, Gordon, and Reverby, *America's Working Women*, pp. 137–38.

14. See Rosalyn Baxandall and Linda Gordon, with Susan Reverby,

America's Working Women: A Documentary History 1600 to the Present, rev. and updated (New York: W. W. Norton & Co., 1995), pp. 200–201.

15. Susan Strasser, *Never Done: A History of American Housework* (New York: Pantheon Books, 1982), p. 170. See also, for example, Lynn Y. Weiner, *From Working Girl to Working Mother: The Female Labor Force in the United States, 1820–1980* (Chapel Hill: University of North Carolina Press, 1985).

16. Quoted in David M. Katzman, *Seven Days a Week: Women and Domestic Service in Industrializing America* (New York: Oxford University Press, 1978), p. 31.

17. Katzman, *Seven Days*, p. 163.

18. Frances A. Kellor, *Out of Work: A Study of Employment Agencies: Their Treatment of the Unemployed, and Their Influence Upon Homes and Business* (New York: B. P. Putnam's Sons, 1904).

19. Ibid., pp. 8–9.

20. Ibid., pp. 316–37.

21. Ibid., pp. 144, 147.

22. On women's work, see especially Alice Kessler-Harris, *Out to Work: A History of Wage-Earning Women in the United States* (New York: Oxford University Press, 1982). It is interesting to note that Irish women immigrants boasted high literacy rates and "were more literate than were either their counterparts at home or the men and women in most other immigrant groups." Nolan, *Ourselves Alone*, p. 69.

23. I am grateful to Barbara Therese Ryan, at the University of Michigan, for her thoughtful comments about domestic servants and cooks and where they were likely to live.

24. Offspring, "Petition."

25. *New York World*, July 20, 1909, p. 18.

26. George A. Soper, "The Curious Career of Typhoid Mary," *Bulletin of the New York Academy of Medicine* 15 (1939): 698–712. Drayton told Soper that "when it was over he had been so grateful to Mary for all the help she had given him that he rewarded her with fifty dollars in addition to her full wages" (p. 703).

27. Ibid., p. 702.

28. George A. Soper, "Typhoid Mary," *The Military Surgeon* 45 (July, 1919): 7.

29. George A. Soper, "The Work of a Chronic Typhoid Germ Distributor," *JAMA* 48 (1907): 2022.

30. Stanley Walker, "Profiles: Typhoid Carrier No. 36," *New Yorker* 10 (January 26, 1935): 21.

31. See, for example, "The Tragedy of Vacation Typhoid," *American Journal of Public Health* 5 (1915): 204–5.

32. Soper, "Curious Career," p. 705.

33. Ibid., p. 699.

34. Ibid., p. 709.

35. On average wages, see Katzman, *Seven Days*, app. 3, pp. 303–14. Mallon's wage is given in Soper, "Curious Career," p. 701.

36. Soper, "Typhoid Mary," p. 7.

37. Soper documents investigations into the cause of previous outbreaks of typhoid fever in homes in which Mallon worked in "Chronic Typhoid Germ Distributor," pp. 2019–22; see also his "Typhoid Mary" and "Curious Career."

38. Soper, "Curious Career," p. 705.

39. See ibid., p. 706, for Baker quotation.

40. S. Josephine Baker, *Fighting for Life* (New York: Macmillan, 1939), p. 75.

41. Although Soper and Baker give essentially the same account of Mallon's capture, there are some discrepancies. For example, Soper wrote that Mallon was finally cornered in an "outside closet" (privy?) in the rear of the next-door house; Baker (who was there) said she finally found Mallon in an "areaway closet under the high outside stairway leading to the front door." See Soper, "Curious Career," p. 706 and Baker, *Fighting for Life*, p. 75.

42. Baker, *Fighting for Life*, pp. 75–76. This was not an unreasonable worry, given the risks of abdominal surgery in these years.

43. Soper, "Typhoid Mary," p. 7.

44. Soper, "Curious Career," p. 705.

45. The description is Soper's, from "Curious Career," p. 709. He does not say how he gained Briehof's confidence, nor if any money was involved in the bargain.

46. Ibid., pp. 704–5.

47. Cecil K. Blanchard, "Typhoid Carriers: Their Detection and Control," *Public Health News* (Trenton) 9 (1924): 250–58, quotations from p. 251.

48. On Riverside Hospital, see New York City Department of Health, *Annual Reports*, passim. See also "Local Island-Hopping," *New York Times*, July 24, 1994. My thanks to Bert Hansen for calling the article to my attention. The island's history is told also by Dee Wedemeyer, "City Selling Parcels to

Bidders with Better Ideas," *New York Times*, August 15, 1982, sec. 8, p. 7. The island was a private residence before 1871, when it became part of Morrisania and the Bronx. Riverside Hospital was built in 1885 and used until 1943 as a tuberculosis and contagious disease hospital. Then it was leased to the state and, in 1951, transformed into an institution for teenage drug rehabilitation. That function ceased in 1963. See also *New York Times*, August 11, 1960, p. 16.

49. The Hoffman/Marr Collection contains a 1944 list of the thirty-two buildings on the island which provides the date and type of construction, the cubic feet, and the cost.

50. Emma Rose Sherman studied the plot plan and identified for me which building Mary Mallon occupied. When Sherman came to the island in 1929, she set up the bacteriology laboratory on the second floor of the chapel, directly across from Mallon's cottage. Sherman, Interview, July 16, 1993.

51. Sherman, Interview, July 16, 1993. See accounts in the New York newspapers for June 15 and 16, 1904, about the heroic rescues of steamboat passengers by Riverside Hospital patients.

52. The (New York) *Sun*, June 30, 1909. The *New York Times* essentially repeated the story: "She was treated like a leper and compelled to occupy a house by herself, with a dog as her only companion. Food was brought to her three times a day by a nurse, she said, who left it at the door and turned away" (July 17, 1909, p. 3).

53. *New York American*, June 30, 1909, p. 3. It is interesting that Mallon explicitly distinguished herself from other infected people; she did not question that people with leprosy should be isolated.

54. The family of Dr. John Cahill, who was head of the island hospital for many of the years of Mallon's stay, assures me that he left no papers, and they do not know of any patient records extant. The city and state health departments confirm that no hospital records survive.

55. *New York World*, July 20, 1909, p. 18.

56. Quoted in the *New York World*, July 20, 1909, p. 18.

57. Offspring, "Petition." The context of the passage where Offspring refers to Mallon's visitors leaves it slightly ambiguous whether this applied to the years of Mallon's first or second incarceration. Offspring was born in Canada and immigrated to the United States either in 1895 or 1901. She was twenty-three years old when she first became acquainted with Mallon. Offspring is listed in the Thirteenth Census and Fourteenth Census of the United States, 1910 and 1920, enumeration for Riverside Hospital. Mallon did not appear in the census listing of hospital patients in either year. The first enumeration was taken on April 15, 1910, and Mallon had already been released in Feb-

ruary. According to the Civil List (New York Municipal Archives), Offspring began employment as a nurse at Riverside Hospital on July 9, 1906.

58. Mary Mallon, Part Seven of her Last Will and Testament, Offspring inherited the amount of $3,572.05, residuary from the total estate value of $4,172.05.

59. Quoted in *New York World*, July 20, 1909, p. 18. There is no clear evidence that Mary Mallon connected the injustice she felt specifically with her Irish background, nor that she strongly identified with, and was spurred on by, the Irish National Movement, a connection posited by Mary McLaughlin, "Mary Mallon: Alias Typhoid Mary," *The Recorder* 40 (1979): 44–57, and repeated by Alan Kraut, *Silent Travelers*, p. 101. I am grateful to Dr. McLaughlin for consulting with me about her statements that Mallon was hired by the Bryant family of Marblehead, Massachusetts, sometime during the years of her release between 1910 and 1915 (not confirmed by Soper's speculations about her jobs during those years). The Bryants' grandson told McLaughlin that his family had employed "Typhoid Mary" and that the cook had ties to the Irish movement, and that a petition in the Irish press raised money to gain Mallon's release. This information could not be confirmed. I have reason to question it because of the frequency with which people named any Irish-born cook who might be associated with illness as "Typhoid Mary." A close reading of the New York Irish newspapers in this period revealed no petition, nor even mention of Mary Mallon's case, her initial isolation, her release, or her reincarceration. I am grateful, too, to John Concannon, Historian of the Ancient Order of Hibernians in America, for his help in tracing Mallon's Irish connections, and to the many others who answered my query in the Irish *Echo*.

When I questioned Emma Sherman (Telephone interview, July 13, 1994) about whether Mallon felt discriminated against because she was Irish, Sherman indicated that Mallon did not. Many of the nurses and some of the doctors on the island were Irish.

60. I am grateful to Susan Lederer for alerting me to antivivisectionists' writing on Mallon, Moersch, Barmore, and other healthy typhoid fever carriers. Antivivisectionists remained disbelievers. See, for example, *The Starry Cross* 37 (1928): 85, 148; 31 (1922): 93–94; 35 (1926): 44; 43 (1935): 101–3; and 46 (1938): 164. The quotation is from 45 (1937): 148.

61. *New York World*, July 20, 1909. Mallon did not name the family. The *Brooklyn Daily Eagle* quoted Mallon when she named another family for whom she had worked: "I was cook for Mr. Stebbins' family and for other families and nobody fell sick while I was there" (June 29, 1909, p. 1).

62. See the entry for George Albert Ferguson in *Who's Who in America*, vol. 1 (1897–1942), p. 392. Ferguson was the author, with Arthur Henry Elliot, of *A System of Instruction in Qualitative Chemical Analysis*, 3d ed. (New York:

the Authors, 1899). He was professor of analytical chemistry and mathematics at the New York College of Pharmacy beginning in 1896 and chemist to the New York State Board of Pharmacy. I am grateful to Greg Higby for consulting with me about the New York College of Pharmacy and for his guidance in the history of pharmacy collection at the University of Wisconsin.

63. *New York World*, July 20, 1909.

64. The handwritten letter survives in In the Matter of the Application for a Writ of Habeas Corpus for the Production of Mary Mallon, New York Supreme Court (June 28–July 22, 1909) in the New York County Courthouse. Warren Boroson published major parts of the letter pseudonymously in Gilbert Wersan, "The Truth (For a Change) About Typhoid Mary," *MD*, September, 1985, p. 109.

65. This is the same Dr. R. J. Wilson, superintendent of hospitals for the New York City Health Department, who had investigated one of the household outbreaks of typhoid fever that Soper later traced to Mallon.

66. Another interpretation of this remark might emphasize Mallon's naiveté or foolishness in refusing to make such a statement. I see her description of it as an effort to portray herself as a woman of integrity.

67. William H. Studdiford, a gynecologist on the Bellevue Hospital staff, who consulted on female patients at Riverside Hospital. Mallon misspelled his name.

68. Soper had attributed only one death to Mallon, that of a child in the Bowen home on Park Avenue where he found Mallon in 1907.

69. In the Matter of . . . Mary Mallon (1909), Mallon's letter.

70. Affidavit and letter from Ernest J. Lederle to Mayor Gaynor, February 26, 1910, in the New York Municipal Archives, "Welfare" Box GWJ-95, William J. Gaynor Papers. A reference to O'Neill's letter is at the top of the letter. Mallon agreed, also, to let Lederle know her whereabouts every three months.

71. *New York Times*, February 21, 1910, p. 18. See also the *New York Daily Tribune*, February 21, 1910, p. 5. When Mallon and George Francis O'Neill began a suit to recover damages for false imprisonment in December, 1911, the health department listed her address as 147 W. 143rd Street, Manhattan, a different address from the one she shared with Briehof. It was possibly an employer's address. I have been unable to locate Mary Mallon at this address in the City Directory for these years. See *Minutes*, Board of Health of the City of New York, New York Municipal Archives, Box 3933, vol. 1, December 12, 1911.

72. *New York American*, February 21, 1910, p. 6. See also *New York Call*, February 21, 1910, p. 1, and *New York Herald*, February 20, 1910, p. 1.

73. Two and one-half years after giving Mary Mallon her liberty, while describing her case and her release to a meeting of the International Hygiene Congress, New York City Health Department officials justified releasing her and did not indicate any problems with keeping abreast of her activities. See *New York Times*, September 26, 1912, p. 6.

74. *New York Times*, December 3, 1911, p. 9. See also *New York American*, December 3, 1911, sec. 4, p. 6, and *New York World*, December 3, 1911. Official notice of the pending suit can be found in the *Minutes*, Board of Health of the City of New York, Box 3933, vol. 1, December 12, 1911, p. 8.

75. By 1914 S. S. Goldwater was commissioner of health, and Lederle would not have been in a position to help.

76. Soper, "Curious Career," p. 709. This exaggeration leads us to question Soper's account of Mallon's whereabouts for the years 1910–1914.

77. *New York Times*, Editorial, November 29, 1914, sec. 3, p. 2.

78. Soper, "Typhoid Mary." The health department believed the woman cooking in a New Jersey inn was Mary Mallon and traced five cases to that inn, but it cited "indirect channels" for the identification and provided no evidence to make the connection convincing. Also it claimed her employment began in January, 1912, but in September, 1912, Biggs confidently stated that her release was working. See M. L. Ogan, "Typhoid Fever in New York City," *Monthly Bulletin of the Department of Health* 5 (April, 1915): 104–5; and *New York Times*, September 26, 1912, p. 6.

It is possible, even probable, that these instances involved a cook other than Mary Mallon. The term "Typhoid Mary" came to be used generally to refer to any Irish woman cook in the vicinity of a case of typhoid fever, and the name Mary Mallon itself was a common one. See, for example, Mary McLaughlin's case of a cook in the Marblehead, Massachusetts, for which there is no independent confirmation. See also the cook fired from a Philadelphia, Pennsylvania, orphan home in 1932, after an outbreak of typhoid, who was referred to as "Typhoid Mary." I am grateful to Jack Taub, who lived in the home in those years and became sick himself, for calling my attention to this incident. Jack Taub to author, January 20, 1994 and March 4, 1994.

79. The Sloane Hospital outbreak is discussed in M. L. Ogan, "Immunization in a Typhoid Outbreak in the Sloane Hospital for Women," *New York Medical Journal* 101 (1915): 610–12.

80. See accounts in *New York Times*, March 28, 1915, sec. 2, p. 11; *New York Tribune*, March 28, 1915, p. 7, and Editorial, March 29, 1915, p. 8; *New York World*, March 28, 1915, Classified section, p. 1; and *New York American*, March 28, 1915, p. 1, and March 31, 1915, p. 5. Official notification is in *Min-*

utes, Board of Health of the City of New York, Box 3939, vol. 1, March 30, 1915.

81. Soper reported, "One day her best friend, a man whose name she often went by, sent for her. He was ill with a bad heart. Mary got him into a hospital, where he died" ("Curious Career," p. 709). Unfortunately, Soper did not say when this occurred. I have not been able to find a death notice for Briehof (or Breshof) in this period of time.

82. This conclusion would hold for other healthy carriers I have seen traced and described in the literature. As the St. Louis health officers concluded, referring to healthy carriers of typhoid fever, "As the average man is not a wilful murderer at heart, he would, undoubtedly, be anxious to follow instructions and would be glad to find himself pronounced a non-carrier." C. W. Gould and G. L. Qualls, "A Study of the Convalescent Carriers of Typhoid," *JAMA* 58 (1912): 545.

83. I am indebted to Sarah Pfatteicher for this suggestion.

84. Riverside Hospital building list, 1944. See also, for example, NYCDH, *AR*, 1926, p. 111, describing the hospital's capacity.

85. George Edington to author, January 18, 1944, in response to my Author's Query, *New York Times*, Book Review sec., January 16, 1994, p. 16.

86. Adele E. Leadley to Surrogate's Court of Bronx County, January 17, 1939. (Copy in the Hoffman/Marr Collection.) None of the letters Leadley referred to exist today.

87. Charles-E. A. Winslow, *The Life of Hermann M. Biggs, M.D., D.Sc., LL.D.: Physician and Statesman of the Public Health* (Philadelphia: Lea & Febiger, 1929), p. 199; Baker, *Fighting for Life*, p. 76. Unfortunately, neither Winslow nor Baker indicated the dates of these letters, and we cannot determine if Mallon wrote them during her first or second isolation (or during both). There is no evidence that Mallon actually tried to contact either Biggs or Baker during the years she was not isolated, 1910–1915.

88. Mallon, Last Will and Testament. I have tried to trace the Lempe family in the Census and in various city directories, but cannot locate them with certainty. A Lempe family with these names lived for a while at 33rd street and 3rd avenue, near where Briehof and Mallon lived, and Mallon's friendship with them might have dated from the years she and Briehof shared rooms.

89. Sherman, Interview, July 16, 1993.

90. Department of Health Employment Record for Mary Mallon, in Hoffman/Marr Collection. The form provides the following information:

3/1/18	Appointed "Domestic" at a salary of	$240/year
1/1/19	Continuing as Domestic	$300/year
1/1/20	Continuing as Domestic	$400/year
8/20/20	Continuing as Domestic	$500/year
3/1/21	Continuing as Domestic	$588/year
1/1/22	Continuing as Domestic	$588/year
8/1/22	"Nurse" (Change of Title)	$588/year

Somewhat confusing this issue, and also in the Hoffman/Marr Collection, is a typed reference to a Civil List 1926, in which Mary Mallon is said to be a "Senior Hospital Helper" beginning March 1, 1918, with a salary of $612, which increases to $630 (no date) and then to $690, also no date provided.

The Civil List on microfilm at the Municipal Archives provides the following additional information about Mallon's employment:

1929	Domestic	$588/year
1931	Senior Hospital Helper	$630/year
1932	Senior Hospital Helper	$690/year

91. The board of health considered her day trips to the mainland as recorded in the *Minutes*, Board of Health of the City of New York, Box 3943, vol. 30, June 11, 1918, p. 20.

92. Clerk, Division of Epidemiology, to the Director of the Bureau of Preventable Diseases, January 6, 1919. See also letter from J. W. Crawford, Superintendent, to H. G. MacAdam, Chief, Division Institute of Inspection, January 3, 1919. During these years, too, George Soper tried to keep informed about Mallon's infective state, and on May 9, 1919, the clerk of the division of epidemiology wrote the director a memo about "Information for reply to Dr. Soper's inquiry re: Mary Mallon," that her stools continued to test positive. Copies of these letters and memo are in the Hoffman/Marr Collection. Mallon was not alone in her refusal to submit stool samples. In 1922, for example, four carriers "refused absolutely to give stool specimens when requested, making it necessary for us to resort to the exercise of police power to procure compliance." NYCDH, *AR*, 1922, p. 92.

93. Sherman, Interview, July 16, 1993.

94. Soper reported that Mallon visited a family on Long Island on some of her day trips off of North Brother Island, although he thought that "they were not particularly glad to see her." This family was probably the Lempes, the only family mentioned in her will with a Long Island address. "Curious Career," p. 712.

95. According to the 1925 AMA Physician Directory, Plavska was born in Russia in 1895, attended medical school at the University of Moscow, later called the Moscow Medical Institute, graduating in 1917. Sometime between

then and 1925, when she is listed in the city and AMA directories as being at Riverside Hospital, Plavska came to this country and may have pursued further medical training. For most of her career, she practiced on Riverside Drive in Manhattan. Her daughter provided John Marr with the information that she had a private practice of gynecology. Plavska is mentioned two times in *Minutes*, Board of Health of the City of New York: on February 11, 1924 (Box 3949, vol. 46), when she was temporarily assigned to Willard Parker Hospital as an Interne, and on June 11, 1926 (Box 3952, vol. 55), when she received her diploma and certificate of service following her internship at Riverside Hospital. In the former instance, her name was spelled "Alexandra Plavskaja," and in the later instance, her name was given as "Alexander [*sic*] Plavska."

96. Sherman, Interview, July 16, 1993.

97. John Marr and Ida Peters Hoffman spoke to Mrs. Efros, Plavska's daughter, November 25, 1976. Their notes are in the Hoffman/Marr Collection. Sherman confirmed Mallon's visits to Plavska. Sherman, Interview, July 16, 1993.

98. Sherman's official title was "laboratory technician," but she performed all the bacteriological work on the island during her years there. She was first employed on October 17, 1929. See the Civil Lists, 1929–1935, microfilm, New York Municipal Archives. At the time she began work on North Brother Island, her name was Emma Rose Goldberg, which changed to Emma Rose Sherman on her marriage. Her family prefers that her married name be used in this book. (Telephone conversation with niece, Bubbles Yadow, October 25, 1995.)

99. Sherman, Interview, July 16, 1993. See also follow-up telephone interview, June 26, 1994.

100. Soper, "Curious Career," p. 711.

101. Sherman, Interview, July 16, 1993.

102. See, for example, Milicent L. Hathaway and Elsie D. Foard, *Heights and Weights of Adults in the United States*, Home Economics Research Report No. 10 (Washington, D.C.: United States Department of Agriculture, 1960), p. 4. Weight—like height, age-dependent—ranged from 127.9 pounds to 145 pounds.

103. C. E. Banker, Chief, Division of Epidemiology, to Kenneth Mitchell of Elyria, Ohio, February 15, 1932. See also John L. Rice, Commissioner of Health, to Paul A. Teschner, American Medical Association, September 20, 1938, in which he describes Mallon: "She continues to have positive stools; is bedridden, but is otherwise cheerful and resigned to her lot." Copies in the Hoffman/Marr Collection.

104. One indication of Mallon's resignation to her life on North Brother Island, and continuing employment there, was that she volunteered to join the New York City employees retirement system and have proper deductions made from her salary. See *Minutes*, Board of Health of the City of New York, Box 3946, vol. 35, November 23, 1920.

105. Walker, "Typhoid Carrier," p. 24.

106. Sherman, Interview, July 16, 1993.

107. See, for example, John A. Cahill, Medical Superintendent of Riverside Hospital, to Samuel Frant, Director of the Bureau of Preventable Diseases, November 12, 1938, which repeats the December 24, 1932, date that Soper claimed. Copy in the Hoffman/Marr Collection. Emma Sherman remembered the day, but not the date. The October, 1933, date was suggested in "I Wonder What's Become of—'Typhoid Mary,'" *Daily Mirror*, Sunday Magazine sec., December 17, 1933, p. 19. Mary Mallon's death certificate says she was admitted to the hospital (following the stroke) on December 4, 1932, a date I am most inclined to trust. (The Hoffman/Marr Collection contains a copy of Mallon's death certificate.)

108. Quotations from Mallon's Last Will and Testament, and from the attorney's statement, filed with the will at the Bronx Surrogate's Court. Sherman thought the choice was made to put Mallon with the children because they were hospitalized with all sorts of illnesses, rather than place her with only tuberculosis patients. Interview, July 16, 1993.

109. Offspring, "Petition."

110. Ibid. The Catholic Charities received $250; Michael Lucy, $200; Alexandra Plavska, $200; Willie Lempe, $200; Mary Lempe, "clothing and personal effects"; Adelaide Jane Offspring, residuary estate, $4,172.05.

111. Sherman, Interview, July 16, 1993.

CHAPTER SEVEN: "Misbegotten Mary"

I am extremely grateful to the writers whose generosity in sharing published and unpublished material and joining into the spirit of my endeavor made this chapter possible. I wish to thank especially Tanya Contos, Barry Drogin, Joan Schenkar, Marc Sherman, and Mark St. Germain.

1. Roueché's writings won him the Raven Award by the Mystery Writers of America for the best book in a mystery field outside the regular category of crime novels and reporting. His obituary can be found in the *New York Times*, April 29, 1994, p. B8.

2. Berton Roueché, "A Game of Wild Indians," *New Yorker* 28 (April 5, 1952): 84–95, quotation from p. 84. Roueché used the widely accepted figure

of fifty-three cases traced to Mary Mallon. See chap. 1 for the corrected figure of forty-seven. His title referred to a children's game that led to a pipe stoppage, which fomented the epidemic.

3. Roueché, like many medical writers who published accounts of Mallon in the period following her death, described her case in the context of the high incidence of disease and large numbers of typhoid carriers at the same time that he separated Mallon from the pack and referred to her by the objectifying phrase Typhoid Mary. See, for example, Bayard S. Tynes and John P. Utz, "Factors Influencing the Cure of Salmonella Carriers," *Annals of Internal Medicine* 57 (1962): 871–82, an article that begins with "Typhoid Mary" and studies the treatment of twenty-seven adult chronic carriers, but also maps the 3,637 chronic carriers then known to state health departments. (Map is p. 873.)

Medical writers, too, often repeated the story of Mrs. X, first traced by Wilbur A. Sawyer in 1914. She was implicated in transmitting typhoid fever to ninety-three people who ate the food she prepared for a church supper in Hanford, California. See Wilbur A. Sawyer, "Ninety-Three Persons Infected by a Typhoid Carrier at a Public Dinner," *JAMA* 63 (1914): 1537–42. See also Sawyer's account of his most famous case, H. O.: "A Typhoid Carrier on Shipboard," *JAMA* 58 (1912): 1336–38; and his "Late History of a Typhoid Carrier," *JAMA* 64 (1915): 205–53. For a similar case in Washington, D.C., see James G. Cumming, "Should the Barriers Against Typhoid be Continued?" *JAMA* 98 (1932): 93–95. Mrs. X's story is retold in Paul F. Clark, *Pioneer Microbiologists of America* (Madison: University of Wisconsin Press, 1961), pp. 298–300. See also, Burnet MacFarlane and David O. White, *Natural History of Infectious Disease*, 4th ed. (Cambridge: Cambridge University Press, 1972), p. 126: "The most famous (or notorious) carrier was an American cook, 'Typhoid Mary.'"

4. Madelyn Carlisle, "The Strange Story of the Innocent Killer," *Coronet*, December, 1957, pp. 38–42, quotations from pp. 38, 41, 42. There are some interesting misstatements in the article. Carlisle credited Soper with finding fourteen families who suffered from typhoid in Mary Mallon's wake (a dozen plus two), when the total was seven (see chap. 1). She wrote that there was "no epitaph on her grave," and there was one, "Jesus Mercy." Both statements add to the pile of guilt the author attributes to Mallon.

5. M. F. King, "Typhoid Mary's Secret," *American Mercury* 91 (August, 1960): 124–28.

6. John Lentz, "The Malady of Mary Mallon," *Today's Health*, April, 1966, pp. 34–36.

7. Gordon W. Jones, "The Scourge of Typhoid," *American History Illustrated* 1 (1967): 22–28.

8. The probable source was Milton J. Rosenau, *Preventive Medicine and Hygiene*, 6th ed. (New York: D. Appleton-Century Co., 1935). On p. 142, Rosenau wrote, "A subsequent study of her career showed that . . . she may have given rise to the well-known water-borne outbreak of typhoid in Ithaca, New York in 1903, involving over 1300 cases." Soper, who conducted the most thorough study of the Ithaca outbreak, did not consider Mallon its cause. See George Soper, "The Epidemic of Typhoid Fever at Ithaca, N.Y.," *Journal of the New England Water Works Association* 18 (1905): 431–61. See also Heather Munro Prescott, " 'How Long Must We Send Our Sons Into Such Danger?' Cornell University and the Ithaca Typhoid Epidemic of 1903," Paper presented at the Conference on New York State History, June 11, 1988. For a similar connection of Mary Mallon with the Ithaca epidemic, see the *Guiness Book of World Records* (New York: Sterling Publishing Co., 1971–1987).

9. Jones, "The Scourge," pp. 25, 26.

10. Mark Sufrin, "The Case of the Disappearing Cook," *American Heritage* 21 (1970): 37–43.

11. The caption is on p. 39, the picture on p. 38.

12. Mark Sufrin, "They Called Her 'Typhoid Mary,' " Illustration by Gary Viskupic, *Newsday*, September 9, 1979, pp. 27, 36, 40.

13. Mary C. McLaughlin, M.D., "Mary Mallon: Alias Typhoid Mary," *The Recorder* 40 (1979): 44–57.

14. Ibid., p. 55.

15. I want to thank all the people who answered my query about these points in the *Irish Echo*, November 20, 1993, most especially F. T. O'Brien, James N. O'Connor, John Concannon, Nora Finger, John O'Connor, and Kevin Cahill. An Irish political connection for Mallon was very intriguing, but outside of McLaughlin's one informant, Joel Bennett (now deceased), there is no evidence to support it. In this regard, I am also grateful for the reminder from Jack Taub, in response to my Author's Query, *New York Times*, Book Review sec., January 16, 1994, who said that when the cook in an orphan home in Philadelphia in 1932 was found to be a carrier she was referred to as "a typhoid Mary." Thirty children came down with typhoid fever as a result of her cooking, and she was fired. Jack Taub to author, January 20, 1994, and March 4, 1994.

Another reference to a countess in Mallon's story is revealed by Julia Efros in the BBC production, "Typhoid Mary," written and produced by Jonathan Gili, shown on the History Channel, September 24, 1995. Efros is the daughter of Alexandra Plavska, the physician who first employed Mary Mallon in the laboratory at North Brother Island. She told the BBC that her mother was a countess, although she always preferred to be addressed as "Dr.," the title she earned.

16. Shirley Gee, *Typhoid Mary*, The Monday Play, *Best Radio Plays of 1979* (London: Eyre Methuen/BBC Publications, 1980), pp. 7–49.

17. The Irish song, "Cockles and Mussels" or "Molly Malone," has the familiar refrain: "She wheeled her wheelbarrow, / Through the streets broad and narrow, / Crying cockles and mussels, / Alive alive oh." These are the last words of Gee's play. See James F. Leisy, *The Folk Song Abecedary* (New York: Hawthorne Books, 1966), pp. 61–62.

18. Vermont Royster, "Tests vs. Rights: The Story of Mary Mallon," *Wall Street Journal*, September 18, 1986, p. 32. I am grateful to Ann Carmichael for this reference and for her discussion of the contemporary issues raised by Mary Mallon's experiences.

19. J. F. Federspiel, *The Ballad of Typhoid Mary*, trans. Joel Agee (New York: E. P. Dutton & Co., 1983), originally published in 1982 by Suhrkamp Verlag, Frankfurt am Main, under the title *Die Ballade von der Typhoid Mary*.

20. Possibly because of the verisimilitude of the novel, reviewers believe as fact considerably more than is warranted. See, for example, John Calvin Batchelor, "Death Dogged Her Footsteps," *New York Times*, Book Review sec., February 12, 1984, p. 11. See also Samuel G. Freedman, ibid., March 18, 1984, p. 24.

21. "The Tale of Typhoid Mary," *Current Health*, January, 1984, pp. 20–21.

22. Another article in the same period, this one putting Mallon into the context of food-borne disease outbreaks, is Catherine Carey, "Mary Mallon's Trail of Typhoid," *FDA Consumer*, June, 1989, pp. 18–21. See also Joseph McNamara, "A Justice Story: The Long Search for Typhoid Mary," *New York Daily News*, November 3, 1985, p. 53; and Dick Donovan, "Typhoid Mary Served Death on a Platter!" *Weekly World News*, January 7, 1990, p. 41. I am grateful to Jeff Stryker for sending me a xerox of this article in response to my Author's Query, the *New York Times*, Book Review sec., January 16, 1994.

23. Tanya Contos, *Typhoid Mary*, Produced at the Cambridge Multicultural Arts Center, June, 1985. I am grateful to Tanya Contos for allowing me to read her play, which has not been published, and for her permission to quote from it. The play was reviewed by John Engstrom in the *Boston Globe*, June 20, 1985, p. 35.

24. Joan Schenkar, *Fulfilling Koch's Postulate*, 1986. I am grateful to Joan Schenkar for sending me a copy of the play, which remains unpublished, al-

though it was excerpted in *Drama Review*, and for her permission to write about it. See Elin Diamond, "Crossing the Corpus Callosum: An Interview with Joan Schenkar," *The Drama Review* 35 (Summer, 1991): 99–128. The play ran in New York and London.

25. Diamond, "Corpus Callosum."

26. Vivian M. Patraka, "Mass Culture and Metaphors of Menace in Joan Schenkar's Plays," in *Making a Spectacle*, ed. Linda Hart (Ann Arbor: University of Michigan Press, 1989), pp. 25–40, quotation from p. 36.

27. For other reviews, see D. J. R. Bruckner, "Science of Cooking," *New York Times*, February 12, 1986, p. C21; Michael Feingold, "Play-Doh's Cave," *Village Voice*, February 18, 1986, pp. 99–100.

28. Barry J. Drogin, *Typhoid Mary*, 1988. Music and dance piece. Original production with the Bicycle Shop Dancers, choreographer Peg Hill, September 30–October 9, 1988, Nikolai/Louis ChoreoSpace, New York City. A tape of the production is available from Not Nice Music, which holds the copyright. I am grateful to Barry Drogin for corresponding with me about this production, for allowing me to hear the tape, and for providing me with a copy of the original production notes.

29. Barry J. Drogin to author, February 5, 1994, in response to Author's Query, *New York Times*, Book Review sec., January 16, 1994.

30. Julinda Lewis, *Dance Magazine* 63 (February, 1989): 98.

31. Ibid.

32. Gus Solomons, Jr., "Branded," *Village Voice*, October 25, 1988, p. 94; Lewis, *Dance*.

33. Mark St. Germain, *Forgiving Typhoid Mary*, 1989. Produced at the Long Wharf Theater, New Haven, January 3–22, 1989; George Street Playhouse, New Brunswick, March, 1991; Contemporary American Theater Festival, Shepherd College, Shepherdstown, West Virginia, July 6–24, 1994, and Refreshment Committee Theatre Company, Minneapolis Theater Garage, March 2–4, 8–11, 15–18, 1995. I am grateful to Carolyn G. Shapiro for first calling this play to my attention and for arranging with Mark St. Germain for me to read it in final draft form, and to Mr. St. Germain for his permission. I also would like to thank University of Wisconsin Drama Professor Robert Skloot for helping me locate various theater materials and Elaine Tyler May for alerting me to the Minneapolis production of St. Germain's play.

34. As cited in Refreshment Committee Theatre Company, 801 Dayton Avenue, St. Paul, Minn., ticket advertisement for the March, 1995, production in Minneapolis.

35. Ibid.

36. Carolyn Gage, *Cookin' With Typhoid Mary* in *The Second Coming of Joan of Arc and Other Plays*, Copyright 1994 by Carolyn Gage, Printed by Mc-Naughton and Gunn, pp. 127–39, quotations from pp. 129, 130, 133, 136, 138.

37. John Steele Gordon, "The Passion of Typhoid Mary," *American Heritage* 45 (1994): 118–21, quotation from p. 120.

38. John Steele Gordon, National Public Radio, May 24, 1994, interviewed by Alex Chadwick. My thanks to Vanessa Northington Gamble for taping the interview for me, and to Gerard Fergerson and Lauren Bryant for quickly calling my attention to it. Gordon assumes that most cooks did not change jobs very often, but the evidence (see chap. 6) does not support that conclusion. See also John F. Wukovits, "Destroying Angel," *American History Illustrated* 25 (1990): 68–72, who sees Mallon as "a victim at least in part of circumstances beyond her control."

39. Jane E. Brody, "Personal Health," *New York Times*, August 24, 1994, p. B8.

40. *The American Heritage Dictionary of the English Language* (Boston: Houghton Mifflin Co., 1992), p. 1934; *Webster's Third New International Dictionary* (1986).

41. Willard J. Lassers to author, February 19, 1994, in response to Author's Query, *New York Times*, Book Review sec., January 16, 1994. The legal cure for such Typhoid Marys is to build a "Chinese wall" between the new lawyer and the attorneys working on the case. Lassers's search of the literature turned up thirteen cases between 1977 and 1994. I am very grateful to Judge Lassers, Circuit Court of Cook County, Chicago, for this information.

42. Anthony Lewis, "Good Old Reliable Nixon," *New York Times*, March 15, 1976, p. 31.

43. "Grand New Party?" *Wall Street Journal*, August 16, 1988.

44. Bill Powell, "America's Bad Example," *Newsweek*, April 11, 1994, p. 39.

45. "Saturday Night Live," NBC, April 17, 1993.

46. Arthur M. Schlesinger, Jr., "Memo to the 1993 Crowd: Believe in Yourselves," *Newsweek*, January 11, 1993, p. 39.

47. Patricia D. Cornwell, *Body of Evidence: A Kay Scarpetta Mystery* (New York: Avon Books, 1991), p. 335. See also a reference to "Typhoid Jenny" in Nancy Pickard, *Bum Steer* (New York: Pocket Books, 1990), p. 27.

48. Marge Piercy, *The Longings of Women* (New York: Fawcett Crest, 1994), p. 349.

49. Bernie Lincicome, "Spare us the Scoop on Rodman," *Wisconsin State Journal*, May 26, 1995, p. 1D.

50. Symantec Advertisement, *Byte*, January, 1994.

51. I want to thank Stacie Colwell, an M.D./Ph.D. student at the University of Illinois, for the suggestion about jump rope rhymes and Len Berlind for responding to an internet request for the words. I was unable to locate or date the rhyme in a text, for example, in Roger D. Abrahams, ed., *Jump-rope Rhymes, a Dictionary* (Austin: University of Texas Press, 1969).

At least one version of the rhyme includes this second line: "Typhoid Mary, what do you carry?/Homo Harry, who will you marry?" The juxtaposition more than suggests the theme of social deviance.

Another example of the story's spread through American culture is its appearance as a comic, "Sickness Unto Death: Typhoid Mary," in Bronwyn Carlton, *The Big Book of Death* (New York: Paradox Press, 1995), pp. 74–75. I am grateful to David Bordwell for calling this example to my attention.

52. Russell Baker, "The Diversity Cuisine," *New York Times*, July 8, 1995, p. 15.

53. See, for example, a "Q&A" in the *Wisconsin State Journal*, June 13, 1993, in which she was referred to as "an immunological marvel," as if she were the only healthy carrier known.

54. Lawrence K. Altman, in a *New York Times* article about a carrier, wrote: "Though many people think of 'Typhoid Mary' as a nickname for a mythical spreader of typhoid fever, she made her presence known in New York early in this century as the most famous typhoid carrier." "Typhoid Carrier Tied to Epidemic," *New York Times*, October 26, 1970, p. 16.

55. Marc L. Sherman, "A Diptych," *The Belletrist Review* 1 (Fall, 1992): 15–23. I am grateful to Marc Sherman for sending me a copy of this story, March 2, 1994, in response to my Author's Query, *New York Times*, Book Review sec., January 16, 1994.

CONCLUSION

1. See, for example, Peter Brooks, *Reading for the Plot: Design and Intention in Narrative* (New York: Alfred A. Knopf, 1984); Morton W. Bloomfield, ed., *The Interpretation of Narrative: Theory and Practice* (Cambridge: Harvard University Press, 1970); W. J. T. Mitchell, ed., *On Narrative* (Chicago: University of Chicago Press, 1981); and Barbara Herrnstein Smith, "Narrative Versions, Narrative Theories," *Critical Inquiry* 7 (1980): 213–36. For application of this work to history, see Hayden White, "The Value of Narrativity in the Representation of Reality," *Critical Inquiry* 7 (1980): 5–27; Hayden White, *The Content of the Form: Narrative Discourse and Historical Representation* (Baltimore: Johns Hopkins University Press, 1987); Robert H. Canary

and Henry Kozicki, eds., *The Writing of History: Literary Form and Historical Understanding* (Madison: University of Wisconsin Press, 1978); and Dominick LaCapra, *Rethinking Intellectual History: Texts, Contexts, Language* (Ithaca: Cornell University Press, 1983).

I am particularly grateful to Susan Stanford Friedman for consulting with me on this project and helping me see how narrative structure influences understanding. See her "Making History: Reflections on Feminism, Narrative, and Desire," in *Feminism Beside Itself*, ed. Diane Elan and Robyn Wiegman (New York: Routledge, 1995), pp. 11–53.

2. The quotation of James C. Scott is from p. 169 of his "History According to Winners and Losers," *Senri Ethnological Studies* 13 (1984): 161–210; see also his *Domination and the Arts of Resistance: Hidden Transcripts* (New Haven: Yale University Press, 1990). I have quoted Paul Farmer's *AIDS and Accusation: Haiti and the Geography of Blame* (Berkeley: University of California Press, 1992), p. 21.

The idea that situation affects perceptions and functions is not new. It is what literary critics call "positionality" and philosophers call "standpoint theory." See, for example, Sandra Harding, *Whose Science? Whose Knowledge? Thinking from Women's Lives* (Ithaca: Cornell University Press, 1991), especially pp. 119–33; and Linda Alcoff, "Cultural Feminism Versus Post-Structuralism: The Identity Crisis in Feminist Theory," *Signs* 13 (1988): 405–436. Historians, too, have been sensitive to relative points of view, and some interesting recent work has focused on seeking out multiple perspectives on historical events. See, among medical historians, for example, Steven M. Stowe, "Obstetrics and the Work of Doctoring in the Mid-Nineteenth-Century American South," *Bulletin of the History of Medicine* 64 (1990): 540–66; and among labor historians, Alice Kessler-Harris, "Treating the Male as 'Other': Redefining the Parameters of Labor History," *Labor History* 34 (1993): 190–204. One of my own examples of how positionality affects our interpretation of the past is " 'A Worrying Profession': The Domestic Environment of Medical Practice in Mid-Nineteenth-Century America," the Fielding H. Garrison Lecture, *Bulletin of the History of Medicine*, 69 (Spring, 1995): 1–29.

3. George Soper, "The Curious Career of Typhoid Mary," *Bulletin of the New York Academy of Medicine* 15 (October, 1939): 704.

4. George Soper, "Typhoid Mary," *Military Surgeon* 45 (July, 1919): 7.

5. Timothy F. Murphy, *Ethics in an Epidemic: AIDS, Morality, and Culture* (Berkeley: University of California Press, 1994), p. 14. See Randy Shilts, *And the Band Played On: Politics, People, and the AIDS Epidemic* (New York: St. Martin's Press, 1987). Another review of Shilts's book made explicit the connection between Mary Mallon and Gaetan Dugas: "An airline steward

from Montreal may have been the 20th century's equivalent of Typhoid Mary, responsible for introducing AIDS in North America." "Man Linked to AIDS Invasion," *Atlanta Constitution*, October 8, 1987, p. 39.

6. Another factor to weigh when considering testing programs is cost. As we saw in chap. 2, New York's expensive program of testing food handlers was discontinued in the 1930s. Given limited resources, all the programs that might be tried need to be weighed with regard to cost effectiveness.

7. "Preface," *The Impact of Homophobia and Other Social Biases on AIDS* (San Francisco: Public Media Center, 1995), p. 3. See also, for example, study of the use of the term "AIDS Mary" as it applies to women infected with HIV who purposefully seduce partners, in Gary Allen Fine, "Welcome to the World of AIDS: Fantasies of Women's Revenge," *Western Folklore* 46 (1987): 192–97. I am grateful to Vanessa Northington Gamble for giving me these references.

8. *New York World*, July 20, 1909, p. 18.

9. Ramon Perez is quoted in Rosanne Pagano, "Quarantine Considered for AIDS Victims," *California Lawyer* 4 (March, 1984): 17. See also, for example, Nancy Rabinowitz, "Hospitals Revive Quarantine of TB Patients," (Madison, Wisconsin) *Capital Times*, November 29, 1992, p. C1. For a discussion of various states' practices see Harlon L. Dalton, Scott Burris, and the Yale AIDS Law Project, eds., *AIDS and the Law: A Guide for the Public* (New Haven: Yale University Press, 1987).

10. Stephen C. Joseph, "Quarantine: Sometimes a Duty," *New York Times*, February 10, 1990, p. 15.

11. Sandor Katz, "HIV Testing—A Phony Cure," *The Nation*, May 28, 1990: 738–42. On this sort of dilemma applied to other issues, see, for example, Tamar Lewin, "Debate in Philadelphia on Forced Vaccinations," *New York Times*, February 24, 1991, p. 17; and James J. Kilpatrick, "Fluoridation is Abomination," *Wisconsin State Journal*, March 5, 1990.

12. Nancy Scheper-Hughes, "AIDS, Public Health, and Human Rights in Cuba," *Lancet* 342 (1993): 966. See also Karen Wald, "AIDS in Cuba: a Dream or a Nightmare?" *Z Magazine*, December, 1990, pp. 104–9. I am grateful to Allen Hunter for calling the latter to my attention.

13. Scheper-Hughes, "AIDS," p. 967. See also the same author's "Commentary: AIDS, Public Health and Human Rights in Cuba," *Anthropology Newsletter*, October, 1993, pp. 48, 46.

14. Wald, "AIDS in Cuba," p. 104.

15. Ibid., p. 106, 105. If they are considered to be adequately educated about how to avoid infecting others, Cuban HIV-positive isolated individuals are now permitted day or weekend passes to go back to their homes and fami-

lies. Also there are examples of families moving with their infected relative into the AIDS compound.

16. Tim Golden, "Patients Pay High Price in Cuba's War on AIDS," *New York Times*, October 16, 1995, pp. 1, 4. Quotations from p. 4.

17. Ibid.

18. Barron Lerner has explored the ways in which the public health measures that were developed to control tuberculosis early in the twentieth century should be understood as custodial rather than health promoting in his paper "Negotiating Medical, Social, and Public Health Imperatives: Detention of Tuberculosis Patients in Seattle, 1949–60," presented to the American Association for the History of Medicine 67th Annual Meeting in New York City, May 1, 1994.

19. Johan Giesecke, "AIDS and the Public Health," *Lancet* 342 (October 16, 1993): 942.

20. Charles McClain, "Of Medicine, Race, and American Law: The Bubonic Plague Outbreak of 1900," *Law and Social Inquiry* 13 (1988): 447–513. See also Philip A. Kalisch, "The Black Death in Chinatown, Plague and Politics in San Francisco," *Arizona and the West* 14 (1972): 113–36, and Alan Kraut, *Silent Travelers: Germs, Genes, and the "Immigrant Menace"* (New York: Basic Books, 1994), pp. 79–96.

21. James Jones, *Bad Blood: The Tuskegee Syphilis Experiment—A Tragedy of Race and Medicine* (New York: Free Press, 1981); and Vanessa Northington Gamble, "A Legacy of Distrust: African-Americans and Medical Research," *American Journal of Preventive Medicine* 9 (1993): 35–38.

22. Kraut, *Silent Travelers.*

23. See, for example, Katie Leishman, "A Crisis in Public Health," *Atlantic Monthly*, October, 1985, pp. 18–41.

24. Evelynn Hammonds, "Race, Sex, AIDS: The Construction of 'Other,'" *Radical America* 20 (1986): 28–36, quotation from p. 29. Hammonds effectively explores how the "white media's silence on the connections between AIDS and race; the black media's silence on the connections between AIDS and sexuality/sexual politics, [and] the failure of white gay men's AIDS organizations to reach the communities of people of color" exacerbated this critical public health issue.

25. *New York Tribune*, March 29, 1915, p. 8.

26. Robert J. T. Joy, M. D., to author, July 29, 1994. I am grateful to Bob Joy for his insightful comments on my work and for his permission to quote from this letter.

27. Gilbert Wersan [pseud. for Warren Boroson], "The Truth (For a

Change) About Typhoid Mary," *MD*, September 1985, p. 109. See, for example, Barry Blackwell, "Compliance," *Psychotherapy and Psychosomatics* 58 (1992): 161–69.

28. A. J. Chesley, "Give Typhoid Carriers a Square Deal and Eliminate Typhoid," *Health*, February, 1922, pp. 22–25.

29. Ibid., p. 23.

30. Ibid., p. 24. Similar compassion for carriers' "mental anguish and depression" can be found in, for example C. B. Sylvester and A. W. Sylvester, "A Typhoid Carrier," *JAMA* 85 (July 11, 1925): 111.

31. Chesley, "Square Deal," pp. 24, 25.

CREDITS

Figure 1.1 Originally appeared in George A. Johnson, "The Typhoid Toll," *Journal of American Water Works Association* 3 (June 1916): 249–326, p. 308.

Figure 2.1 From the Prints and Photographs Collection, History of Medicine Division, National Library of Medicine, Frame 2220, Side B.

Figure 4.1 *New York Times*, April 4, 1915, sec. 5 (magazine sec.), p. 3.

Figure 4.2 *New York American*, June 20, 1909, p. 6.

Figure 4.3 Reprinted courtesy of the Bettmann Archive.

Figure 5.1 *New York American*, June 20, 1909, p. 6.

Figure 5.2 *New York American*, June 20, 1909, pp. 6–7.

Figure 5.3 *New York American*, June 20, 1909, pp. 6–7.

Figure 5.4 *New York American*, June 20, 1909, p. 7. Reprinted courtesy of Brown Brothers.

Figure 5.5 *New York American*, June 20, 1909, p. 7.

Figure 5.6 *New York American*, June 30, 1909, p. 7.

Figure 5.7 *New York Daily Mirror*, December 17, 1933, Sunday Magazine sec., p. 19.

Figure 5.8 Drawing by P. Barlow; Copyright 1935, 1963, The New Yorker Magazine, Inc. Published in *New Yorker* 10 (January 26, 1935): 21.

Figure 6.1 New York City Municipal Archives, Department of Public Charities Collection, Image no. 1924.

Figure 6.2 New York City Municipal Archives, Department of Public Charities Collection, Image no. 2000.

Figure 6.3 Courtesy of Ida Peters Hoffman and John S. Marr.

Figure 6.4 Courtesy of Emma Rose Sherman.

Figure 6.5 Letter in Mary Mallon's hand, accompanying In the Matter of the Application for a Writ of Habeas Corpus for the Production of Mary Mallon, New York Supreme Court (June 28–July 22, 1909), New York County Courthouse.

Figure 6.6 Courtesy of Emma Rose Sherman.

Figure 6.7 Courtesy of Ida Peters Hoffman and John S. Marr.

Figure 7.1 *Coronet*, December 1957, p. 38.

Figure 7.2 *Today's Health*, April 1966, p. 34. Published with permission of Thomson Healthcare Communications.

Figure 7.3 Sketch by Lawrence DiFiori, *American Heritage* 21 no. 5 (August 1970): 38. Reprinted by permission of the artist, Lawrence DiFiori.

Figure 7.4 *American Heritage* 21, no. 5 (August 1970): 40. Reprinted by permission of the artist, Lawrence DiFiori.

Figure 7.5 *American Heritage* 21, no. 5 (August 1970): 42. Reprinted by permission of the artist, Lawrence DiFiori.

Figure 7.6 Illustration by Gary Viskupic, originally appeared in *New York Newsday*, Nassau Edition, September 9, 1979, sec. L1, p. 27. Published by permission of Los Angeles Times Syndicate International.

Figure 7.7 *Current Health*, January 1984, p. 20. Reprinted by permission from Weekly Reader Corporation. Copyright 1984 by Weekly Reader Corporation. All Rights Reserved.

Index

Ebola virus, 215, 238
Edington, Edmund, 192
Edington, George, 192–93
Epidemics, 21–22, 23, 52, 246
Erlanger, Mitchell L., 34, 76, 78, 90
Ethnicity considerations in typhoid
    carriers, 97, 100, 101, 118, 124,
    125

Farmer, Paul, 233
Federspiel, J. F., *The Ballad of
    Typhoid Mary*, 217–18
Ferguson, George, 32, 74
Ferguson Laboratories, 32, 33, 36–
    37, 73–74, 87, 184, 201
Filth theory of disease, 22, 23, 24,
    26, 29
Food handlers, 119, 122; examina-
    tion of, 52–53, 54; isolation of,
    89–90; as typhoid carriers, 56,
    57–58, 60, 64
Foreign birth considerations in
    typhoid carriers, 97, 100, 118,
    124, 125
Fourteenth Amendment, 79
Fowler, Gene, 154
Frant, Samuel, 99
Friedman, Stephen M., 52, 56, 63–
    64

Gage, Carolyn, *Cookin' with
    Typhoid Mary*, 225
Gallbladder, 30, 107, 144, 173, 175,
    201; surgical removal of, 34–
    35, 92, 186–87
Garbage disposal problems, solu-
    tions to, 23
Gee, Shirley, *Typhoid Mary*, 215–
    16
Gender considerations in typhoid
    carriers, 97–100, 124, 125

General Slocum steamboat, 179
"Germ-Carrier, The" (O.S.), 147–
    48
Germ theory of disease, 6
Giegerich, Leonard, 76
Giesecke, Johan, 245
Gilsey, Henry, 17, 77
Golden, Tim, 242
Goldwater, S. S., 67
Gordon, John Steele, 225–26
Gostin, Larry, 77
Gray, Reuben, 142–43
Greater New York Charter (city
    code), 71, 79–80, 81
GRID (Gay-Related Infectious Dis-
    ease), 235

Habeas corpus hearing, Mary Mal-
    lon's, 72–90 *passim*, 94, 128,
    144, 145, 168, 180; *New York
    American* on, 138–41
Hanta virus, 215
Harlan, John M., 78
Harrington, Charles, 128
Harvard University, 49
Haymarket riots, 217
Hearst, William Randolph, 73, 74,
    75, 128, 142, 161; his brand of
    journalism, 131–32
Hell's Kitchen, 115
Helms, Jesse, 240
Hill, Peg, *Typhoid Mary*, 222–
    23
Hispanics, 247
Hitler, Adolf, *Mein Kampf*, 240
HIV, 2, 4, 11, 21, 95, 202; Cuba's pol-
    icy about, 240–42, 246; infec-
    tion, isolation of people with,
    69; parallels between "Typhoid
    Mary" and, 215, 219, 221; stig-
    matizing of persons with, 237–

13, 231–33; habeas corpus hearing of, 72–90 *passim*, 94, 128, 138–41, 144, 145, 168, 180; identified as healthy typhoid carrier, 29–30; isolations of, 2, 6, 7, 11, 20–21, 36, 38, 47, 52, 138; laboratory studies of, 30–38, 39, 86–87; legal authority surrounding isolation of, 8–9, 70–95; media and cultural construction of, 10, 12, 126–61; her own perspective on loss of liberty and personal misfortune, 11, 162–201; and public health policy, 7–8, 39–69; release of, from isolation, 65–67, 145, 188–90; retellings of story of, 11–13, 202–30; second isolation of, 67–69; social expectations and prejudices about, 9–10, 96–125; suit against city, 190; her work as cook, 14–19, 100–101, 163–71

Mann, Jonathan, 237

Marital status considerations in typhoid carriers, 97, 100, 101

Markiewicz, Countess, 212–14

Marshall, John, 79

Massachusetts State Board of Health, 128

Meader, F. M., 55–56

Media's perspective on Mary Mallon, 10, 12. *See also* Chapter Five

Medical perspective on Mary Mallon, 6–7. *See also* Chapter One

Medical Record, 107

Medico-Legal Society, 75

Miasmas, 6, 22

Microorganisms, 26; as single cause of disease, 23, 24

Milk controls, 63

Minnesota State Board of Health, 251, 252

Moersch, Frederick, 121–24, 153, 155–56, 157, 228

Moscow, University of, school of medicine, 194

Municipal Court, 94

Murphy, Timothy, 235

Nation, The, 239

National Basketball Association, 227

National Historian of the Ancient Order of Hibernians, 214

National Hygienic Laboratory, 49

New England Hospital for Women and Children, 44

New Jersey, number of typhoid carriers in, 49

Newsday, 212

Newsweek, 227

New York Academy of Medicine, 128

New York American, 65–66, 71, 83, 154, 185; articles on Mary Mallon in, 73, 74–75, 128–29, 130, 131–41, 142, 143, 146, 160, 180–81, 182, 189

New York Call, 143, 183

New York City, number of typhoid carriers in, 50, 52, 56, 88

New York City Department of Health, 7, 20, 33, 44; "extraordinary and even arbitrary" powers of, 42, 69, 71, 82; and habeas corpus hearing, 76–77, 79–83, 85, 87–90; leadership of, in American public health policy, 40, 42; on necessity of isolating Mary Mallon, 97; and

Library of Congress Cataloging-in-Publication Data

Leavitt, Judith Walzer.
    Typhoid Mary : captive to the public's health / Judith Walzer Leavitt.
      p.   cm.
    Includes bibliographical references and index.
    ISBN 0-8070-2102-4
      1. Typhoid Mary, d. 1938.   2. Typhoid fever—New York (N.Y.)—History.
    3. Quarantine—New York (N.Y.)—History.   I. Title.
    RA644.T8L43   1996
    614.5′112′097471—dc20   95-43486